PROMOTING REPRODUCTIVE SECURITY IN DEVELOPING COUNTRIES

ISSUES IN WOMEN'S HEALTH

Series Editors: Ralph J. DiClemente and Gina M. Wingood
Emory University
Rollins School of Public Health
Atlanta, Georgia

HANDBOOK OF WOMEN'S SEXUAL AND REPRODUCTIVE HEALTH
Gina M. Wingood and Ralph J. DiClemente

INTIMATE PARTNER VIOLENCE
Societal, Medical, Legal, and Individual Responses
Sana Loue

PROMOTING REPRODUCTIVE SECURITY IN DEVELOPING COUNTRIES
Maurice I. Middleberg

PROMOTING REPRODUCTIVE SECURITY IN DEVELOPING COUNTRIES

Maurice I. Middleberg
Engender Health
New York, New York

KLUWER ACADEMIC / PLENUM PUBLISHERS
New York, Boston, Dordrecht, London, Moscow

Library of Congress Cataloging-in-Publication Data

Middelberg, Maurice I., 1953–
   Promoting reproductive security in developing countries/by Maurice I. Middleberg.
      p.   cm. — (Issues in women's health)
   Includes bibliographical references and index.
   ISBN 0-306-47449-2
     1. Reproductive health—Developing countries. 2. Human reproductive
technology—Developing countries. I. Title. II. Issues in women's health (Kluwer
Academic Publishers)

RG133.5 .M535 2003
362.1'96692'0091724—dc21

2002034145

ISBN 0-306-47449-2

©2003 Kluwer Academic / Plenum Publishers, New York
233 Spring Street, New York, New York 10013

http://www.wkap.nl/

10 9 8 7 6 5 4 3 2 1

A C.I.P. record for this book is available from the Library of Congress

All rights reserved

No part of this book may be reproduced, stored in a retrieval system, or transmitted in any form or by any means, electronic, mechanical, photocopying, microfilming, recording, or otherwise, without written permission from the Publisher, with the exception of any material supplied specifically for the purpose of being entered and executed on a computer system, for exclusive use by the purchaser of the work.

Printed in the United States of America

Preface

For twenty years, it has been my privilege to be part of an extraordinary transformation—the evolving human encounter with sexuality and reproduction. Sex and childbearing are often linked to our most intense and joyful moments—the discovery of one's identity, the wonder of intimacy, the miracle of holding a child in one's hands for the first time. Sex and reproduction can and should be profoundly *healthy*—physically, emotionally and spiritually. This includes the ability to make free and informed choices in matters of sex and reproduction, healthy pregnancy and healthy sexuality.

It is sadly the case that intimacy and its aftermath are often blighted by illness and trauma. In the course of working in dozens of countries over this period, I have witnessed some heartbreaking moments. There was the young woman in Togo, only in her early twenties, who was in despair over her sixth pregnancy. I can still see the men's AIDS ward in a hospital in Haiti, filled with haunted, skeletal figures. I can hear the voice of the woman in Kenya, who feared she would beaten by her husband. There was the taxi driver in Cameroon who shared his worries about being able to care for his children, while feeling pressured by his extended family to have more offspring. I remember watching a woman in agony from eclampsia on the floor of a tiny rural clinic in Cambodia that was bereft of the simple medication that could help her. My colleagues and I put her in a car to be driven into the city, where she might receive treatment. I never learned what happened to her, but the image of her on the floor of that clinic returns to me frequently.

These vignettes are more than offset by testimonies of hope and progress. In the remote village of Cuschcandahy, Peru, the home of the village health worker is adorned with a sign that reads, "Family planning here". In India, a group of men allowed me to sit in on their discussion of the dangers of encouraging their adolescent daughters to marry. In a Nepali village, the women's group proudly talked about their efforts to gain control over their bodies and their lives. In Zambia, I watched a group of doctors and nurses undertake a stunning effort to change the quality of reproductive health care offered to the communities they served. In Haiti, community health workers and a women's group developed songs and dances to teach the danger signs of pregnancy. In Bolivia, police, sex workers and the gay community agreed to set aside suspicions and hostility to join in an HIV/AIDS prevention program. In more places than I can recount, I have seen clients and health providers exhibit enormous courage, skill, and determination in the pursuit of reproductive health. These experiences have left me an optimist.

On a global level, much has been accomplished. Twenty years ago, the percentage of women using a contraceptive method in the less developed world was only about 38 percent.

By the late 1990s, contraceptive prevalence in the less developed countries rose to 60 percent. By any estimation, this is one of the most important demographic and public health changes to ever occur in a comparable period of time. Population growth is much slower than it would otherwise have been. The evolution of birth rates and birth spacing has been an important contributor to the global decline in child mortality. Fewer pregnancies have also reduced the likelihood that a woman will die from complications of pregnancy and childbirth. Much has been learned about what makes for effective HIV/AIDS programming and there are excellent models on which to build.

Conversely, the catastrophe of HIV/AIDS has been beyond anything that I imagined twenty years ago and the global response remains woefully inadequate. Prevention and management of other sexually transmitted diseases remains woefully inadequate. Once a woman becomes pregnant, very little progress has been made in assuring her of life saving care. Too many women and households suffer from sexual violence, which is still shamefully neglected. Scores of millions of women still lack access to the family planning services they want.

At this point in my career, I would like to encourage and prepare others to work in reproductive health. This book is therefore primarily aimed at students of public health, though I hope it will prove useful to others seeking a survey of the field. The need for skilled, dedicated professionals is great: to provide high quality family planning services, to reduce maternal death and illnesses, to combat HIV/AIDS, and to reduce sexual violence. Beyond the very real health benefits to those who are served, advancing reproductive health has profound social consequences, reflecting and affecting a wide range of issues, including the relationship between women and men, economics, politics, law, and values. Those who choose to pursue the discipline are promised an endlessly rewarding and absorbing profession that will touch upon the most intimate aspects of people's lives, while reverberating globally.

Acknowledgments

This book was made possible through the joint support of CARE and the Rollins School of Public Health of Emory University. They jointly funded a sabbatical year that I spent at the Rollins School, during which the bulk of this book was developed and written. I am particularly grateful to Peter Bell, the President of CARE; Pat Carey, the CARE Senior Vice President for Programs; Dr. James Curran, the Dean of the Rollins School; and, Dr. Reynaldo Martorell, Chair of the Department of International Health at the Rollins School. This book would never have been started without their support and I am profoundly grateful to all four and to the two institutions they lead. The book was completed while working at EngenderHealth and I would like to thank the EngenderHealth President, Dr. Amy Pollack, for her support and encouragement.

Dr. Ralph DiClemente, also of the Rollins School, served as Women's Health Series editor on behalf of the publisher, Kluwer Academic. He reviewed the entire first draft of the manuscript in detail, making many helpful suggestions. Reynaldo Martorell reviewed early efforts and provided useful guidance and encouragement. Dr. Amy Pollack critically reviewed the chapter on contraception.

Much of this book reflects my experience during my ten years with CARE. I benefited enormously from my interaction with my colleagues in the CARE Health and Population Unit, as well as with the health staff in the CARE Country Offices. I would like to express my appreciation and gratitude to my CARE colleagues.

I was very fortunate to have wonderful colleagues at the Rollins School, especially in the Department of International Health. They were very gracious and supportive and I learned a great deal from spending a year with such sterling scholars and teachers.

Teresa Krauss at Kluwer was very helpful during the latter stages, providing gentle but insistent prodding to complete the book.

I am more grateful than I can express to my wife, Fran Middleberg, who, in addition to being endlessly supportive, meticulously went through every page of the manuscript, catching and correcting many errors. Thank you.

Over the years, I benefited from the insights and experiences of hundreds of health workers, analysts and managers in developing countries. Most of all, I want to thank the many people who allowed me into their homes and communities to share part of their lives. It is to them this book is dedicated.

Disclaimer

The views and opinions expressed in this book are solely those of the author and do not necessarily reflect those of CARE, Emory University, EngenderHealth or any of the reviewers. While the author is grateful for helpful reviews, any remaining errors are solely the responsibility of the author.

This book is intended only as a source of general information and reference. It is not intended as a guide for patient care or as a substitute for professional medical training or professional medical guidance. Readers who wish to use the information contained herein for purposes of medical care should always consult with a qualified health or medical professional.

Contents

1. Purpose and Conceptual Framework 1
   Purpose 1
   An Historical Perspective on Reproductive Health 3
      Drawing Lessons from History...................................... 5
   Reproductive Health and Managing Risk 11
   The Locus of Risk Management: Individuals, Couples, and Households 16
   Gender and Reproductive Health 17
   Reproductive Risk Analysis 18

2. Epidemiology of Reproductive Health 25
   Magnitude and Impacts of Reproductive Insecurity 25
      Unintended and High Risk Pregnancies............................. 25
      Maternal Mortality and Morbidity................................. 29
      Induced Abortion 32
      HIV/AIDS and Other Sexually Transmitted Diseases 36
   Key Lessons from the Epidemiology of Reproductive Health 40
      Rapid Declines in Fertility Are Possible 40
      Obstetrical Emergencies Are the Key to Reducing Maternal Mortality 43
      HIV and STD Prevention Efforts Must be Targeted to Achieve
      Maximum Impact 46

3. Behavior Change 53
   Theoretical Basis for Behavior Change 55
      Working with Pre-Contemplators: Fostering the Saliency of Health
      Reproductive Behaviors 57
      From Contemplation to Preparation: Paving the Path to Action 58
      From Preparation to Action: Following through on Commitment 60
      Action and Maintenance: Sustaining New Behaviors over the Long Term 61
      Summing Up: Applying Behavior Change Concepts 62
   Translating Theory into Practice: Communication for Behavior Change 62
      Analyzing the Population.. 62
      Setting Objectives.. 66
      Guidelines for Communication 67
   Assessing Behavior Change 72

4. Community Empowerment 75

How Community Variables Influence Reproductive Health 75
The Meaning of Community 76
The Confusing Language of Community Participation 78
Community Empowerment for Reproductive Health 80
The Community Empowerment Cycle 82
Community Empowerment Requires Participatory Approaches 83
Developing a Facilitation Team 84
Defining and Describing the Target Community 84
Assessing Needs through Participatory Appraisal 86
    Synthesizing the Findings. 91
Mapping and Mobilizing Community Resources 91
    Mapping Assets: Associations and Organizations. 92
    Mapping Assets: Individuals 93
    Building Relations among Organizations and Individuals 94
    Mobilizing Cash 96
    Seeking External Resources 98
Building Organizational Capacity 99
Leadership Development 100
Assessing Community Empowerment 101

5. Building Institutional Capacity 103

Essential Services for Reproductive Health 104
Maximizing Access to Services 106
    Mapping the Network of Health Providers. 106
    Matching Providers to Services. 108
    Strengthening Clinical Services 111
    Supporting Community Health Workers 113
    Using the Commercial Sector Effectively 116
Improving the Quality of Care 118
    Quality Standards 118
    Quality Processes. 120
Strengthening Management Systems 124
    Defining Management Systems 125
    Assessing Management Capacity 128
    Designing and Implementing A Management
    Development Plan. 128
    Case Study: Improving Institutional Capacity in Bangladesh 128

6. Contraception 133

The Biology of Contraception 133
    The Menstrual Cycle. 133
    Male Reproductive System 134

- Contraceptive Technology 135
  - Abstinence 136
  - Withdrawal 137
  - Fertility Awareness Methods 138
  - Male Condoms 140
  - Spermicides and Female Barrier Methods 141
  - Combined Oral Contraceptives 144
  - Progestin-Only Oral Contraceptives 147
  - Progestin Injection Contraceptives 150
  - Contraceptive Implants 151
  - Intrauterine Devices 153
  - Female Sterilization 156
  - Vasectomy 159

7. Maternal Health Care 161
   - Prenatal Period 161
     - Maternal Adaptation and Fetal Growth 161
     - Objectives of Prenatal Care 162
     - Monitoring Progress during Pregnancy 164
     - Complications of the Prenatal Period 164
     - Helping Households Plan for Obstetrical Emergencies 169
     - Nutrition and Pregnancy 170
   - Intrapartum Period 173
     - Physiology of Normal Labor 173
     - Care during Labor and Delivery 174
     - Use of a Trained Birth Attendant 175
     - Complications of the Intrapartum Period 176
     - Intrapartum Complications of the Fetus 180
   - Postpartum Period 181
     - Changes in the Postpartum Period 181
     - Care in the Postpartum Period 182
     - Complications in the Postpartum Period 183
   - Induced Abortion 186
     - First Trimester Methods 186
     - Second Trimester Methods 187
     - Managing Complications of Unsafe Abortion 187
     - Post-abortion Contraception 188
   - Newborn Care 189

8. HIV/AIDS and Sexually Transmitted Diseases 191
   - A Quick Guide to Sexually Transmitted Diseases 191
   - Case Detection and Management 194
     - Detecting People with an STD 195
     - Managing Patients in Resource Poor Settings 198

Syndromic Management	199
STD Treatment and HIV Control	203
Care for People Living with HIV/AIDS	204
Alleviating Stigma and Strengthening Social Support	204
Palliative Care and Opportunistic Infections	205
Antiretroviral Treatment	206
Maternal to Child Transmission of HIV and STD	209
HIV	209
Syphilis	211
Gonorrhea	212
Chlamydia	212
Blood Screening for HIV	213
HPV and Cervical Cancer	214
9. Policy and Politics	219
Why Policy Matters	219
The Many Faces of the Reproductive "Problem"	220
Reproduction as a Problem of National Power	221
Reproduction as an Economic Problem	222
Reproduction as a Health Problem	225
Reproduction as a Human Rights Problem	226
Reproduction as a Religious or Moral Problem	227
Summing Up: Different Definitions, Different Prescriptions	228
The Manager as Policy Advocate	229
Clarifying Policy Objectives	230
Identifying the Relevant Decision-makers and Political Actors	230
Different Audiences, Different Arguments	231
Notes	235
Notes for Chapter 1	235
Notes for Chapter 2	236
Notes for Chapter 3	238
Notes for Chapter 4	239
Notes for Chapter 5	240
Notes for Chapter 6	241
Notes to Chapter 7	243
Notes to Chapter 8	245
Notes to Chapter 9	249
References	251
Index	261

1

Purpose and Conceptual Framework

PURPOSE

Let us imagine a newly promoted health manager in a developing country. The manager, a physician by training, has been successful as a clinician and clinic manager. She has recently been selected by the district health manager to lead the reproductive health program. Enthusiastically embracing her new role, she sits down at her first staff meeting and asks, "What are the most important issues? What do you think we need to work on?" She is dismayed to receive the following array of responses:

"Many women would like to use contraception, but there is a real problem with access to services."

"People are not organized and they expect us to do everything for them. We have to mobilize the communities."

"We have had a high number of maternal deaths. The problem is that women show up at the clinics too late and they die on the table."

"People have the wrong attitudes and there is a lot of ignorance. We have to change behavior."

"There is a serious AIDS crisis in this district."

"The staff aren't trained and our facilities lack equipment and supplies. We need to strengthen our capacity."

"The quality of care is often poor."

"The real problem that nobody will talk about openly is the abuse of women in our district."

"We are very constrained by government policy and the governor is very reluctant to speak out on these issues for fear of a political backlash."

Undaunted, but now confused, the manager tries to define the seemingly innocuous term "reproductive health care" so she knows what to include in her evolving program. The United Nations source document to which she refers says that, "... reproductive health care is defined as the entire constellation of methods, techniques and services that contribute to reproductive health and well-being by preventing and solving reproductive health problems. It includes sexual health, the purpose of which is the enhancement of life and personal relations, not merely counseling and care related to reproduction and sexually transmitted diseases.[1]" This is not much help to a new manager struggling to craft a coherent program in the face of multiple demands and meager resources.

The confusion felt by our intrepid manager is reflected at the global level. The 1994 International Conference on Population and Development (ICPD) concluded that the presumed focus on fertility and family planning that had marked earlier programs should be replaced by a comprehensive, integrated approach to reproductive health. The definition of reproductive health care encountered by the manager reflects this comprehensive approach. The move to a reproductive health approach created a huge conceptual and practical dilemma. Managers are faced with the challenge of deciding what specific interventions to include in reproductive health programs and how to set priorities in the allocation of resources. Moreover, as the responses to our manager's innocent query suggests, effective reproductive health programming requires drawing on diverse bodies of knowledge and deploying a wide array of skills.

The purpose of this book is to provide a guide or road map for public health students aspiring to manage reproductive health programs or clinically trained managers needing a broader public health perspective. After reading this book the student or manager should have a grasp of the core knowledge, tools and skills needed to oversee a reproductive health program. I am suggesting that there are six core competencies that will be needed by the manager—reproductive risk analysis, behavior change, community empowerment, institutional capacity building, health technologies, and policy advocacy. Within the definition of key health technologies I include contraception, maternal health care, and management of HIV/AIDS and other sexually transmitted diseases. Principles and applications in each of these domains are explored. As often as possible, examples are given of effective programming, many of which are drawn from CARE, which helped support the writing of this book.

The plan of the book is as follows:

- The remainder of this chapter sets forth the general framework, which I call reproductive security. The emphasis is on helping households identify, prevent and manage risks to reproductive health.
- Chapter 2 reviews the epidemiology of reproductive health, with an emphasis on drawing general lessons that can help guide programming. The chapter concludes with a procedure for making choices and setting priorities among reproductive health problems.
- Chapter 3 addresses the issue behavior change. We look at how a few key constructs—stages of change, decisional balance and self-efficacy—can be of enormous utility in shaping interventions. The characteristics of good communication programs are also reviewed, with examples from the field.
- Community empowerment is the subject of Chapter 4. The meaning of community empowerment is explored and participatory approaches to appraisal, resource mobilization, capacity building, and leadership development are described.
- Chapter 5 is devoted to the issue of institutional capacity building, which encompasses expanding access to services, improving the quality of care and strengthening management systems.
- Chapters 6–8 are more biomedical in orientation. Chapter 6 is a guide to contraception. Chapter 7 discusses key interventions to promote maternal health. Chapter 8 describes essential services to prevent and manage sexually transmitted diseases, with a special emphasis on HIV/AIDS.
- Chapter 9 concludes the book with an exploration of reproductive health policy and the role of the reproductive health manager as policy advocate.

AN HISTORICAL PERSPECTIVE ON REPRODUCTIVE HEALTH

Every culture, for as long as history is regarded, prominently features reproduction in its stories and norms. Statuary dating back 25,000 years suggest consciousness of the unique status of the pregnant woman[2]. Depictions of birth dating back to the ice age have been uncovered in caves in France. Conception, sexual relations and childbirth have always played a powerful and central role in human affairs. Efforts to apply social regulation and medical technology to reproduction are as old as recorded history. The act of human reproduction has been central to the evolution of family and social structure, religious and ethical norms, social controversy, scientific inquiry, medical technologies, polemics, literature and art.

Midwifery may well be the oldest form of medicine. By 6000 B.C.E. women were helping each other deliver babies. Scenes of childbirth are found on Egyptian tombs dating back to 2350 B.C.E.[3,4] Guidelines for obstetrical care can be found in ancient Egyptian texts, including the Kahun papyrus (1900 B.C.E.) and the Ebers papyrus (1550 B.C.E.). The god Bes served as protector of women during pregnancy and delivery and women prayed to the goddess Hathor for a pain free delivery. The cause and duration of pregnancy was known. In an early version of the pregnancy test, women urinated on wheat and barley seeds—if they germinated the woman was deemed pregnant. Childbirth was attended by women only, which may explain the relatively scant descriptions of technique in the texts written by men. It is known that a birthing stool was usually employed. The Ebers papyrus describes uterine prolapse and proposes a treatment. A passage in the Kahun papyrus suggests that there was use of stitching to close perineal lacerations. Early writings from India (c. 1500 B.C.E.) tell of the use of physicians rather than midwives as birth attendants. This may reflect the relatively high status accorded women during the period of greatest Buddhist influence. The practice of dissection helped the ancient Indians develop a detailed knowledge of female reproductive anatomy. Vedic texts in India dating to 1500 B.C.E. describe obstetric instruments for removing the fetus. At childbirth, women were removed to a clean hut, where labor was "hastened" through the use of gruel and inhaling the smoke of burning snakeskins. In cases of intrauterine demise, the dead fetus was dismembered and extracted vaginally. Shaking, emetics and pressure were prescribed for retained placenta. Chinese treatises on obstetrics and gynecology were in evidence no later than the 6th century B.C.E. Management of childbirth was reserved exclusively for midwives and physicians were forbidden to intervene. Hemorrhage was treated with a solution made of dried nettles. Retained placenta were extracted by placing a weight on the end of the severed umbilical cord. Potions and astringents were applied to correct transverse and breech lies. Midwives would, *in extremis*, manipulate the position of the fetus or dismember it in instances of obstructed labor. Ceremonial rituals surrounded pregnancy and childbirth among the Aztec[5]. The pregnant woman was visited on a regular basis by the *ticitl* or midwife. The midwife would attend the birth, giving the woman massage, food, teas and baths in the hope of provoking a quick and painless birth. She would monitor fetal movement and the duration of labor. If she concluded that the fetus was dead or labor hopeless, a sharp stone was used to dismember the fetus. Labor and birth in ancient Greece took place in the home, with the assistance of midwives. Different types or levels of midwife were recognized, according to their sophistication in nutrition, drugs and surgical technique. A birthing chair was typically used. Hippocrates and Aristotle advocated breathing exercises to relieve pain. Dystocia was recognized and instruments were devised to deliver breech births and stillbirths. Obstetrical knowledge in Western antiquity reached its high point in the writings of Soranus, who practiced in Rome during the second century[6]. He provided descriptions of the external female genitalia and attempted to depict the uterus, as well as fetal positions. His writings included essays on the anatomy of the uterus, signs of pregnancy, hemorrhage and uterine prolapse. Arab physicians appear to have used an early form of forceps for delivery no later than the tenth century.

The desire for safe births has been accompanied by an equally ancient and fervent effort to control the timing and number of births[7]. Egyptian papyri dating back to 1850 B.C.E. refer to vaginal suppositories for preventing pregnancy. These were concocted of such ingredients as crocodile feces, fermented dough, honey and saltpeter. The Berlin Papyrus from about 1300 B.C.E. suggests a purported oral contraceptive made of oil, celery and sweet beer. The Book of Genesis makes explicit reference to withdrawal as a method of contraception. In Genesis 38:8–10, Onan is commanded to "join" with his deceased brother's wife Tamar, so that she can bear an heir in accordance with the custom of levirate. Unwilling to take responsibility for another child, Onan spills his seed on the ground. The Talmud states that, "There are three women that must cohabit with a sponge: a minor, a pregnant woman and one that nurses her child." As is clear from subsequent commentaries, the sponge was quite literally an absorbent material, such as cotton or wool, intended to block passage of sperm. The seventh century C.E. Chinese physician, Master Tung-hsuan, discussed both *coitus reservatus* and *coitus obstructus*, which served to prevent the release of semen during intercourse. Though contraceptive in effect, the purpose may have been preserving the man's *yang* rather than avoiding pregnancy. During the same period, a text by Sun Ssu-mo describes the "Thousand of Gold Contraceptive Prescription", consisting of oil and quicksilver fried together for a day and then taken orally to induce sterility. The *I Ching* contains the following passage, "... married women have difficulties at the time of childbirth. Some bear offspring unceasingly but desire to stop this, therefore prescriptions are written so that they may be prepared for use." In a thirteenth century commentary on this passage, Hsieh Chi recommends a potion made of the ashes of paper on which silkworm eggs have hatched. As far back as a thousand years ago, Indians used a variety of contraceptives, including a potion made of powdered palm leaf and red chalk and vaginal suppositories made of honey, clarified butter, rock salt or the seeds of the *palasa* tree. Indian texts such as the twelfth century *Ratirahasya* ("Secret of Love") and *Pancasayaka* ("The Five Arrows") and the sixteenth century *Anangaranga* ("The Stage of the God of Love") describe no fewer than nineteen contraceptive prescriptions, consisting largely of mixtures of herbs and other plants. Contraception also appears early in Islamic history. During the late ninth or early tenth century C.E., the Persian physician, Muhammed ibn Zakariya al Razi, described three forms of contraception: withdrawal, preventing ejaculation and application of suppositories blocking the cervix. He described a variety of such suppositories, ranging from elephant dung to cabbages to pitch, used singly or in combination. During roughly the same period, Ali ibn Abbas al-Majusi wrote *The Royal Book*, in which he discusses treating women for whom a pregnancy would be dangerous with vaginal suppositories made of rock salt. During the early years of the tenth century, Abu Ali al-Husain ibn Abdallah ibn Sina, known in Europe as Avicenna, produced his medical encyclopedia *The Canon*, which includes a chapter on contraception describing twenty different methods for preventing conception. Works by Hippocrates refer to contraceptives. Soranus, the second century C.E. authority on gynecology, provided recommendations for vaginal suppositories and gave the recipe for four oral contraceptives. During the first century C.E., Discorides proposed the use of solutions made of white willow bark, white poplar bark, cabbage flowers, pepper and ivy as oral contraceptives. He further suggested that a paste made of juniper berries be placed on the penis or used as a vaginal suppository to prevent conception.

The suffering associated with sexually transmitted diseases (STD) has marred the pleasures of sex and conception. Many STD have afflicted the human race since antiquity, while others have emerged more recently. Gonorrhea is described in the Book of Leviticus, appears in the writings of Hippocrates and has probably been present in Africa for at least 2,000 years[8,9]. Pubic lice afflicted Bar Kochba's soldiers in the Jewish revolt against Rome in the second century CE[10]. Chlamydia and genital warts are also described in ancient Greek and Roman writings[11,12]. There is considerable evidence that syphilis returned to Europe from the Americas with Columbus' sailors. Called "a most presumptuous pox" by Erasmus, it ravaged the Old World, spreading rapidly and manifesting a virulence much greater than the modern variant[13]. Syphilis was reported in Uganda in 1863[14] and in Ethiopia by the beginning of the twentieth century[15]. A French physician described genital herpes in 1763[16], while chancroid was identified as a separate disease in 1850[17] and trichomoniasis in 1836[18]. Almost 400,000 U.S. soldiers were diagnosed with syphilis, gonorrhea or chancroid between 1917 and 1919[19].

Drawing Lessons from History

Three themes emerge from the historical record. The first is that there has been a strong tendency to deny, ignore or suppress the contours of reproductive health. The second has been the necessary but not sufficient role played by advances in medical technology to improve reproductive health. Third, public policy and public health approaches have been keys to improving reproductive health.

It is clear, for example, that knowledge of contraception deteriorated in the West during the Middle Ages[20]. As the Church grew in influence and hardened its position on birth control, knowledge of contraception was increasingly restricted among the two groups who were its transmitters: physicians and midwives. Profound social pressures were brought to bear on both these groups that worked against preserving the contraceptive knowledge gained over centuries. Physician training became increasingly concentrated in the universities, which were expected to be centers of Christian thought. Though Avicenna's *Canon* was the standard text for training physicians, the chapter on contraception in this massive text received less and less attention until it was eventually ignored. During the same period, the professionalization of medical training yielded increasing disdain among physicians and surgeons for the knowledge of midwives, who were also seen as competitors. The exclusion of women from medical training certainly contributed to declining interest in contraception. Midwives, meanwhile, were being subjected to a terrifying onslaught. The fifteenth century saw the apogee of the Inquisition. Part of the ideology of the Inquisition was the confluence of witchcraft, birth control and midwifery. Witches were deemed to have special powers over sexuality, using magic to induce impotence, sterility, abortion and transfer of children to control of the devil. Hence, knowledge of contraceptives and abortifacients coincided perfectly with the definition of a witch. As many as 500,000 witches were burned by the Inquisition, most of them women; an equal number were persecuted as witches, though not executed. It would be a foolhardy midwife who would advertise her knowledge of contraception and risk being charged with witchcraft. While folk knowledge of traditional contraceptives was always retained to some degree, open discussion of contraception was largely suppressed and certainly little advancement of knowledge occurred. Despite technological advances beginning in the nineteenth century, contraception remained a taboo in large swathes of the world until very recent years. Laws suppressing access to contraception in the United States were in effect until the middle of the twentieth century; the U.S. Supreme Court did not assert the constitutional right to contraception until 1965.

Open discussion of sexually transmitted diseases has been subject to similar pressures. Allan Brandt has remarked that when AIDS first emerged as a global health problem, "Not surprisingly, early socio-political responses were characterized by denial.[21]" Unlike virtually any other disease (with the possible exception of addiction), there is a strong tendency to blame the victim of a sexually transmitted disease. Though lifestyle plays a decisive role in the etiology of many illnesses, STD carry a unique degree of stigma. This has engendered denial at both a personal and social level. Political and social leaders have, with rare exception, been unwilling to publicly address STD as a public health priority until a crisis has been reached. Acknowledging a high prevalence of STD is to also openly state that a significant portion of the population engages in sexual behavior that violates ostensible social norms. Hence, social and political leaders have usually avoided the issue altogether or offered odd interpretations that skirted the truth. In Victorian England and nineteenth century United States, for example, cases of syphilis were widely ascribed to non-sexual causes, a phenomenon termed 'syphilis of the innocent'.

To the extent that the link to sexual intercourse was acknowledged, there has been an urge to suppress the offending behavior. From the emergence of syphilis in Renaissance Europe to the appearance of AIDS, religious and social leaders have labeled STD as the "natural" consequence of immoral behavior. 'Education', exhortation and the suppression of offensive public discourse were then used to return the population to the path of virtue. This has been accompanied by efforts to single out for quarantine, punishment and ostracism sub-groups believed to be the locus of infection. Laws aimed at controlling and isolating sex workers in the U.S., the United Kingdom and Thailand are examples of this misplaced strategy. Homophobia was part of the reaction to AIDS in the United States and elsewhere. An alternative strategy has been to blame 'foreigners' of one ilk or another and seek their expulsion. In the sixteenth century, European nations routinely blamed each other as the source of syphilis; the English called the disease the French pox, while the French called it the Italian illness. The response to AIDS in much of the world has been similar, with the political finger pointing to external sources, which only served to delay useful domestic policy.

The social stigma attached to STD has served as a major barrier to care. Shame, embarrassment and the fear of public disclosure have inhibited persons afflicted with the disease from seeking treatment.

Obstetric care has been less of an "underground" movement than some other aspects of reproductive health. However, one may plausibly argue that the secondary status of women has contributed to according lesser priority to maternal health. Greater power and prominence among women might have resulted in attention and resources being directed earlier to making essential obstetric care widely available. In a famous article published in 1985, Allan Rosenfield and Deborah Maine argued cogently that the obstetric, medical and public health communities had neglected maternal mortality.[22] Maternal and child health programs had in fact focused on child survival to the exclusion of saving women's lives. The silence of the health community had been matched by that of international organizations and national governments. To this must be added what John Paxman and his colleagues termed the "clandestine epidemic" of abortion.[23] They argued that in Latin America there reigned a prevailing fiction that abortion, being illegal, was not practiced. Consequently, public discussion of the reality of widespread clandestine abortion was rare. The same observation might be made of other regions of the world. Legal and social strictures served to veil the actual practice of unsafe abortion and the consequences for women's health.

The phenomenon of denial has been particularly acute in the field of sexual violence. The norms of many societies legitimize violence against women, granting men the explicit or implicit right to coerce women through the actual or implied use of force. Sexual violence commonly occurs within the household, where it is shielded by closed doors and the presumption of privacy. Both health providers and law enforcement officers are often unwilling, unsupported or untrained to intervene in domestic violence. Sexual violence has been increasingly used as a tool for terrorizing populations in civil wars. The taboos against open discussion of child sexual abuse are often more stringent than those affecting sexual violence against women. Women are often ashamed or unwilling to discuss being victimized by sexual violence and children are usually prevented from articulating their experience. Advocacy organizations and protective institutions, such as women's and children's shelters, are all too rare in traditional and resource poor settings. All of these circumstances have served to obscure the dimensions and realities of sexual violence.

Over time, the urgency and legitimacy of interventions to improve reproductive health has grown. Determined advocacy has helped overcome the tendencies to denial and neglect. But the underlying social tensions remain. Abortion, contraception, STD and sexual violence remain controversial issues about which public discourse is often difficult, emotional and strained.

Fortunately, biomedical advances have provided an increasing array of effective tools for improving reproductive health. In the early twentieth century, maternal mortality remained very high in most Western countries[24]. Levels were comparable to today's developing countries; i.e., about 600 deaths per 100,000 births in the United Kingdom and Australia and between 700 and 900 deaths per 100,000 births in the United States. Rates in Sweden were somewhat lower, at 250–300 deaths per 100,000 births because, as shall be discussed shortly, an effective maternal health strategy had been introduced around 1870. The major causes of death were also similar to those in developing countries—hemorrhage, eclampsia, obstructed labor and infection.

Widespread use of modern obstetrical methods was an essential precursor to the decline in maternal mortality[25]. Obstetrics benefited from the more general progress of medicine, including a detailed understanding of anatomy, the introduction of asepsis, improved surgical techniques, diagnostics procedures with wide applicability (e.g., blood pressure), antibiotics and blood transfusion. The importance of asepsis to preventing puerperal infection had been known since the mid-nineteenth century. It was adopted quickly in Sweden but was not widely practiced in the United Kingdom and the United States until well into the twentieth century. Equally important was the introduction of antibiotics, particularly the sulphonamides in the 1930s and penicillin in 1941. Mortality from infection dropped precipitously as asepsis was joined to antibiotic drugs. The big breakthrough in treating eclampsia came in 1930, when Vasilii Stroganoff developed an anti-convulsive therapy using morphine and chloral hydrate. This led to a dramatic decline in deaths from eclampsia, which was reinforced by the later development of combined anticonvulsive/antihypertensive therapy. The successful management of obstructed labor required the confluence of three streams of medical innovation—forceps to aid labor, induction of labor and Cesarean section. The first two would prove critical to facilitating vaginal labor, while Cesarean sections would provide the needed alternative. A major advance was made during the seventeenth century, when the Chamberlen family of Essex, England developed forceps that were curved to fit the fetal head. The design and use of forceps underwent a series of innovations over the next 300 years. The introduction of anesthesia in obstetrics made possible the advent of the Kielland forceps in 1915, which facilitate rotation of the fetal head. Successful stimulation of labor became possible after 1935, when J. Chassar Moir isolated ergometrine. While ergometrine did not prove to be an appropriate drug for stimulating labor, subsequent research led Moir to the development of synthetic oxytocics. In 1876, the Italian physician Eduardo Porro integrated anesthesia, asepsis and new surgical techniques to carry out a successful Cesarean section free of hemorrhage and infection. In 1882, Max Sanger introduced new techniques that preserved the uterus and further reduced infection, resulting in a decline in mortality subsequent to Cesarean section. Asepsis in Cesarean section was enhanced after 1890, as the use of rubber gloves became commonplace. John Kerr and Edward Holland further refined the procedure in 1921, including the switch to incision in the lower segment of the uterus, which carries many advantages in reduced risk to the mother. The control of hemorrhage brought together the innovations described above with blood transfusions. Prenatal hemorrhage due to placenta previa could be prevented with Cesarean section by the 1920s. The likelihood of uterine rupture declined as the number of excessively long labors decreased. Ergometrine could be used after birth to hold postpartum hemorrhage in check. Blood transfusions became safe and feasible after 1900 when methods for ensuring blood group compatibility were developed. This dramatically reduced maternal deaths due to hemorrhage. After 1914, blood banks were relatively common in Europe and the United States as the technique for blood storage was introduced.

Widespread use of modern contraceptive methods did not begin until the vulcanization of rubber in 1844 permitted mass production of the modern condom[26]. Condom production from natural materials was tedious and expensive. With the advent of the rubber condom, production soared into the millions by the turn of the century. By the 1930's sales in the United States alone exceeded 300 million condoms per year. The sponge was introduced to France and England by the early 1800's. In 1832, Dr. Charles Knowlton, an American, published the first of what was to be many editions of *Fruits of Philosophy*, in which he provided an elaborate rationale for contraception, as well as a discussion of methods. He focused chiefly on douching using a syringe, a technique he claimed to have invented. He proposed a variety of presumed spermicides – aluminum phosphate sulfate, zinc sulphate, salt, vinegar, liquid chloride of soda – that could be mixed with water in specified proportions and injected via the syringe immediately after intercourse. Contraceptive douches became increasingly popular, but were renamed "feminine hygiene" products after the passage in 1873 of the first Comstock Laws, which severely restricted lawful access to contraception. By the middle of the twentieth century, more than 500 "feminine hygiene" products had been marketed, many of which were of highly dubious utility and/or dangerous. As early as 1838, F.A. Wilde recommended the use of a rubber cervical cap made from a wax impression of the client. By the 1880's the rubber diaphragm and cervical cap were in use. The Mesinga diaphragm was in use in

Holland and Germany by this time, while the cervical cap was being advertised in England. One of the more popular publications in late nineteenth century England and America was the *Wife's Handbook* by Dr. Henry A. Allbutt, in which he introduces the rubber cervical cap, along with discussions of the "safe period", douching, the diaphragm and withdrawal. In 1928, Ernst Grafenberg introduced the modern intrauterine device (IUD), which consisted of a ring made of a silver alloy. T. Ota developed a similar device in Japan around the same time. The Grafenberg and Ota IUDs were used sparingly due to fears of perforation and infection. Advances in IUD technology by W. Oppenheimer in Israel and Atsui Ishihama in Japan during the 1950's greatly relieved medical concerns and significantly advanced the popularity of the IUD. Many variants of the IUD followed, using a range of materials and shapes. The popularity of the IUD device suffered a blow in the 1970s and 1980s due to the association of pelvic inflammatory disease with the Dalkon Shield version of the IUD. Today, IUDs are widely used and generally considered safe and effective. The roots of modern female sterilization techniques can be traced to the late nineteenth century, when S.S. Lungren of Toledo, Ohio ligated the fallopian tubes in the course of a Cesarean section. Multiple techniques of female sterilization were essayed during the early twentieth century, but it was not until 1928 that Ralph Pomeroy developed a safe and effective means of tubal ligation. Laparoscopy as a technique for sterilization was introduced in 1937, but became more widely applied in the 1960s and 1970s as the techniques for abdominal insufflation, electrocoagulation and mechanical occlusion of the tubes evolved. Vasectomy was available during the early part of the twentieth century, but it did not become a widely used method until the 1960s with the introduction of new occlusion techniques. More recently, the field has seen the advent of "no scalpel" vasectomy, which further limits the degree of surgical intrusion. The most dramatic modern change in contraceptives was the introduction of hormonal methods, beginning with the approval of the combined oral contraceptive (COC) by the U.S. Food and Drug Administration in 1960. The COC consists of a combination of the hormones estrogen and progestin. Over the years, the dosage of hormones in commonly used COCs has been progressively decreased to very low levels without loss of efficacy. Over the next twenty-five years a variety of progestin-only methods were developed. The progestin-only pill was released in 1966 and Depo-Provera, an injectable progestin, was introduced in 1967. The 1980s saw the introduction of long term, subdermal implants consisting of small rods that continually release low levels of progestin. A hormone releasing IUD has also been developed, thus combining two contraceptive approaches.

Developing a treatment of syphilis was one of the landmark achievements in all of medicine. In the early twentieth century Paul Ehrlich developed an arsenic based compound known as salvarsan that he called "a magic bullet". It was the first time that a specific drug had been successfully developed to attack a specific infectious agent. Salvarsan, because of its toxicity, proved a difficult and dangerous drug to administer. Nonetheless, it created the path to customizing drugs for specific diseases. The next big breakthrough came with the development of antibiotics, beginning in the 1940s. Penicillin and its derivatives proved extremely effective at combating syphilis, leading to a period of euphoria in which it was predicted the disease would be eradicated. Treatments for gonorrhea and other bacterial and fungal STD soon followed. The emergence of antimicrobial resistant strains of STD has led to increasing concern about the long term efficacy of drug therapies. However, modern medicine now has at its disposal a wide range of safe, effective and relatively inexpensive antibiotics that can be used to cure a wide range of STD. Viral STD have remained a major hurdle. Until the advent of HIV, viral STD, though potentially debilitating, were not deadly. Antiviral drugs, focused initially on genital herpes, were developed during the 1970s and became the subject of frenetic activity as the AIDS pandemic took hold. These drugs do not cure viral disease, but basically serve to inhibit replication of the virus. Anti-retroviral drugs that can control HIV are now available. However, they are complex and, with some exceptions, extremely expensive.

Medical advances, however important, have not been enough to bring about substantial improvements in reproductive health in either developed or developing countries. The combination of denial, traditional practices and resistance from the medical community to new approaches has invariably delayed using the available techniques. Major advances in reproductive health status have involved the confluence of multiple events or trends:

- Zealous advocates and political action have been needed to raise public awareness of a specific problem, demonstrate the feasibility of solutions and attract public and private resources. Private citizens, non-governmental organizations and government bureaucrats have served as pioneers in marshaling the evidence, coalescing allies and launching programs, often in the face of fierce opposition. In both the West and developing countries, the advent of programs in family planning and HIV/AIDS resulted from vigorous, politically astute and often risky efforts by advocates to place reproductive health issues on the agenda and obtain government support.
- Nations must build the institutional capacity to deliver services reflecting best practice. Technical advances are of little use unless systems are developed that permit easy access to essential services and goods, including drugs. The advancement of maternal health is a clear case in point. Re-training of health professionals and institutionalization of new standards by professional and accrediting bodies played an important role. The use of untrained birth attendants was systematically de-legitimized among health providers and the general public. New laws and regulations increased health provider accountability for maternal health outcomes, including penalties for poor performance. In Sweden, for example, training and certification of a large cadre of professional midwives began relatively early in the nineteenth century[27]. By 1861, 40 percent of births were attended by trained midwives; this figure rose to 78 percent by 1900. By this time, 80 percent of all Swedish midwives had received professional training. New techniques were promptly diffused within the midwifery corps. Maternal mortality in Sweden began to decline in 1870 and reached 300 per 100,000 birth by the turn of the century, half that of other Western nations. Declines in the United States and the United Kingdom did not manifest until after 1930, largely because these two countries delayed introducing the necessary policies. Training of physicians and midwives in modern obstetrical techniques did not really take effect until the 1930s. Concurrently, well-publicized inquiries into the state of maternal health brought public attention to bear on obstetrical practice. Improvements in hospital asepsis and ability to manage obstetrical emergencies also played a major role in reducing maternal mortality. In both countries, public authorities took a hand by promulgating regulations enforcing better maternal health care.
- Change in reproductive behavior and community norms must accompany or precede technological advances for substantial gains in health status to be achieved. The health benefits of contraception for women and children can only be realized when there is a widespread desire to space births and have smaller families. Reductions in maternal health occurred only as women turned away from the use of untrained attendants and begin to demand access to professional care. The spread of STD is directly linked to risky sexual behavior. Sexual violence must be socially de-legitimized for women to receive protection. There is an interaction between organized reproductive health programs and changes in behavior and norms. Programs are sometimes responding to latent demand, making it easier for people to exercise

new choices. For example, there is a large unmet need for family planning. Easy access to high quality services facilitates the adoption of contraception among those already predisposed. Organized programs also serve to promote new behaviors either through educational efforts or by modeling new behaviors and new possibilities.

In sum, a public health approach combining health technologies, behavior change, reinforcement of new norms, capacity building and public policy has been needed for substantial gains in reproductive health to be achieved.

REPRODUCTIVE HEALTH AND MANAGING RISK

Reproductive health is fundamentally a *social phenomenon*, intricately linked to the wider social and economic circumstances of individuals and households. The state of reproductive health in a community reflects the more general health status, which in turn responds to the broader development setting. Hence, our thinking about reproductive health should emanate from a broader perspective on health and development issues.

Poor people are extremely sensitive to risk. By this I mean that small changes in their immediate environment can make the difference between attaining or not attaining basic needs, including food, clean water, shelter, health care, education and participation in the decisions that affect their lives. The difference between the poor and the secure is the possession of assets. The secure control economic, social, physical and intellectual assets that allow them to weather losses in income, illness, political change or other alterations in circumstance without losing the ability to meet basic needs. Among the vulnerabilities of the poor are:[28]

- *Physical weakness*: Essential labor, such as farming, carrying water and fetching firewood, is physically demanding. Households are composed of a high proportion of children and, often, elderly or disabled relatives. The ability to prevent or care for illness is often very limited. Poor health, inadequate nutrition and a low proportion of working age adults diminish over-all labor productivity. Any change that increases physical weakness, such as illness or accident, decreases the labor available to meet basic needs.
- *Low income and few material goods*: Even in the best of times, the poor have a very thin surplus above the income level required to meet basic needs and very few fungible goods. Hence, even small perturbations—such as the illness of a child or a reduced harvest—can drain available resources, depriving the family of basic needs or forcing reliance on moneylenders or patrons.
- *Limited knowledge and skills*: While the poor have an intense knowledge of the local environment that must be respected, they frequently lack the schooling or technical knowledge that can help them increase productivity or fend off risks to health and welfare.
- *Tenuous natural resources*: The rural poor are especially susceptible to degradation of natural resources or changes in weather patterns. Pressures on land and water resources reduce access to the means by which poor families secure their livelihoods.
- *Little political power*: Poor families are subject to abuse stemming from lack of political power. In its most egregious forms, near feudal conditions exist that keep poor families in thrall to local elites. Poor families are particularly vulnerable to politically motivated violence. Even in more stable settings, poor families in non-democratic settings often lack the political power to secure essential services and foster policies that direct resources towards their needs. Government health budgets, for example, often disproportionately benefit the relatively well off at the expense of the poor.

- *Isolation*: Poor people are often physically, economically or socially cut off from contact with the wider society. This inhibits access to essential services, such as health care, and renders them vulnerable to exploitation by middlemen. Brokers and mid-level bureaucrats are often in a position to profit from the isolation of poor families.

In sum, poor people struggle to meet basic needs. They possess few economic, intellectual, political and social assets that can help them respond to risks to sustaining their livelihoods. While the poor are often remarkably ingenious and creative in developing coping strategies, their options are usually limited and they are easily driven further into poverty. Small perturbations—bad weather, a poor harvest, illness, loss of very small amounts of cash—can threaten access to basic needs. As should be evident, the risks facing the poor are linked; each dimension of vulnerability feeds the others. A down turn in any aspect tends to drain resources in other areas. As a consequence, poor people are often faced with very difficult choices in deploying scarce resources. One basic need must be traded against another. A poor person must ask questions such as: Do I pay for antibiotics to treat an STD or food? Do I invest in contraceptives or tools? Should I borrow from the money-lender to pay for obstetrical care or sell one of the animals? In practice, the poor make sophisticated and rational calculations in light of available knowledge to secure basic needs. For our purposes, we must recognize that investing time and money in health, including reproductive health, is an option that the poor must weigh against other basic needs.

The foregoing analysis suggests a basic approach to development, which emphasizes increasing the assets of the poor so as to sustain their ability to meet basic needs. To use the social science jargon, we call this achieving *livelihood security*, which is defined as adequate and sustainable access to the income and other resources needed to meet basic needs, including food, water, health, shelter, education and participation in civil society.[29] Livelihoods are sustainable when an individual or household can cope with and recover from stress and shocks, maintain capabilities and assets and provide sustainable livelihood opportunities for the next generation. A useful development strategy helps build the assets that buffer the poor from risk. Assets include good health, income, labor power, technical skills, equipment, land, capital, access to food and water, shelter, protected natural resources, education and training, and participation in collective decision-making. Each of these helps protect the poor against perturbations in the environment and changes in circumstance. Moreover, the assets are mutually supportive. Just as vulnerability in one area tends to increase vulnerability in others, so, too, does an increase in assets in one domain tend to reinforce progress across sectors.

It follows from our preceding discussion that we must really think of health in two ways, as an end and as a means. All of us seek good health. A state of robust vitality, absent illness and disability, is a desired state regardless of its specific ancillary consequences. Improved health among clients is often considered a sufficient goal for health providers and managers. Certainly, there is much worth in setting health goals in terms of reduced morbidity and mortality. Yet the analysis of vulnerabilities suggests that health must be considered as a means as well as an end. Health is an asset in the struggle of the poor to meet basic needs. This gives us a particular optic through which to view the allocation of scarce public health resources. Health programming, in the context of reducing risk, needs to focus on reducing the costs to the household – in cash and labor productivity – of morbidity and mortality. Viewing good health as an end and as a means suggests that the focus of health programming should be on promoting *health security, which is defined as the ability to identify, prevent and manage risks to health.*[30]

The foregoing analysis suggests a basic approach to health and development programming that informs the conceptual framework for this book. Both the poor and the secure are subject to risk. What differentiates the two groups is that the secure possess economic, social and intellectual assets that help them weather risk. The secure can draw on savings in the event of a loss of income; the poor cannot. The secure are able to prevent illness through greater knowledge, whereas the poor are more prone to unhealthy behaviors. Both savings and knowledge are assets used to enhance security and reduce vulnerability to risk. *The objective of development programming is, therefore, to increase security by accumulating assets.* The asset accumulation approach has five major elements:

1. *Understanding and influencing the web of inter-related risks that determine decisions*: Because they are acutely aware of their vulnerability, poor households are highly sensitive to risk. A seemingly simple act, like prolonged breastfeeding or safe sex or a visit to a clinic, may entail risks to income or physical safety that exceed the tolerance of a poor person. In many instances, women cannot simply say no to sex, postpone the next pregnancy or insist the partner use a condom because the consequences for meeting basic needs are too great. Choices by poor people are rarely simple or easy. Altering the risk calculation by changing the objective degree of risk and the perception of risk is essential to effective programming. The poor cannot risk new choices; the secure can experiment with new paths.

2. *Increasing the intellectual assets for managing risk*: The secure differ from the poor in the repertoire of behaviors they can deploy to identify, prevent and manage risks to well-being. The secure have a more accurate understanding of the causality of risk. A secure woman has a better understanding of how and why pregnancy can imperil her life than a poor woman. A secure person has a better understanding of how to prevent or forestall risk, such as the practice of safer sex. A secure person has a better understanding of how to manage risk, such as using contraception to space births or end childbearing. A secure person has a repertoire of skills and behaviors for managing complex scenarios, such as negotiating condom use or fending off sexual violence. Building intellectual assets increases security.

3. *Increasing the capacity for collective action*: Risks to individuals are often most effectively offset through collective action. The poor are disorganized; the secure are able to mobilize together to obtain what they need. Community norms and the sanctions that accompany adherence or violation of those norms can powerfully influence individual behavior. The posture of community leaders can be determinative of the choices and risks that people encounter. Services and goods that may be beyond the means of an individual or household can become accessible when resources are pooled. Communities that are organized into a collective voice are usually more effective at negotiating with external authorities and resources than individuals operating on their own. Community competence at accurately assessing shared risks and devising an appropriate strategy for collective action is a critical asset in meeting basic needs, including health.

4. *Increasing access to essential services*: The poor cannot obtain essential services in time of need; the secure are able to do so. Health services provide an exemplary case in point. Access to health services among the poor is often very difficult. Long walks, insufficient income to pay for goods and services, social and cultural taboos and bad information pose formidable obstacles. Such services as may be accessible are often inappropriate to the priority health needs in a community. The quality of care is often poor. The transformation from poor to secure involves identifying the interventions that will have the greatest impact, obtaining access to these essential services and ensuring the appropriate standards of quality in service delivery are respected.

5. *Increasing the ability to affect public policy choices*: The poor lack political power; the secure are able to exercise influence over the decisions that impact their lives. One of the strategies for managing risk is shaping the allocation of public sector resources and other decisions by government officials. Health resources in developing countries are often disproportionately distributed to urban populations and tertiary care, with those in higher income brackets receiving a disproportionate share of public sector resources. Skills at policy advocacy are an asset in achieving greater security. The ability to clearly define a policy goal, identify the key decision-makers, build a supportive coalition and deflect opponents can elicit needed government responses.

We can now apply this general framework to the special problem of reproductive health. Individuals and households are subject to a wide range of reproductive risk—unwanted or mistimed pregnancies, diseases and disorders of the reproductive system, maternal morbidity and mortality, sexual violence in all its forms, and psychosexual dysfunction. Some of these risks can be prevented from manifesting, while others must be managed as they appear. The objective of reproductive health programs is *reproductive security, which is achieved when individuals and households are able to identify, prevent and manage significant risks to their reproductive health*. Reproductive security means that people are reasonably knowledgeable about the most salient risks to reproductive health in their lives, manifest behaviors that help prevent reproductive diseases and disorders and have an effective strategy for coping with illness that does not drain resources from other basic needs. Reproductive security is enhanced through a supportive environment at the community, institutional and policy levels. This conceptualization of reproductive health—the ability to identify, prevent and manage reproductive risks—embodies a causal model that is depicted graphically in Figure 1-1 on page 19. The reproductive security approach defines the six critical elements of effective reproductive health programs:

1. *Reproductive risk analysis*: The first step in fostering reproductive security is ensuring that the salient risks to reproductive health in a given context have been properly identified and prioritized. This simply means that all the actors in a health system—individuals, communities, health providers, and managers—*are focused on the right problems*. The most important reproductive health problems are those which most affect the ability of the poor to secure basic needs. The perceptions of the poor are therefore critical in selecting priorities. Reproductive risk analysis is used to identify reproductive risks and sets priorities among reproductive health problems. Reproductive risk analysis combines the tools of epidemiology with participatory approaches that take into account the perceptions of the poor as to the problems they view as of greatest significance. Reproductive risk analysis includes criteria and procedures for making choices among reproductive health problems in the face of limited resources. At a global level there are three types of reproductive risk that most dramatically affect the security of the poor—unwanted, mistimed or risky pregnancies; maternal morbidity and mortality; and, sexually transmitted diseases (STD), especially HIV/AIDS. These three topics are the focus of much of this book, though their relative importance will depend on the context and other issues, such as sexual and gender based violence, also weigh heavily on reproductive security.
2. *Encouraging healthy reproductive behaviors*: Reproductive security is enhanced through the practice of appropriate behaviors. The specific behaviors of concern in a given context are derived from the risk analysis. The risk analysis will normally have clear implications for the behavior changes needed to manage risks to health, e.g., contraceptive use, safe sex, birth planning, nutritional practices, etc. Reproductive health programs can encourage healthy behaviors by using appropriate behavior change models and communication strategies. There are four key

concepts that can be used in shaping behavior change programs: stages of change, decisional balance, processes of change, and self-efficacy. Stages of change refers to the fact that behavior change is not an on-off switch. Change takes place incrementally with movement from lack of awareness of risk to experimenting with new behaviors to adopting and sustaining healthier behaviors over the long term. The changes occur as the perceived benefits exceed the perceived costs; that is, the decisional balance changes. Change processes are the cognitive and emotional factors that lead to a new decisional balance. Self-efficacy is the degree of confidence that people have to undertake change. Effective behavior change programs make use of these concepts to increase intellectual assets for reproductive risk management; i.e., the repertoire of behaviors that are used to achieve greater reproductive health.

3. *Community empowerment*: Fostering the ability to undertake collective actions that mitigate risk is a critical part of improving reproductive health. These actions include sustaining community health workers, community based distribution of contraceptives, rapid transport of obstetrical emergencies, blood donation, ensuring access to essential drugs, support to people living with AIDS, community health education, emergency health loan funds, and refurbishing and equipping local health facilities. These actions emanate from a process of community empowerment that includes participatory appraisal of needs, mobilizing community resources, building the capacity of community based organizations and leadership development. Effective reproductive health programs work in partnership with communities to build community competence for collective action.

4. *Institutional capacity building*: Reproductive security can be achieved only if essential health services are available. Reproductive security means, at minimum, access to contraception, obstetric care, and management of sexually transmitted diseases, especially HIV/AIDS. In many contexts, programs that prevent and treat sexual and gender based violence will also be critical to fostering reproductive security. One of the basic responsibilities of reproductive health managers is to increase the capacity of health institutions to deliver essential services. The term "institutions" must be understood broadly, covering the range of suppliers of health services, including public, private not-for-profit, traditional and for-profit providers. There are four essential, inter-connected elements to capacity building: (1) selecting the interventions most responsive to the priority health needs of the population being served; (2) increasing access to services; (3) improving quality; and, (4) strengthening management systems.

5. *Use of optimal health technologies*: Associated with each of the major reproductive risks are what experience and research tell us are the optimal health technologies, which may be either preventive or curative. One of the major challenges facing developing country health providers is ensuring that the health interventions selected reflect the evidence as to their efficacy. Given the very limited resources available, managers must focus their efforts on the core technologies that will have the greatest impact. Contraception, STD case detection and management, and essential obstetric care are among the core health technologies for mitigating reproductive risk.

6. *Public policy advocacy*: Health managers are always political actors. By this I mean they influence, if only by inaction, the choices made by governmental bodies ranging from village councils to ministries of health. Public policy can affect all the other elements of reproductive security. It can change the range of health technologies available, encourage or discourage behavior change, support or stifle community empowerment, expand or limit access to services, reward or ignore quality of care and support or undermine good management. Effective managers learn how to identify critical policy issues, map the array of relevant political actors and influence the outcome of government decisions.

Let us return now to our heroine, the manager of the reproductive health program. Our advice would be as follows, "We suggest that the goal of your program should be advancing reproductive security, which is defined as the ability to identify, prevent and manage risks to reproductive health. There are six essential steps to achieving this end: reproductive risk analysis, encouraging health reproductive behaviors, community empowerment, institutional capacity building, using optimal health technologies, and public policy advocacy. The rest of this book is a series of essays that can help you undertake these tasks."

THE LOCUS OF RISK MANAGEMENT: INDIVIDUALS, COUPLES, AND HOUSEHOLDS

One key issue for health managers and providers is choosing the appropriate focus or target for their interventions. Reproductive health care typically involves an encounter between health provider and a client, with women constituting the large majority of clients. The provider may prescribe a course of treatment or suggest a change in behavior. This behavior by the provider implicitly assumes that (a) the risk to reproductive health stems from the woman's behavior; and, (b) that she is free to make choices and changes that would reduce reproductive risk. Decisions about reproductive health often involve both partners and other members of the household. Understanding how decisions about managing reproductive risk are made is one of the keys to effective programming.

Let us assume the following scenario. A woman decides that she wishes to postpone or end childbearing and a clinic offering high quality family planning services is within easy walking distance. Can we then assume she adopts family planning? The answer to this question depends a great deal on who is making decisions and how decisions are made. If she is married or in some form of long-term union, as is true for the vast majority of women in developing countries, she is likely to need the acquiescence of her husband. Acting without her husband's assent may incur significant costs and risks. An individual choice has now become a decision by a couple, which will in turn reflect the degree to which the husband and wife have the same reproductive goals and the relative power of the woman and the man in making decisions. If scarce cash must be spent to purchase reproductive health care, then the decision will almost certainly involve both the husband and wife, but may also draw in other household members. If the marriage is polygamous, the woman's decision may also be conditioned by the behavior of other wives, with whom she may be competing for the favor of the husband. In many societies, parents and in-laws will also play an important role in decision-making. In South Asia, the mother or mother-in-law often plays a powerful role in choices about family size or obstetric care. In some parts of Latin America, the father encourages risky sexual behavior by adolescent sons as a rite of passage to manhood. In many parts of Africa and Asia, a woman cannot travel outside the home unless an adult male relative accompanies her. In all these instances, the decision rests not with the individual or with the couple but with the household. There is a complex interplay of the individual, the sexual partners and the household that yields the pattern of reproductive risk management.

An interesting twist on the complexity of household decision-making is choice in the *absence* of communication about reproduction and sexuality. Sexuality and reproductive health are often taboo subjects. Conversation on these issues may be very difficult or intensely strained. As a result, decisions are made by individuals on the basis of an assumption about the likely reaction of the spouse or other household member(s). Women may fear raising the issue of contraception or safe sex with their husbands, which may or may not be warranted. Contraceptive behavior is then predicated on a presumption about the reaction of the husband, whereas there is ample research that spouses are more likely to agree than disagree about fertility goals.[31] Pregnancy is frequently off-limits as a topic of household discussion, which complicates the problem of making good decisions about maternal health care. Poor communication within the household can distort individual behavior in ways inimical to reproductive security.

This complexity poses practical problems for the manager in terms of targeting services and communication. Who is the target: the individual, the couple or the household? Each might be important for a specific purpose and contexts differ, but I would argue for the primacy of the household as the starting point for analysis and programming. "Household" is defined as a small grouping of people who share residence, assume joint responsibility for producing and distributing the necessities of life and who engage in reproduction and socialization of the young[32]. The specific meaning of household clearly varies by culture and its definition remains a subject of debate, but it is a widely applicable concept.

Reproductive health programs have tended to focus on women as individuals, but decision-making about reproductive health is rarely a solo event. The household focus is a useful corrective to the tendency to define reproductive health as synonymous with women's health, rather than fully involving the male partner or recognizing the role other household members play in reproductive decision-making. The household focus certainly allows for analysis of different roles, resources and behaviors within the household. Services and communications can be targeted to women, men, couples, mothers-in-law and youth. But understanding the differing roles and interplay of these actors in decision-making can very usefully inform the content of programs. An analysis of the household dynamics of reproductive decision-making is usually very helpful in crafting effective programs.

GENDER AND REPRODUCTIVE HEALTH

Gender is a powerful force in reproductive health. The complexity of household decision-making in reproductive health is largely derived from the differences in roles ascribed to men and women. Gender discrimination compounds the vulnerability induced by poverty. Gender discrimination has negative consequences for both women and men, but women suffer disproportionately. Gender affects reproductive health in at least the following ways:

- *Access to assets*: Gender differences inhibit access by girls and women to assets that have a positive affect on reproductive security. Girls are less likely to be able to attend school, which is a powerful determinant of fertility behavior and other health outcomes. Women are less likely to have access to income and capital goods that can be used to obtain health care. Girl children in a household typically receive less food than their brothers, which results in small stature and chronic anemia. Girls and women are less likely to access health care for any reason than males.
- *Decision-making about reproductive health*: Girls and women are usually dependent on the agreement of a husband, father or other significant male to make reproductive decisions or secure reproductive health care, even when they have access to resources. They cannot independently

insist on contraception, safe sex practices or obstetric care. They may not be able to travel without the accompaniment of a male relative, thereby limiting access to care. Women are far less likely than men to influence collective decision-making at the household or community level, which serves to obscure their health needs and block appropriate action.
- *Value placed on women's health and life*: Girls and women may be viewed as chattel with relatively little intrinsic worth. This negatively influences the willingness to invest household resources in saving women's lives.
- *Expectations about reproductive behavior*: For both men and women, gender expectations can work against reproductive security. Women may be expected to have a large number of children, especially sons. This multiplies the risk of an unwanted or dangerous pregnancy. There may be substantial social pressures on men to engage in risky sexual behavior, such as having multiple partners or visiting sex workers. Women seeking reproductive health care may be subject to ridicule or other forms of pressure from family members and/or neighbors. The same problem often afflicts men, who are subject to scorn from their peers and health services poorly designed to accommodate the reproductive health needs of men.
- *Violence and the threat of violence*: Girls and women are subject to many forms of violence that have direct and indirect affects of reproductive health. Rape, abuse and female genital cutting are the most egregious and obvious forms of violence. Violence and the threat of violence also act indirectly by influencing pregnancy outcomes, use of contraception and safe sex practices.

Enhancing reproductive security almost invariably requires modulating the negative impacts of gender discrimination. This reinforces the importance of understanding and addressing the dynamics of household decision-making. Behavior change programs can be directed at couples and other household members to change the pattern and process of reproductive choice. Community norms and structures also play a role in gender bias, since women are often excluded from decision-making. Reproductive security is enhanced by community empowerment exercises that raise consciousness about reproductive health needs, help women mobilize resources, and support women leaders and women's organizations.

REPRODUCTIVE RISK ANALYSIS

The causal model suggested by Figure 1-1 can be translated into a set of key questions and indicators that allow the manager to draw a portrait of the reproductive security of a community. The model suggests that there are, in fact, a handful of basic questions that should preoccupy the manager, though answering the questions can take a bit of work. Drawing upon the reproductive security framework, the key questions are:

1. *Is the behavior of individuals and households consistent with preventing and managing risks to reproductive health?* Do they have adequate knowledge of reproductive risks? What is their attitude towards key reproductive behaviors, such as contraception, safer sex, sexual violence or use of trained birth attendants? What is the current pattern of reproductive behavior? Do they express intention or desire for changed behavior? Do they have confidence in their ability to undertake new behaviors? How do couples and households communicate and make decisions about reproductive behavior?
2. *Does the community manifest the capacity to undertake the collective actions needed to improve reproductive security?* Who makes up the community and what are its boundaries and physical attributes? What are the social networks within the community? Has the community arrived at an

PURPOSE AND CONCEPTUAL FRAMEWORK

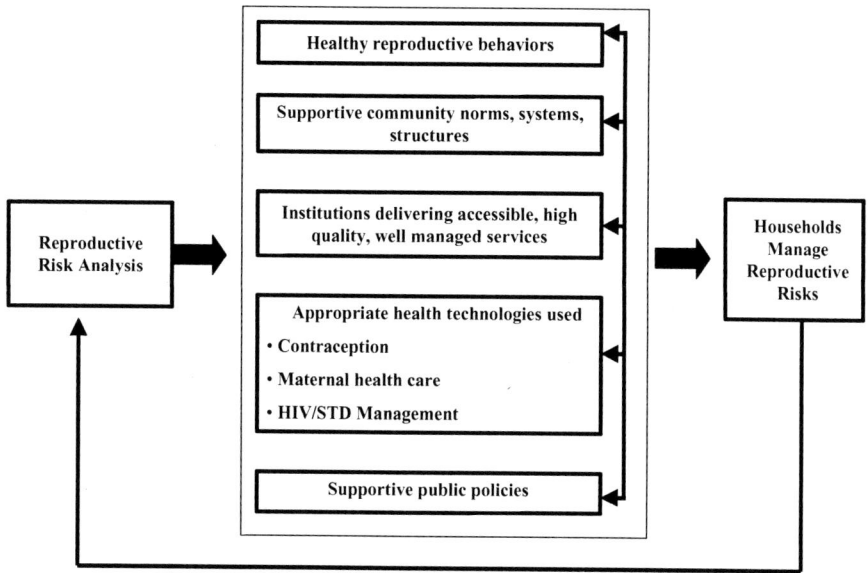

FIGURE 1-1. Achieving reproductive security.

agreement as to the frequency, severity and priority of reproductive health problems through a participatory process? Has the community mapped and mobilized its own resources to advance reproductive security? What community organizations exist that might support reproductive health programs and what is their capacity? Are community leaders supportive of reproductive health programs? What collective actions have been taken to advance reproductive security?

3. *What are the strengths and weaknesses in institutional capacity to deliver essential reproductive health services?* Is there an inventory of service providers and service delivery points? What are the barriers to accessing care? Is the service delivery strategy maximizing access to care? What is the quality of care? What are strengths and weaknesses in the management system supporting care?

4. *Are appropriate health technologies being used?* Is the current array of interventions optimal relative to the health needs of the populations? Are technologies suitable to the context being used? Are they sustainable and cost-effective?

5. *Is there political and policy support for reproductive health programs?* Are political leaders supportive? What is the degree of political opposition to the reproductive health program? What is the level of public resource allocation? Are laws, regulations and decisions by government officials advancing reproductive security? Are government officials rewarding health officials for progress in reproductive health? Are there informal, unwritten rules that are hurting or helping reproductive health programs?

Table 1-1, which presages much of what will be presented in the remainder of this book, summarizes the key questions and indicators to be used in carrying out a reproductive risk analysis. Carrying out such an analysis may seem daunting, but the manager should not feel intimidated. This book suggests a number of practical tools, methods and techniques for carrying out the analysis as we take up various topics. In addition, doing a complete risk analysis is not a necessary precursor to programming. Rather, the manager might make

TABLE 1-1. Key Elements of a Reproductive Risk Analysis

	Family planning	Maternal health	HIV/STD	Sexual violence
Individual/ Household Variables	• Knowledge/attitudes about contraception • Perceptions of personal cost/benefits of additional children • Unmet need for family planning • Intentions regarding use of family planning • Confidence in ability to use contraceptives • Couple/household communication about family planning • Couple/household decision-making about family planning • Median length of birth intervals • Distribution of population in terms of "readiness to change" • Contraceptive prevalence	• Knowledge of maternal health risks and danger signs of pregnancy • Perception of personal vulnerability to maternal mortality/morbidity • Intentions regarding birth attendant/place of birth • Confidence in ability to control circumstances of birth • Couple/household communication about maternal health • Couple/household decision-making about maternal health • Mean number of prenatal care visits • % of households with a pregnant woman that have a birth plan • % births attended by trained personnel • % women receiving 2 visits during first 5 days post-partum • % births receiving emergency obstetrical care	• Knowledge/attitudes about HIV/STD transmission • Perceived level of personal vulnerability to HIV/STD • Intentions regarding "safer sex" behavior • Confidence in ability to control exposure to STD • Couple/household communication about safer sex • Couple/household decision-making about safer sex • Number of sexual partners: Identity of "core" and "bridge" populations • % adults (>15) practicing high risk behavior for HIV/STD • % sexually active adults reporting current, consistent use of condoms • % adults seeking health care to reduce HIV/STD infection • Prevalence of major STD	• Gender specific attitudes towards use of violence in household relations (e.g., approval of wife beating) • Gender specific reports of various forms of sexual violence: psychological abuse, forced sex, other forms of sexual abuse, physical abuse • Help seeking behavior by abused women and reasons for not seeking help • Prevalence of child sexual abuse • Incidence of sexual violence recorded by health providers and law enforcement officials

TABLE 1-1. (*Continued*)

	Family planning	Maternal health	HIV/STD	Sexual violence
Technology variables	• Temporary/supply contraceptive methods • Surgical/permanent contraceptive methods	• Emergency obstetrical care • Prenatal care • Intrapartum care • Postpartum care • Safe abortion services	• Case detection • Case management, including appropriate use of syndromic management • Laboratory services • Prevention of maternal to child transmission • Blood screening • Care for people living with AIDS	• Detection and documenting of cases of sexual violence* • Assessing for immediate danger and taking counter-measures • Physical and psychological treatment of abuse • Helping women develop safety plans • Counseling as to legal rights and protections • Referral to community resources
Community variables	• Members, boundaries and physical attributes of the community • Social networks within the community • Type and degree of participatory processes used to identify and prioritize reproductive health problems. • Degree of agreement within the community as to frequency, severity and priority of reproductive health problems. • Mapping of resources to support reproductive health • Type and magnitude of community resources devoted to reproductive health • Number, type, size and capacity of community organizations addressing reproductive health issues. • Knowledge, attitude and actions of community leaders with regard to reproductive health • Type and degree of collective actions undertaken to support reproductive health			

(*continued*)

TABLE 1-1. (Continued)

Institutional variables	• Number and type of service providers and service delivery points
	• Degree to which available services align with reproductive health needs and priorities of population served
	• Service delivery strategy: community based, clinical, commercial, public, private
	   — Effectiveness of each service delivery component
	• Barriers to access to essential services: physical, monetary, sociocultural
	• Quality of care
	   — Availability of essential drugs, equipment and supplies
	   — Information and counseling
	   — Client involvement in decision-making
	   — Technical competence of providers
	   — Interpersonal relations
	   — Continuity of care
	• Management systems
	   — Community liaison
	   — Planning
	   — Human resource management
	   — Management information system
	   — Commodity management
	   — Financial management
	   — Facilities and equipment management

Policy variables	• Degree of open, public support for reproductive health programs from government officials • Level of public resources allocated to reproductive health • Laws/regulations/decisions governing the type of services that can be provided • Laws/regulations/decisions governing the range of authorized service providers • Laws/regulations/decisions governing the type/range of drugs and contraceptives that can be distributed • Laws/regulations/decisions governing communication and advertising • Incentives/disincentives from government officials for performance of public health officials and providers

*Interventions adapted from Heise, L., Ellsberg, M., and Goetemoeller M. "Ending Violence Against Women" *Population Reports* Series L., No. 11. Baltimore: Johns Hopkins University School of Public Health, Population Information Program, December 1999.

a reasoned judgment as to an appropriate starting point, such as institutional capacity or community empowerment. Research and programming could focus for a period on one or two elements of the framework. Once adequate progress has been achieved, the manager could begin strengthening additional elements of reproductive security. Over time, additional components of the framework could be added as objects of analysis and programming until gains in the entire system have been realized.

2

Epidemiology of Reproductive Health

MAGNITUDE AND IMPACTS OF REPRODUCTIVE INSECURITY

Unintended and High Risk Pregnancies

Between 20 percent and 40 percent of births in the developing world are the result of either mistimed or unwanted pregnancies[1]. Figure 2-1[2] shows both the actual number of births and the number of children that would be born if women's fertility desires were being realized in Latin America and the Caribbean (LAC), sub-Saharan Africa and Asia, based on Demographic and Health Survey (DHS) data. For all 29 countries surveyed, actual fertility exceeds wanted fertility, ranging from a low of 0.4 children per woman to a high of 2 children per woman in Bolivia, Kenya and Rwanda. Unwanted fertility averages 1.4 children per woman in the Latin American countries surveyed, 1.1 children in Africa and 0.9 children in the three Asian countries surveyed. Only about half of all births in the developing world are the result of planned pregnancies, with 20 percent of pregnancies ending in induced abortion and 16 percent leading to unintended births[3].

The high level of unwanted fertility is largely attributable to a high level of unmet need for family planning. A woman with an unmet need for family planning is a woman who is fecund, exposed to the risk of pregnancy (i.e., in sexual union), does not wish to have a child within the next two years and is not using any method to prevent conception. By this measure, at least 120 million women in the developing world have an unmet need for family planning, including 26 million in Africa, 8 million in the Near East and North Africa, 12 million in Latin America and the Caribbean, 2 million in the Asian Newly Independent States (NIS) and 72 million in Asia (excluding China, Japan and the Asian NIS)[4]. Using DHS data from the 1990s, Table 2-1 shows that the unmet need for family planning is quite high in a large number of countries.

The level and pattern of fertility is a crucial determinant of child mortality. Hence, regulating fertility through family planning is a critical part of the armamentarium of public

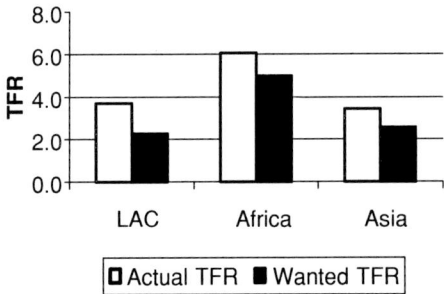

FIGURE 2-1. Wanted and unwanted fertility by region of the world (weighted averages using countries for which DHS data are available).

health practitioners seeking to improve child survival. Infant and under five mortality is more likely when:

1. the mother is an adolescent;
2. the birth of the child takes place less than 36 months after a preceding birth;
3. the child is of higher parity; i.e., the fifth or higher birth;
4. the birth is to an older women; i.e., aged 35 or older; or,
5. the birth is the result of an unwanted pregnancy.

Every year, about 15 million births occur to teenagers in the developing world[5]. Of these births, about 7 million occur in Asia, the Near East and North Africa, 5.4 million in sub-Saharan Africa and 1.4 million in Latin America and the Caribbean. Teenage births constitute about twelve percent of total births in the developing world. Data from 28 countries show that the percentage of urban adolescents who had their first child by age 19 ranged from 5 percent to 29 percent, while among rural women the percentage of teens who have had a child ranged from 7 percent to 40 percent. In general, the rate of adolescent child bearing is declining as women increasingly postpone the birth of their first child. However, the absolute number of births to teenagers will probably remain constant. A projected increase in the number of births to adolescent women in Africa will offset declines in other parts of the world.

There is a consistent and strong association between adolescent childbearing and infant mortality, with the effect most pronounced among younger teenagers[6]. In 41 of 43 countries for which Demographic and Health Survey data are available, the infant mortality rate for 15–19 year old mothers exceeds that of children born to women 20–29 years of age. Children

TABLE 2-1. Unmet Need for Contraception by Region (Number of countries)

Region	% Women with unmet need			
	<10%	10–19%	20–29%	>30%
Africa		3	12	8
Near East & North Africa		3	1	
Asia		3	2	1
Latin America & Caribbean	2	3	2	1

born to teenage mothers are 1.5 times as likely to die in infancy as children born to women aged 20–29. Teenagers are more likely to have premature births, low birth weight babies and babies with congenital anomalies. Children born to women under the age of 17 have a higher mortality rate than either children born to older teens (17–19) or women in their twenties. John Ross and Elizabeth Frankenberger reached the following conclusion:

> Children born to teenagers have 34 percent higher mortality before age five than children born to mothers aged 25–34. Children born to women under age of 18 have 42 percent higher mortality than do children born to women aged 25–34, while the excess mortality for children born to women aged 18–19 is only 13 percent[7].

The reason for the association between young maternal age and child mortality is a matter of debate. Among very young mothers, there may be physiological reasons for the observed association. However, young mothers are also more likely to experience a first birth, which generally carries higher risk than second or third births. Teenage mothers are also less apt to get good prenatal care and generally suffer disproportionately from the ills of poverty, poor education and low status that contribute to child mortality.

Birth interval has been consistently shown to have an important impact on infant and child mortality across a wide range of countries and socioeconomic circumstances[8]. Birth interval—the number of months that elapse between births—is often quite short among women in developing countries. An analysis by Shea Rutstein of DHS data from 17 countries show that the percent of birth intervals of less than 24 months ranges from 15 percent to 36 percent, while the percent of birth intervals of less than 36 months ranges from 36 percent to 70 percent[9]. The Rutstein analysis of Demographic and Health Surveys carried out in 17 countries during the 1990s showed that infant mortality and under-five mortality rise when the interval between births is less than 36 months, even after controlling for a host of potentially confounding variables. The impact on mortality is particularly dramatic for birth intervals of less than 24 months. As compared to a child born 36–47 months after a sibling, children born after a 24–35 month interval have a 31 percent greater risk of dying in infancy. Children born after less than a 24 month interval have a 137 percent greater risk of dying in infancy. The effect of birth interval holds until children reach the age of five. Compared to children born after a 36–47 month interval, children born after a 24–35 month interval have a 41 percent greater risk of mortality and those born after an interval of less than 24 months have a 144 percent greater risk of death.

Short birth intervals have been decreasing as a proportion of total births since the 1970s, contributing the world-wide reduction in infant and child mortality. Further increases in birth intervals could have a significant impact on infant mortality. Rutstein estimated that infant mortality in India would decrease by 29 percent, while under-five mortality would decline by 35 percent if all births were at least 36 months apart. This would decrease the number of child deaths in India by 1.4 million per year.

The exact mechanisms underlying the impact of birth intervals are unclear. However, it is probable that both physiological and social factors are at work. Short birth intervals may mean that the mother is less apt to enjoy an optimal pregnancy, that she is less able to care effectively for the child and/or that childcare resources are strained when children are born in quick succession.

In at least 65 countries, the total fertility rate exceeds 4.0 children per woman. Higher order births—those born fourth or higher—have been consistently associated with a higher risk of infant mortality[10]. Higher order pregnancies (6 or more) are also associated with increased likelihood of stillbirths. Iron deficiency anemia, multiple births, and complications of pregnancy are also associated with high parity. Whether high parity is causally related to infant and child mortality is uncertain. Higher order births tend to be to older women, so the effects of maternal age and parity may be confounded. High parity women may also exhibit less effective childcare behaviors, thus increasing the likelihood of child mortality.

Births to older women are more likely to end in the death of the child, though births to older women constitute a relatively small fraction of total.[11] Infants of older women are more likely to be low birth weight, which in part explains the higher level of mortality. Higher maternal age is also associated with chromosomal abnormalities (especially Down's syndrome) and other birth defects. This probably also contributes to the higher death rate among children of older women. Women over 35 are also more likely to experience complications of delivery.

Whether a pregnancy is intended or not has an impact on the health of the child[12]. In the first place, unintended pregnancies are often high-risk pregnancies, occurring to women who have had more than four children, are very young or older, or gave birth to a child less than 24 months earlier. This may account for the finding that unintended pregnancies are more likely to result in low birth weight babies than intended pregnancies. Reducing these unintended births would reduce the over-all level of child mortality by diminishing the proportion of high-risk pregnancies. Unintended pregnancies also tend to elicit maternal behaviors that are inconsistent with optimal child health. Women with unintended pregnancies are less likely to seek prenatal care, either because these women are also less likely to access health services in general or because of ambivalence towards the pregnancy. Women experiencing an unintended pregnancy are also more likely to engage in risky behavior; in the United States women with an unintended pregnancy are more likely to smoke or drink alcohol. Children of unintended pregnancies are also less likely to receive optimal care and resources from the parents.

High fertility is also an important determinant of maternal mortality.[13] About 585,000 women die every year from complications of pregnancy and labor, mostly in the developing world. Changes in fertility behavior could dramatically reduce the number of maternal deaths. One of the fundamental reasons for the concentration of maternal mortality in the developing world is the high birth rate. Every additional pregnancy increases the likelihood that a woman will experience an additional complication some time during her life. As discussed above, a high percentage of pregnancies are unintended. Reducing the number of unintended pregnancies would decrease the number of maternal deaths. Simply avoiding unintended pregnancies through contraception could prevent thirty percent of maternal deaths.

Many unintended pregnancies result in abortions. Because abortion is illegal and unsafe in many countries, abortion is a leading cause of maternal mortality. As many as 20 million unsafe abortions occur each year leading to approximately 70,000 deaths.[14] Reducing recourse to unsafe abortion through contraception would be a major contribution to maternal health.

Maternal mortality is also associated with pregnancy at the extremes of the reproductive cycle and among high parity women. In addition, there are a number of underlying medical conditions—hypertension, diabetes, heart disease, and malaria—that are exacerbated by pregnancy. Limiting pregnancy among these high-risk women would serve to reduce maternal mortality rates.

Maternal Mortality and Morbidity

A maternal death is defined as the death of a woman while pregnant or within 42 days of the end of her pregnancy from any cause related to or made worse by the pregnancy, regardless of the duration of pregnancy. Every year, about 585,000 women die from complications of pregnancy and childbirth[15]. These deaths are overwhelmingly concentrated in the developing world; 90 percent occur in Asia and sub-Saharan Africa. Maternal mortality accounts for between a quarter and a third of all deaths to women of reproductive age. A majority of the deaths can be found in just eight countries—Bangladesh, Ethiopia, India, Indonesia, Nepal, Nigeria, Pakistan and Uganda.

A woman's lifetime risk of dying in childbirth is a function of two factors: the number of pregnancies she experiences and the probability of her experiencing a life threatening obstetrical complication. As a consequence, the lifetime risk of maternal mortality is greatest where fertility is highest. As the number of pregnancies increases over the course of a lifetime the likelihood of experiencing a complication grows correspondingly. Among women who do become pregnant and experience a complication, access to quality obstetric care largely determines the likelihood of mortality. Hence, the lifetime risk of maternal mortality is greatest where fertility is highest and the maternal health care is weakest.

Correspondingly, there are two key measures of maternal mortality: the maternal mortality rate and the maternal mortality ratio. The maternal mortality *rate* is the number of maternal deaths per 100,000 women in the population. It is sensitive to the fertility rate for the reasons given earlier—as the average number of births per woman declines the number of maternal deaths per 100,000 women will also decrease. The global decrease in fertility has yielded a decline in the maternal mortality rate. However, unintended pregnancies continue to be a major contributor to maternal mortality. If no women experienced unintended pregnancy, about 30 percent of all maternal deaths—175,000 women—would be prevented. Expanding the use of contraceptives would be a major contribution to reducing maternal mortality. The maternal mortality *ratio* is the number of maternal deaths per 100,000 live births. The maternal mortality ratio is therefore an indicator of the accessibility and quality of maternal health care. By and large, maternal mortality ratios in the developing world have not improved. The declines in the lifetime risk of maternal death have resulted from fertility decreases rather than improved maternal health.

Regional disparities in fertility and obstetric care are reflected in Table 2-2[16], which shows the lifetime risk of maternal mortality by region of the world.

The countries with the highest levels of maternal mortality include Afghanistan, Angola, Bhutan, Chad, Guinea, Mozambique, Sierra Leone, Somalia and Yemen. In these countries, the maternal mortality ratio exceeds 1500 maternal deaths per 100,000 births and the lifetime risk of maternal death is 1 in 9 or greater.

Maternal mortality has serious implications for surviving children. The loss of the mother robs children of their primary caregiver, often without meaningful replacement. The risk of mortality is significantly escalated among children under 5 whose mother has died as compared to those with a living mother. The World Bank estimates that the risk of mortality among children under 5 in developing countries who have lost their mother may be as high as 50 percent[17].

There are five proximate causes that account for 75–80 percent of maternal mortality: hemorrhage, puerperal infection, hypertensive disorders of pregnancy, especially eclampsia,

TABLE 2-2. Lifetime Risk of Maternal Mortality by Region, 1990 Estimates

Region	Maternal deaths	Lifetime risk of maternal mortality	Maternal mortality ratio
Africa	235,000	1 in 16	870
Asia	323,000	1 in 65	390
Latin America & Caribbean	23,000	1 in 130	190
Europe	3,200	1 in 1,400	390
North America		1 in 3,700	
All developing countries	581,000	1 in 48	480
All developed countries	40,000	1 in 1,800	27
World	585,000	1 in 60	430

obstructed labor, and complications of unsafe abortion, which include hemorrhage, sepsis and shock.[18]

- *Hemorrhage* accounts for about a quarter of all maternal deaths. Most of these deaths are the result of post-partum hemorrhage, which is defined as a blood loss of greater than 500 ml. after delivery. Death from hemorrhage can occur very rapidly and demands immediate intervention (control of the bleeding and blood transfusion) by a trained health provider. Bleeding in early pregnancy may result from spontaneous abortion or ectopic pregnancy. Hemorrhage during late pregnancy (after 20 weeks) may be due to placenta previa, placenta abruptio, lesions of the cervix or vagina, or vasa previa.
- *Puerperal infection* is responsible for 15 percent of maternal deaths. Infections can usually be traced either to failure to observe asepsis during delivery or untreated sexually transmitted diseases. Prenatal management of STD, proper hygiene during delivery and use of antibiotics are needed to prevent maternal deaths due to infection.
- *Hypertensive disorders of pregnancy* cause approximately 12 percent of maternal deaths. Women may have pre-existing hypertension, which is exacerbated by pregnancy, or, more commonly, suffer from pregnancy induced hypertension, which is also called pre-eclampsia. Hypertension in pregnancy (blood pressure greater than 140/90) can escalate, leading to convulsions and death. Monitoring of women for hypertension during the prenatal period is one component of detecting and managing hypertensive disease. However, eclampsia (convulsions due to hypertension) can occur without prior evidence of hypertension or any prior symptoms. Eclampsia requires immediate treatment with anti-convulsives, drugs to control hypertension and ensuring the woman's airway remains unobstructed.
- *Obstructed or prolonged labor*, more properly termed dystocia, accounts for 8 percent of maternal deaths. Dystocia results from malpresentation of the fetus, failure of the uterus to contract properly or when the baby is too large for the pelvis. In some instances, malpresentation can be corrected through gentle external manipulation of the fetal position. However, dystocia will usually require a Cesarean section or other medical intervention.
- *Complications of unsafe abortion* cause another 13 percent of maternal deaths world-wide. Hemorrhage, infection and shock can result from poor abortion technique. Preventing unwanted pregnancies through contraception and access to safe abortions are the most appropriate responses to this problem. Women suffering the consequences of an unsafe abortion need prompt medical treatment.

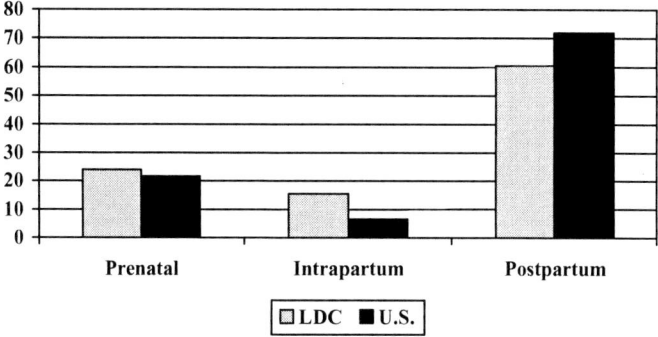

FIGURE 2-2. Distribution of maternal deaths by time of death.

Another 20 percent of maternal deaths occur because pregnancy exacerbates other health problems. Very high proportions of women in the developing world suffer from anemia. Pregnancy, which places a tremendous toll on iron stores, may therefore result in heart failure. Other cardiovascular disorders, malaria, hepatitis, diabetes and HIV/AIDS can combine with the stresses of pregnancy to yield mortality.

Maternal mortality is largely concentrated in the post-partum period. Figure 2-2 shows the distribution of maternal deaths by time of death for the U.S. and the developing world[19]. As can be seen, 60 percent of deaths in the developing world occur during the post-partum period, with 24 percent during the prenatal period and just under 16 percent during labor and childbirth.

Post-partum deaths occur largely within the first few days following childbirth. Forty-five percent occur within the first 24 hours and 68 percent within the week immediately following delivery. Ninety-six percent of deaths have occurred by 30 days following childbirth.

Hemorrhage accounts for 50 percent of all postpartum deaths and over 90 percent of deaths due to hemorrhage happen during the seven days after delivery, with an average interval of only twelve hours from onset of hemorrhage to death. Mortality due to eclampsia, which is responsible for 13 percent of postpartum deaths, is concentrated in the immediate postpartum period, with an average span of two days following onset. Infection is responsible for 30 percent of postpartum deaths and a fifth of these deaths take place during the first week.

The incidence of serious maternal illness is a large multiple of maternal mortality. Approximately 15 percent of all pregnancies yield a life threatening complication. In 1998, there were approximately 120 million births in the less developed countries, which translates to *18 million* cases of serious maternal illness. UNICEF estimates that as much as 40 percent of pregnancies manifest some form of complication[20].

In some instances the complication resolves with the pregnancy. However, millions of women are subject to long term disabilities as a consequence of pregnancy. Of particular concern are two widespread, chronic conditions: obstetrical fistula and genital prolapse. Obstetric fistula are lacerations resulting from labor and childbirth that yield a passage between the vaginal canal and bladder (vesico–vaginal fistula) and/or rectum (recto–vaginal fistula). They are most likely to occur among young women having their first child since the vaginal wall has not been stretched from prior births. If the woman survives the resulting hemorrhage, she suffers a serious chronic disability with urine or feces passing uncontrolled through the vaginal canal. In addition to the medical complications, obstetric fistula have grave social consequences; the woman is apt to lose her husband and become socially ostracized due to the continuing leakage, foul odor and inability to bear children.

Genital prolapse is the collapsing of the uterus or vagina below their normal position. Uterine prolapse can be life threatening, causing hemorrhage and/or infection. Women who have had multiple pregnancies are more apt to experience prolapse due to the weakening of the muscles of the uterus and vagina. Women with genital prolapse are prone to infection, painful intercourse, urinary problems, backache and loss of any succeeding pregnancies.

Though precise estimates are unavailable, it appears likely that millions of women are affected by fistula and prolapse. One estimate places the number of women with vesicovaginal fistula in Africa at 1.5 to 2 million women, with 50,000 to 100,000 new cases per year[21]. Community based studies have commonly found that at least one-third of women suffer from prolapse.

Limited, poor quality obstetric care is a fundamental reality that must be confronted in efforts to reduce maternal mortality and morbidity. Women receive very little prenatal care and attendance at birth is commonly by a relative or untrained traditional birth attendant. Many women receive no prenatal care at all. Table 2-3 shows the proportion of women receiving at least four prenatal contacts with a health professional, which is the minimum recommended by WHO[22]. Approximately 60 million women give birth every year alone, with the aid of a family member or using an untrained traditional birth attendant[23]. Table 2-4 shows those countries for which 50 percent or fewer of births receive the assistance of a trained birth attendant[24].

The limitations on obstetrical care reflect the realities of women's lives and health care in much of the developing world. There are a host of barriers to access to care: physical, economic, social and psychological. Such care as is available is often of poor quality, with badly trained staff, little equipment and scarce drug supply.

Induced Abortion

Induced abortion is defined as "the termination of pregnancy using drugs or surgical intervention after implantation and before the conceptus has become independently viable"[25], which is deemed by the WHO to occur at 22 weeks following the last menstrual period, except where the fetus is lethally malformed. This definition is very helpful in distinguishing contraceptives from abortifacients. Contraceptives prevent fertilization and/or implantation, whereas abortifacients remove the conceptus after implantation.

Each year, between 36 and 53 million abortions are performed worldwide.[26] In 1998 there were 133 million births[27]—meaning one abortion for every 2.4 to 3.7 births. Table 2-5 shows the estimated abortion rate for 1990 (abortions per 1,000 women 15–44) by region of the world[28]. As this table shows, unintended pregnancy and subsequent recourse to abortion remains a major health problem.

Approximately 20 million of the annual abortions are unsafe—performed by the woman on herself or by providers without the requisite training, skills, equipment and/or drugs[29]. Unsafe abortion is therefore responsible for many of the deaths that are labeled "maternal deaths". WHO estimates that about 70,000 maternal deaths are, in fact, complications of unsafe abortion. Poor abortion technique can lead to infection, hemorrhage and trauma to

TABLE 2-3. Percent Women Receiving no Prenatal Care and 4+ Prenatal Visits (pregnancies during 3 years prior to survey, 1990–1996)

Country	% Women receiving no prenatal care	% Women receiving 4+ prenatal visits
Sub-Saharan Africa		
Burkina Faso	40.0	22.5
Cameroon	21.0	49.0
Central African republic	22.1	39.7
Cote d'Ivoire	15.5	28.7
Ghana	12.7	58.8
Kenya	3.8	63.7
Madagascar	13.6	42.6
Malawi	7.2	62.6
Namibia	11.8	55.8
Niger	69.5	8.3
Nigeria	34.7	51.5
Rwanda	5.1	12.0
Senegal	21.1	13.3
Tanzania	3.7	69.3
Uganda	7.5	47.2
Zambia	6.4	68.4
Zimbabwe	5.6	74.1
Asia/Near East/North Africa		
Bangladesh	72.4	5.4
Egypt	60.7	28.3
India	50.1	19.9
Indonesia	12.7	63.1
Jordan	19.2	67.1
Kazakstan	7.3	81.9
Morocco	67.6	7.8
Pakistan	69.7	14.1
Philippines	7.7	52.1
Turkey	36.9	36.1
Latin America/Caribbean		
Bolivia	46.5	31.8
Brazil	13.2	75.9
Colombia	16.8	70.3
Dominican Republic	2.9	84.7
Guatemala	13.7	64.7
Haiti	29.0	35.6
Paraguay	8.7	64.9
Peru	31.8	46.7

the reproductive organs and abdomen. Table 2-6 shows the number of unsafe abortions and number of abortion-related deaths by region[30].

Like the numbers on maternal mortality, the number of abortion deaths is only a fraction of the number of women suffering serious complications from unsafe abortion. WHO estimates that between 10 percent and 50 percent of women experiencing an unsafe abortion need medical care for complications[31].

TABLE 2-4. Countries in which 50% or Less of Births are Assisted by a Trained Attendant, 1996–98

Country	Percent births assisted by trained attendant
Angola	17
Bangladesh	8
Bolivia	46
Burkina Faso	41
Burundi	24
Cambodia	31
Central African Republic	46
Chad	15
Republic of Congo	50
Cote d'Ivoire	45
Egypt	46
Eritrea	21
Ethiopia	8
Gambia	44
Ghana	44
Guatemala	35
Guinea	31
Guinea-Bissau	25
Haiti	20
India	35
Indonesia	36
Kenya	45
Lesotho	50
Mali	24
Mauritania	40
Morocco	40
Mozambique	44
Nepal	9
Niger	15
Nigeria	31
Pakistan	18
Rwanda	26
Senegal	47
Sierra Leone	25
Togo	32
Uganda	38
Yemen	43
Zambia	47

A review of literature on sub-Saharan Africa concluded, *inter alia,* that unsafe abortion constitutes a major health problem, disproportionately affects unmarried adolescents and young women and consumes vast amounts of public health resources in treating complications.[32]

Properly performed, abortion is very safe and pain can be managed through local anesthesia, analgesics and supportive care. The 1990 mortality rate in the United States was 0.3 per 100,000 procedures, largely due to complications of general anesthesia (rarely used) and pulmonary embolism. This is much lower than the U.S. maternal mortality ratio of 10 deaths per 100,000 births. There is no evidence of long term sequelae from abortion.

TABLE 2-5. Abortion Rate by Region, 1990
(abortions per 1,000 women 15–44)

Region	Abortions per 1,000 women 15–44
Latin America and Caribbean	42
Southeast Asia	36
Sub-Saharan Africa	28
South Asia	25
USA and Canada	26
Western Europe	14

Unfortunately, the quality of abortion care, even where legal, varies greatly. Legal abortions often suffer from gaps in provider technical competence, supportive counseling, pain management and post-abortion family planning services[33]. Unsafe abortions use a wide range of very dangerous techniques, including inserting sharp objects through the cervix, deliberately inducing trauma to the abdomen (punching, squeezing, jumping), and ingestion or insertion of drugs and caustics.

Legal status appears to have very little impact on the abortion rate[34]. In Western Europe, for example, abortion is legal and the abortion rate is approximately 14 per 1000, much lower than in Latin America, where abortion is illegal. The effect of restrictive abortion legislation is to increase the proportion of abortions that are unsafe. Restrictive abortion legislation therefore tends to contribute to maternal mortality without reducing abortions.

Legal abortion does not, however, equate to safe abortion. In India, for example, abortion is legal, but custom, low women's status and poor access to competent providers drive many women to use unsafe abortion[35]. That is why South Asia contributes half of the world's unsafe abortions.

Bankole, Singh and Haas explored the reasons for induced abortion.[36] The most common reason for abortion is that women wish to end childbearing or view the pregnancy as mistimed, which speaks to a combination of failing to contracept, using an ineffective method and contraceptive failure. In second place stand socioeconomic reasons, largely having to do with poverty or foregone economic opportunities. Relationship problems also figure into many decisions, notably the partner's objection to the pregnancy and failures to acknowledge paternity. In at least 10 countries, 10 percent or more of the women having abortions cited being young and unmarried as their primary motivation. Risks to maternal health are cited by a relatively small proportion of women as the motivation for abortion, though it is of greater salience in sub-Saharan Africa, where maternal mortality ratios are highest. Fetal malformation or poor fetal health are the least commonly cited

TABLE 2-6. Unsafe Abortions and Abortion-related Deaths by Region

Region	Unsafe abortions	Number of deaths due to unsafe abortion
Latin America	4.6 million	60,000
Asia	9.2 million	40,000
Sub-Saharan Africa	3.7 million	23,000

TABLE 2-7. 2001 HIV/AIDS Statistics by Region

Region	Number people living with HIV/AIDS end 2001	New infections in 2001	Adult prevalence rate	% of HIV positive adults who are women	Main mode of transmission among HIV positive adults
Sub-Saharan Africa	28.5 million	3.5 million	9.0%	58%	Hetero
North Africa & Middle East	500,000	80,000	0.3%	54%	Hetero, IDU
South & Southeast Asia	5.6 million	700,000	0.6%	37%	Hetero, IDU
East Asia & Pacific	1 million	270,000	0.1%	24%	IDU, Hetero, MSM
Latin America	1.5 million	140,000	0.5%	31%	MSM, IDU, Hetero
Caribbean	420,000	60,000	2.3%	50%	Hetero, MSM

Hetero—heterosexual sex; IDU = intravenous drug use; MSM = men having sex with men

reasons for abortion. Sexual coercion or abuse are cited infrequently as the antecedents to abortion.

In sum, a very high proportion of abortions serves to resolve unintended pregnancy, rather than alleviating health problems in an intended pregnancy. Studies across a range of countries consistently demonstrate that the unmet need for family planning underlies the current level of abortion, though unintended pregnancies will occur under any circumstances as a result of contraceptive use failure. Hence, increasing the use and quality of contraceptive services will, in most circumstances, be the most effective policy response to reducing the incidence of abortion, rather than attempts to restrict access to abortion.[37]

HIV/AIDS and Other Sexually Transmitted Diseases

HIV/AIDS extracts a fearsome toll on global health. As of December 2001, 40 million people were infected world-wide with HIV, of which 38.5 million lived in the developing world.[38] There were 5 million new infections in 2001, of which more than 95 percent occurred in the developing world. Of this total, 3.5 million infections occurred in sub-Saharan Africa and 700,000 in South and Southeast Asia. About 25 million people have died from the disease since the beginning of the pandemic, with 3 million deaths in 2001 alone. About 74 percent of the deaths (18.3 million) have occurred in sub-Saharan Africa, with South and Southeast Asia contributing 2 million deaths to the global total. Table 2-7 reproduces estimates from the Joint United Nations Program on HIV/AIDS (UNAIDS), showing key statistics on HIV/AIDS by region of the world[39].

Children have been severely affected by the HIV/AIDS pandemic. In December 2001 there were approximately 3 million children under the age of fifteen infected with HIV, which included 580,000 newly infected during 2001. Since the beginning of the pandemic, there have been 4.7 million child deaths due to HIV/AIDS, including 580,000 child deaths in 2001.

The distinctive regional patterns of HIV transmission have important implications for disease control efforts.[40] As will be described in greater detail below, the dynamics of an HIV epidemic typically involve a relatively small proportion of the population engaging in high risk behaviors (multiple partners, injecting drug use) and a "bridging" population (e.g., customers of commercial sex workers), who pass the disease to individuals who practice low risk behaviors (e.g., monogamous wives of men who use sex workers). Understanding the specific pattern of transmission in a given context is critical to mounting effective strategies for slowing or halting the spread of the disease.

Africa has been the most gravely afflicted by the HIV/AIDS pandemic. In sub-Saharan Africa, the pattern of transmission has been almost exclusively heterosexual. Southern and eastern Africa have been hardest hit, with 8 percent of the adult population infected with HIV in Uganda and Tanzania; 14 percent in Kenya, 20 percent in South Africa and Zambia, 25 percent in Swaziland and 36 percent in Botswana[41]. In west Africa, Cote d'Ivoire is the worst affected, with about 11 percent of the adult population infected. While more men than women were affected during the early stages of the epidemic, it is now certain that more adult African women are infected than adult African men. Both biological and cultural factors are at work in this phenomenon. Adolescent girls are more susceptible to HIV/AIDS than adolescent boys or older women due to the relative immaturity of the cervical lining. There is more and more pressure from older men to have sex with younger women, who are presumed to be infection free. Hence, there is an increasing period of exposure coupled with biological vulnerability.

Though Africa has borne the brunt of the HIV/AIDS pandemic to date, this may change as the disease spreads to the population giants of Asia. India and China, because of their size, dominate any discussion of the future of HIV/AIDS in Asia. As of 2001, the number infected is small relative to population size; about 4 million in India and 850,000 in China.

The Indian situation is highly complex, reflecting the great diversity of that society. Modes of transmission vary by region. In the south and west, transmission is occurring in urban centers with sex workers serving as the core transmitters. In the northeast, the disease is spreading among injecting drug users (IDU), who infect their wives. Prevalence levels also vary significantly by region. The southern states have a higher HIV prevalence level, with high risk groups consistently showing levels above five percent and rates in antenatal clinics exceeding one percent. These levels indicate that the epidemic is poised to spread to the general population. The states of Gujarat, Goa, Kerala, West Bengal and Nagaland have prevalence levels in excess of five percent in high risk groups, but less than one percent among women attending antenatal clinics. In these states the epidemic is still confined to the core transmitters. In the remaining states prevalence is below five percent even among high risk groups.

HIV/AIDS in China was initially largely confined to IDU. However, there are worrisome trends that threaten a wider spread of the disease. The social changes in China have yielded a burgeoning sex industry, with more than 4 million sex workers. Spread of the disease among this group, coupled with the relatively uncommon use of condoms in commercial sex, could induce a more generalized epidemic.

Heterogeneity also marks the rest of Asia. Countries such as Burma and Cambodia have high levels of prevalence. Malaysia and Vietnam have moderate levels of prevalence, but the levels are increasing fairly rapidly. Thailand has a high prevalence level, but is unique in arresting the growth of the epidemic. Bangladesh, Indonesia, Nepal, Philippines and Sri Lanka have low levels of prevalence and slow prevalence growth curves, which means they are poised to arrest an incipient epidemic if action is taken quickly.

Patterns and trends also differ across Latin America and the Caribbean. In South America, multiple, concurrent patterns of transmission are taking place. The epidemic was

TABLE 2-8. Life Expectancy and Child Mortality with and without AIDS, 1998, 2010

	1998				2010			
	Life expectancy		<5 Mortality		Life expectancy		<5 Mortality	
Country	With AIDS	Without AIDS	With AIDS	Without AIDS	With AIDS	Without AIDS	With AIDS	Without AIDS
Botswana	40.1	61.5	121.1	57.4	37.8	66.3	119.5	38.3
Burkina Faso	46.1	55.4	179.1	156.5	45.6	60.7	144.7	108.7
Burundi	45.6	55.4	157.1	131	45.3	60.8	128.6	90.9
Cameroon	51.4	58.6	128.1	109.6	49.8	63.2	108.3	78
Central African Republic	46.8	56.3	162.6	140.2	50.9	61.9	122.7	99.1
People's Republic of Congo	47.1	57.2	166.3	142.5	49	62.4	125.9	97.1
Democratic Republic of Congo	49.3	54.4	152.7	139.3	51.9	59.8	116.2	97.3
Cote d'Ivoire	46.2	56.5	149.2	122.7	46.7	61.8	120.9	84.2
Ethiopia	40.9	50.9	197.6	169.2	38.6	54.7	183.4	136.7
Kenya	47.6	65.6	107	64.9	43.7	69.2	105.2	45.4
Lesotho	54	62	120.2	98.3	44.7	65.9	121.9	70.7
Malawi	36.6	51.1	231.6	190.3	34.8	56.8	202.6	136
Namibia	41.5	65.3	125.5	62.1	38.9	70.1	118.8	37.5
Nigeria	53.6	57.8	139	124.4	46.3	64.9	112.7	68.2
Rwanda	41.9	53.9	181.9	148.5	37.6	59.2	166.4	105.5
South Africa	55.7	65.4	95.5	69.7	48	68.2	99.5	48.5
Swaziland	38.5	58.1	168.1	114.4	37.1	63.2	152.2	77.5
Tanzania	46.4	55.2	160.1	137.8	46.1	60.7	131.3	95.8
Uganda	42.6	54.1	164.5	132.9	47.6	59.5	120.6	92.2
Zambia	37.1	56.2	181.2	125.7	37.8	60.1	160.7	96.9
Zimbabwe	39.2	64.9	123.4	50.5	38.8	69.5	115.6	31.8
Brazil	64.4	71.4	47.3	37.5	67.7	75.5	31.4	20.6
Guyana	62.3	65.7	71.4	61.3	51.1	67.9	86.6	48.7
Haiti	51.4	55.5	155.7	145.9	54.4	58.8	129.1	119
Honduras	65	69.2	61.2	50.4	59.7	73.4	55.2	29.3
Burma	54.5	57.1	113.1	106.4	58.8	62.8	80.3	70.1
Cambodia	48	50.7	179.1	171.9	52.8	56.7	133.9	123.9
Thailand	69	71.3	40.8	36.2	72.9	75.1	25	21.2

initially localized among men having sex with men (MSM), though an increasing proportion is now clearly due to heterosexual transmission. IDU plays an important role in transmission in Brazil, Chile, Uruguay and Paraguay. Among Central American nations, prevalence is still relatively low in Mexico, with transmission due to MSM in urban areas and heterosexual sex in rural areas. Honduras has been particularly affected among the Central American nations, with prevalence in excess of 20 percent among high risk groups and over 4 percent in the low risk adult population in the capital Tegucigalpa. The Caribbean nations have seen soaring prevalence levels. Rates in Haiti are very high, with over 70 percent of high risk groups infected and 5 percent infected among the rest of the adult population. Prevalence is also high among sex workers in the Dominican Republic (6–10 percent) and Guyana (over 40 percent).

HIV/AIDS is having a dramatic impact on mortality rates, as can be seen in the estimates developed by the U.S. Bureau of the Census presented in Table 2-8[42]. In 1998, HIV/AIDS induced lower life expectancy and higher child mortality than would have been the case in the absence of the disease. These trends are continuing and it is likely that an absolute decrease in life expectancy will occur in a number of African nations. Children born to HIV infected mothers in developing countries have a twenty-five to thirty five percent probability of becoming HIV seropositive[43]; HIV can be transmitted *in utero*, during childbirth and through breast milk.

The large number of AIDS orphans is imposing a huge strain on already fragile communities. The United Nations has defined as an AIDS orphan a child under the age of fifteen whose mother has died. The death of the mother often foreshadows or follows that of the father. Children whose mothers die of AIDS are also more likely to die as a consequence of inadequate care in over-burdened adoptive families. By the end of the year 1999, approximately 13 million children under the age of 14 had lost their mothers or both parents since the beginning of the epidemic[44]. The numbers in some countries are staggering. The percentage of children who are AIDS orphans is nine percent in Zambia, seven percent in Zimbabwe, six percent in Malawi and four percent in Botswana. Many of these children are themselves infected, meaning they require intensive care. Those who are not infected are faced with a host of challenges, in addition to lacking the support of a parent. They are more likely to be thrust into an adult role, taking care of younger siblings and/or seeking income for the family. They are less likely to receive education, health care or proper nutrition. They may be emotionally isolated and subjected to the stigma associated with AIDS in many societies. They are particularly vulnerable to sexual abuse and may turn to prostitution as a means of eking out a living.

Sexually transmitted diseases (STD) other than HIV/AIDS also constitute a major disease burden in the developing world and are a co-factor in the spread of HIV/AIDS. Individuals infected with another STD are more susceptible to becoming infected with HIV and are more apt to shed HIV if infected. Hence, the effort to control STD has taken on new urgency. Table 2-9 shows the prevalence and incidence of four curable STD (syphilis, gonorrhea, chlamydia, trichomoniasis) by region of the developing world. As can be seen,

TABLE 2-9. Prevalence and Number of New Cases of Syphilis, Gonorrhea, Chlamydia and Trichomoniasis Population Aged 15–49, 1995

	Adult prevalence	New cases				
		4 STD	Syphilis	Gonorrhea	Chlamydia	Trich.
Sub-Saharan Africa	53 million	65 million	3.5 million	16 million	15 million	30 million
North Africa & Middle East	6.5 million	10 million	620,000	1.5 million	2.9 million	4.6 million
South & Southeast Asia	120 million	150 million	5.8 million	29 million	40 million	75 million
East Asia & Pacific	16 million	23 million	330,000	3 million	6.2 million	13 million
Latin America & Caribbean	24 million	36 million	1.3 million	7.1 million	10 million	18 million
Total	219.5 million	284 million	11.55 million	56.6 million	34.1 million	140.6 million

these four diseases alone affect hundreds of millions of people[45]. About 284 million new cases are acquired each year and approximately 220 million people are infected at any point in time. Global estimates for the other STD are not available.

The regional distribution of these four STD is quite different than that of HIV. Sub-Saharan Africa dominates the HIV statistics, while the absolute number of STD cases is much larger in Asia. If the geographic distribution of HIV were to resemble that of other STD, then the center of gravity of the HIV pandemic would shift markedly.

KEY LESSONS FROM THE EPIDEMIOLOGY OF REPRODUCTIVE HEALTH

Rapid Declines in Fertility Are Possible

Contraceptive use has increased dramatically in most regions of the developing world, though change has been slowest in sub-Saharan Africa. Table 2-10 shows contraceptive prevalence at two points in time for all countries where trend data from the Demographic and Health Surveys are available[46]. The rate of gain in contraceptive prevalence varies considerably, ranging from 0.2 percent per year in Mali to 3 percent per year in Bolivia, with a mean gain of 1.4 per year. If one excludes China, contraceptive prevalence is generally highest in Latin America, followed by roughly equivalent levels in South Asia and the Middle East/North Africa regions, with the lowest levels found in sub-Saharan Africa. As of 1998, about 55 percent of all married women of reproductive age in the developing world are using some form contraception; this means that about 570 million couples are practicing some form of family planning[47].

Contraceptive use varies by age and parity. Younger women just starting families tend to have lower use of contraceptives, with prevalence rising after age 25 and then usually, but not always, declining among women over 40 as their fecundity declines or because older women tend to have more traditional values. The decline with age is not universal—in nine of the twenty-two countries for which DHS data are available, contraceptive prevalence continues to rise among women over 35. The relationship of parity and contraceptive prevalence is much akin to that of age and prevalence. Women with no children tend to use contraception the least in all regions. Contraceptive prevalence tends to rise with the number of living children in Africa but peaks at women with 3–4 children in Latin America. Examples of both the African and Latin American pattern can be found in Asia and the Middle East.

Use of contraceptives is only one determinant of fertility behavior. Figure 2-3 presents a model of the factors that influence fertility behavior, which may be grouped into four general categories: proximate determinants, the demand for fertility control, the characteristics of the family planning program, and the general environment.[48]

- **Proximate determinants**: These are the direct biological determinants of the number of live births. They include the age at which sexual union begins, contraception, abortion, the duration and intensity of breastfeeding (which affects the postpartum return to fertility), coital frequency and infertility. Of these, changes in contraceptive prevalence have been the most important proximate determinant of changes in fertility in the developing world over the last forty years[49].

TABLE 2-10. Percent of Currently Married Women of Reproductive Age and Sexually Active Unmarried Women Using any Contraceptive Method at two Points in Time (Survey dates shown in parentheses)

Country	Earlier prevalence		Later prevalence	
	Any method	Modern	Any method	Modern
Sub-Saharan Africa				
Burkina Faso (1992, 1998/99)	22.2	4	12	5.8
Cameroon (1991, 1998)	19.7	4.2	24	8
Ghana (1988, 1998)	12.3	7.7	18	10.7
Kenya (1989, 1998)	23.2	14.7	29.9	23.6
Madagascar (1992, 1997)	13.3	3.5	16	7.3
Mali (1987, 1996)	4.6	1.2	7.9	5
Niger (1992, 1998)	4.4	2.3	7.6	4.4
Senegal (1986, 1997)	10.1	2.7	10.8	7
Tanzania	9.5	5.9	16.1	11.7
Uganda	5.5	2.7	13.4	7.4
Zambia	11.6	7	19.2	11.2
Zimbabwe	32.2	27.2	35.1	31.1
Near East and North Africa				
Egypt (1988, 1995)	34.9	32.7	44.4	42.2
Jordan (1990, 1997)	38.3	25.8	50.7	36.4
Morocco (1987, 1992)	32.8	26.4	22.9	19.7
Turkey (1993,19988)	60.3	33.3	44.2	26.1
Yemen (1991/92, 1997)	9.1	5.7	19.6	9.3
Asia				
Bangladesh (1993/94, 1996/97)	42.3	34.5	46.6	39.5
India (1993, 1999)	38.4	34.4	45.2	40.4
Indonesia (1987, 1997)	43.8	40.3	53.7	51.2
Philippines (1993, 1998)	24.2	15.1	28.9	17.2
Latin America				
Bolivia (1989, 1998)	19.9	8	31.4	16.5
Brazil (1986, 1996)	43.7	37.2	55.4	51
Colombia (1986, 1995)	38.9	31.9	48.1	39.5
Dominican Rep. (1986, 1996)	31	29.1	44.6	41.3
Guatemala (1987, 1998/99)	16.2	13.4	26.6	21.7
Peru (1992, 1996)	35.7	19.9	40.9	26.4

- **Demand for fertility control**: The decision to use contraception reflects *desired family size* and the *supply of children*. Parents may or may not make a conscious choice as to family size. They may consider family size to be a matter best left to God or fate. Alternatively, they may have a specific goal in mind as to the number of children they desire. The desired family size must be considered relative to the number of children they can have, which is a function of natural fertility and the proportion of children surviving to adulthood. Absent any retarding effect by the proximate determinants, women would have, on average, fifteen children[50]. Societies do not manifest this level of childbearing because of the operation of the proximate determinants (e.g., breastfeeding, taboos on postpartum intercourse) and maternal mortality. High birth rates are more likely to prevail where child mortality is high. Parents attempt to generate a sufficient "stock" of children to ensure the desired number survive. As parents' assurance that children will survive increases, birth rates tend to decline and the demand for contraception goes up correspondingly.

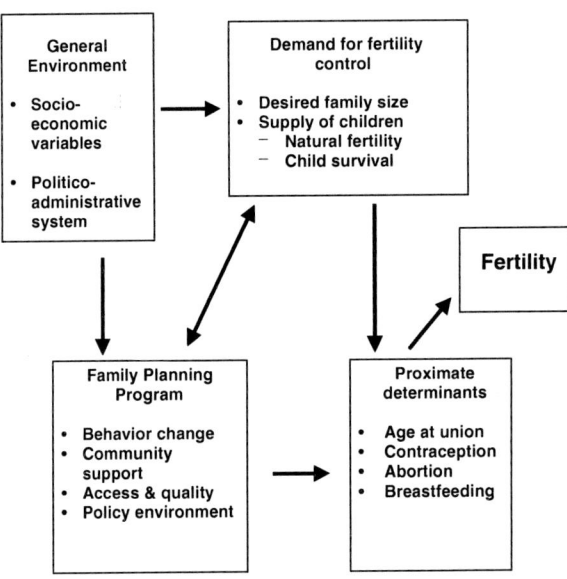

FIGURE 2-3. Fertility and family planning.

- **Family planning programs**: An effective family planning program interacts with the demand for fertility control, as well as directly affecting the use of contraception. Family planning programs can serve to change the desired family size, alter community norms regarding fertility and lower the economic, social and psychological cost of practicing contraception.
- **Status of women**: Both the demand for children and the family planning program are affected by the socioeconomic and political setting. The status of women is a critical determinant of the demand for children. Changes in the status of women increase the opportunity cost of having children. For almost all countries, use of contraceptives rises with female education. Women with a primary education are more likely to use a contraceptive method than women with no schooling and women with a secondary education use family planning most of all. There are a few exceptions to this general pattern. In Egypt and Jordan, contraceptive use among women with a secondary education is slightly lower than that of women with a primary education. In Indonesia and the Dominican Republic, both with over-all levels of contraceptive prevalence in excess of 50 percent, the impact of secondary education on contraceptive use is quite small. Fertility tends to decline as women enter the formal labor force, where time spent on child care must be traded against wages. Urban women also tend to have fewer children than rural women.
- **Government capacity**: The general ability of government to formulate and implement policy will be reflected in the viability of the family planning program. Governments that demonstrate the ability to carry out policies and programs supporting improved health will be well positioned to implement a family planning program. The converse is equally true; a pattern of poorly designed and implemented government programs will probably show up in the family planning program.

Given the complexity of the determinants of fertility, the question emerges as to whether family planning programs have any independent impact. Some authors argue that family planning programs have modest impacts at best, contending that as the demand for fertility control emerges, parents will find the means to curb child bearing without the help of organized programs[51]. Conversely, some family planning optimists seem to believe that family planning can succeed anywhere. The truth probably lies somewhere between these two extremes. There is no specific threshold of socioeconomic development that must be attained before the transition to lower fertility can begin nor have fears that certain cultures are impervious to fertility decline proven correct. Nonetheless, stagnation almost certainly militates against the fertility transition. A process of change in the major socioeconomic determinants—child mortality, female schooling, urbanization, female labor force participation—must probably be in place before the demand for fertility control emerges.

Accompanying these socioeconomic changes is the diffusion of new ideas about fertility. Women and couples begin to crystallize in their minds the notion that child bearing is something they can control. One of the important roles that family planning programs play is to spur discussion of family size and lend legitimacy to the goal of fewer children. Family planning programs have played an important role in engaging political, social and religious leaders in a dialogue about the permissibility and advisability of contraception.

Family planning programs also facilitate the adoption of contraception by reducing costs and barriers. These barriers include lack of knowledge about contraceptive methods, the cost of buying contraceptive goods and services, the social stigma associated with contraceptive use in some cultures, anxieties or fears about contraceptive use and sheer physical lack of access where health services are remote from clients. Through public education, financial subsidy and innovative service delivery mechanisms, family planning programs facilitate the adoption and continuation of contraception.

Measurement of the impact of family planning on fertility while controlling for the other determinants is fraught with methodological difficulties. Not all family planning programs are alike—they vary considerably in terms of resources, ingenuity and skill. Hence, impact assessments must determine whether the *level of program effort* is related to an increase in contraceptive prevalence holding constant other relevant variables. In general, such studies have found that family planning programs do have a significant and independent impact on contraceptive prevalence. One recent study estimated that forty percent of the observed decline in fertility in the developing world from the 1960s to the end of the 1980s is attributable to the impact of family planning programs alone.[52]

What is indisputable is that world fertility has undergone a very rapid decline by historic standards. Figure 2-4 shows the decline in fertility by region of the world[53].

Obstetrical Emergencies Are the Key to Reducing Maternal Mortality

The causes and timing of maternal death have important implications of public health strategy to reduce maternal deaths. The first conclusion that must be drawn is that all pregnant women are susceptible to a life threatening obstetric emergency. Every pregnant woman is susceptible to hemorrhage, infection, obstructed labor or eclampsia. Any woman wishing to terminate a pregnancy in a country where access to safe abortion is restricted is vulnerable to the complications of unsafe abortion. There are no reliable predictors that would eliminate a woman as a possible candidate for an obstetrical emergency. About 15 percent of pregnancies need emergency obstetric care, while 5 percent will require Cesarean section[54].

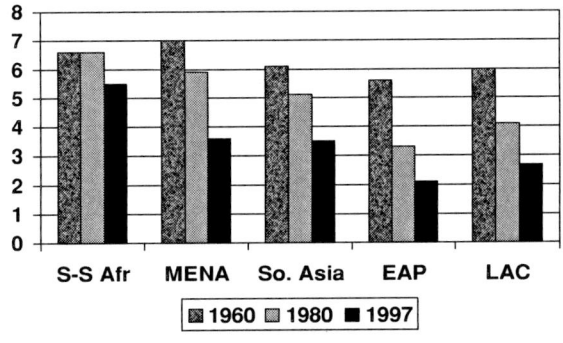

FIGURE 2-4. Total fertility rate by region of the world 1960, 1980, 1997.

Good prenatal and delivery care can prevent some obstetrical emergencies. Treatment of anemia and proper management of labor can help prevent some cases of hemorrhage, though the proportion that could be prevented is unclear. Observing asepsis and prenatal treatment of STD would help prevent many cases of infection. Known hypertension can be managed, but many cases of eclampsia occur without warning signs or symptoms. Cephalopelvic disproportion and abnormal fetal lie can be detected but not corrected during the prenatal period.

However, a strategy based on preventing obstetrical emergencies will not significantly reduce maternal mortality. Obstetrical emergencies will occur even if women have received good prenatal care and have a trained delivery attendant. Most obstetrical emergencies cannot be predicted or prevented. The probability of an obstetrical emergency is enhanced when, as is often the case, prenatal and delivery care are absent or inadequate. Hence, the focus of a maternal health strategy must be on managing obstetrical emergencies.

Because most deaths occur in the immediate and early postpartum periods, particular vigilance is needed at the time of delivery and in the few days following delivery. This focus on the intrapartum and postpartum periods runs counter to the dominant tendency to emphasize prenatal care and birth attendance.

The key to reducing maternal mortality is reducing the delay between onset of an obstetrical emergency and effective treatment. Death from an obstetrical emergency can happen very quickly. Table 2-11 shows the average interval between onset of the emergency and death[55]. As this table vividly demonstrates, quick action is needed if women's lives are to be saved.

Unfortunately, there is often an extended delay between onset of the emergency and action. A schema of the critical delays in maternal health care was first developed by Deborah Maine of Columbia University and has now been widely applied[56].

- **Delays in problem recognition**: Obstetrical emergencies often go unrecognized until an irremediable situation has occurred. Bleeding, pain and labor are normal parts of childbirth and training is needed to understand when safe parameters have been exceeded. Infection often goes unrecognized because care is minimal or absent. Pregnant women, untrained birth

TABLE 2-11. Average Interval from Onset of Emergency to Death

Complication	Interval
Prenatal hemorrhage	12 hours
Postpartum hemorrhage	2 hours
Ruptured uterus	24 hours
Eclampsia	48 hours
Obstructed labor	72 hours
Infection	6 days

attendants and family members are often unable to recognize that a life threatening situation has emerged until it is too late to take effective action.

- **Delays in deciding to seek care**: Once the reality of an obstetrical emergency has been realized, a time consuming decision-making process will often ensue. The woman is usually constrained in her ability to exercise authority, as well as physically and emotionally debilitated by the evolving crisis. Husbands, in-laws, birth attendants and healers—unprepared and uncertain as to how to respond—will engage in a time consuming debate over the appropriate course of action. In some instances, the husband or other authority figure must be fetched from some distance to endorse any course of action. This conversation is usually complicated by the reality of poverty as the decision to seek care implies a major drain on the household's very scarce resources. The upshot is that precious hours can slip by while the family decides whether and how to seek care.

- **Delays in reaching the health facility**: Scores of millions of women live far from a properly equipped health facility. Once the decision to seek care has been made, transport to a health facility becomes the next barrier to care. Access to vehicles is often difficult and the family must pay the vehicle owner for transport. In some instances, vehicle owners and drivers are unwilling to transport an ailing woman for fear she will die in the vehicle. Some areas are bereft of motor vehicles and the woman is placed on a makeshift stretcher that is carried by bearers. Obstetrical care is delayed as a vehicle is sought, negotiations with the driver are concluded and the drive to the facility, which can take hours, is completed.

- **Delays in receiving treatment at the health facility**: Arrival at the health facility does not necessarily mean that care is imminent. Prompt care requires quick processing of the patient through intake and the availability of staff, equipment, drugs and supplies. Any or all of these conditions may be missing. It is commonplace for key medical staff to be absent and for there to be shortages of drugs and supplies. Family members are then in the position of scurrying to find staff and purchase essential commodities on the local market. This process compounds the lapse of time before the woman receives treatment.

To sum up, maternal mortality is largely due to rapid onset obstetrical emergencies that are difficult or impossible to prevent. Prompt, competent treatment is the key to saving lives. The reality confronting many women is that there are systemic barriers to receiving prompt treatment. Hence, the core of an effective public health strategy for reducing maternal mortality is attacking the delays in obstetrical care. The Pathway to Maternal Survival[57], on the following page, provides a framework for addressing maternal mortality that responds to the problem of delayed obstetrical care.

As shall be described in Chapter 7, appropriate care is needed throughout the entirety of the pregnancy cycle. There are essential interventions that should occur at the preconception,

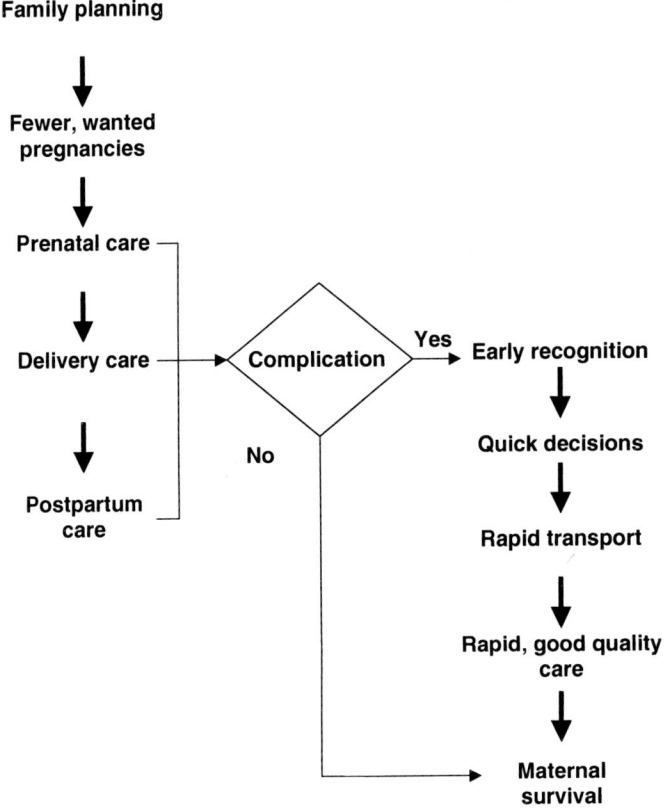

FIGURE 2-5. Pathway to maternal survival.

prenatal, intrapartum and post-partum stages. The special focus on obstetrical emergencies does not vitiate the utility of other steps that can promote maternal and child health, such as improving maternal nutrition and tetanus toxoid injections. The epidemiology of maternal health does, however, lead us to conclude that addressing obstetrical emergencies must have priority if maternal mortality is to be reduced.

Lastly, the option of recourse to safe abortion is an important part of maternal health care. As described above, unsafe abortion is a major contributor to maternal mortality and morbidity. The most effective strategy for preventing recourse to abortion is widespread access to voluntary, high quality family planning services, rather than efforts to criminalize abortion. Safe abortion services are needed, however, for women who do not have access to contraception or who experience contraceptive failure.

HIV and STD Prevention Efforts Must be Targeted to Achieve Maximum Impact[58].

Understanding the dynamic of HIV/STD transmission is essential to effective programming. A very specific chain of events is needed for any STD, including HIV, to spread. This chain of events has been captured in general models of STD transmission. Proper application of the models to specific settings can greatly improve the targeting of limited resources and help break the chain of transmission. The rate of transmission of a sexually transmitted disease within a population is determined by three factors: the probability of transmission, the duration of infectiousness and the number of sex partners.

The Probability of Transmission from an Infected Sexual Partner to a Non-infected Sexual Partner. The per sex act or per partner probability of transmission can vary from very low to quite high depending on the infectious agent, the characteristics of the infected partner and the non-infected partner and the frequency and type of unprotected sex acts between the partners[59]. Empirical estimates show that the probability of transmitting HIV-1 during a single act of penile-vaginal intercourse range from 0.0008 among heterosexual couples in the United States to as high as a 0.13 probability of transmission from a female sex worker to a male client in Kenya. The per partner probability of transmission is higher, since partnership often or usually implies multiple sex acts over time between an infected and uninfected partner. Data from the U.S., Europe and Thailand give an average probability of 0.24 for male to female transmission of HIV and an average probability of 0.12 for female to male transmission. Estimates of the probability of per partner transmission are 50 percent for gonorrhea, 20 percent for chlamydia, 60 percent for syphilis and 80 percent for chancroid.

Gender plays a role in the biological ease of transmission. Transmission from males to females is generally easier than from females to males. This is particularly true during adolescence, but female susceptibility during the reproductive years can also be affected by changes in vaginal acidity, cervical mucus and the phase of the menstrual cycle. In addition, a host of social factors—power imbalances, negotiating skills, sexual practices, and inadequate access to health care—can serve to place women at increased risk.

The presence of one STD can also facilitate the transmission of another STD. It is now well established that presence of gonorrhea, chlamydia or syphilis enhances the transmission of HIV.

The type of sex act affects the probability of transmission. For example, receptive penile-anal sex carries the highest risk of transmission of HIV due to the likely damage to rectal mucosa, which facilitates entry of the virus. Penile-vaginal sex and oral sex are progressively less risky for viral STD transmission, though no method of unprotected intercourse with an infected individual should be considered safe. In some regions of Africa, there is a preference for "dry" sex; women insert herbs vaginally to absorb moisture prior to intercourse. This makes the vaginal walls more liable to abrasion (and hence infection), as well as increasing the probability of condom breakage.

The Average Duration of the Infectious Period. Generally speaking, the longer the infectious period the more likely the disease will be transmitted. A longer infectious period means more sex acts and more partners, which in turn creates more opportunities for the disease to be transmitted. The duration of the infectious period is a function of the natural history of the disease, the biological response of the infected individual and the behavior of the individual. HIV, for example, tends to induce a heavy viral load in the first few months after infection, low viremia for a period of years and then a second period of high viremia as the disease progresses to AIDS. Heavier viral load increases the likelihood of infection, so the longer the period of high viremia, the greater the probability of disease transmission. STD differ in their infectious period and individuals vary widely in their immune response to a disease. For example, gonorrhea typically has an infectious period of six months, while that of HIV lasts for eight to twelve years before mortality sets in.

The behavior of infected individuals is also critical in determining disease transmission. Refraining from unprotected sex during the infectious period or quick treatment of drug susceptible STD serves to reduce the duration of infectiousness. Drug treatment is therefore both protective of the individual treated and the wider community that may be susceptible.

The Number of New Sexual Partners. The greater the average number of sexual partners per unit of time, the greater the likelihood of an infected person encountering an uninfected person and spreading the disease. The importance of understanding the rate and pattern of new partner acquisition as the basis of effective programming cannot be overstated. Individuals with a high rate of partner acquisition play a disproportionate role in launching and sustaining an STD epidemic. They are usually a small fraction of the total population and tend to have sex with other individuals practicing high-risk behaviors. This results in a high prevalence of STD within the group practicing high-risk behaviors. A fraction of the sexual contacts of this group will be with the majority that has few partnerships, transmitting the disease into the general population. The concept of a group of core transmitters has become central to public health thinking about STD control. Commercial sex workers, who have hundreds of clients during the course of a year, are an example of core transmitters.

In discerning the dynamics of HIV/STD transmission in any given setting, it is useful to think of three general groups:

1. Core transmitters who display a high level of risky behavior relative to the general population, such as many sexual partners and/or sharing of needles, and contribute disproportionately to new infections;
2. A bridge population that mixes with the core transmitters and becomes infected.
3. A vulnerable population that does not practice risky behaviors but is susceptible to infection through contact with the bridge group.

One common example of this dynamic would be the chain of infection from sex workers (core transmitters) to male clients (bridge population) to monogamous wives (vulnerable population). The specifics of this dynamic depend very much upon the local context. Understanding the dynamic is essential to targeting prevention efforts.

The rate of transmission from the core group to the general population is determined by the presence of a "bridge" group. For example, in many parts of the world it is common for long distance truck drivers to use commercial sex workers. The truckers serve as the bridge group. The spread into the general population occurs when the truck drivers have sex with their spouses or other partners.

A simple example will help illustrate the utility of understanding sexual behavior patterns[60]. Assume two groups:

(1) 500 commercial sex workers, each of whom has one new, uninfected client per night or 365 per year. Assume 80 percent are infected with HIV, which is a typical level for urban sex workers in Africa, and that the per sex act transmission probability is 10 percent.
(2) 10,000 men, 25 percent of whom are infected, all of whom are married and who have an average of two short-term liaisons each per year. Since multiple acts of coitus occur in such relationships, the likelihood of per partner infection also increases. Empirical studies show the probability of per-partner transmission of HIV-1 ranges from 10 percent to 50 percent, with a mean of 24 percent.

The general formula for calculating the number of new infections would be:

$$D = N \times I \times E \times P$$

D is the number of new cases of the disease; N is the size of the population; I is the percent of the population infected; E is the efficiency of disease transmission and P is the average number of partners per person per year.

The number of new cases generated by the sex workers over one year would be:

$$D_{sw} = 500 \times .8 \times .1 \times 365 = 14{,}600$$

The number of new cases infected by the group of 10,000 men would be:

$$D_{men} = 10{,}000 \times .25 \times .24 \times 3 = 1800$$

The point of this simple example is to demonstrate the relative efficiency of focusing on core transmitters in slowing the spread of an STD epidemic. A campaign aimed at changing the behavior of 500 sex workers would have almost ten times the impact of changing the behavior of 10,000 men. The behavior of all 10,000 men would have to be changed since the identity of those infected is unknown. Changing the behavior of just 50 infected sex workers in this example would have the same impact as changing the behavior of 2500 infected men.

Most societies are bimodal in the distribution of high risk behaviors. That is, a relatively small proportion of the population will have many partners and/or be IDU. Most people have very few partners or only one partner over a given time period and most people do not inject illegal drugs. Moreover, people who practice high risk behaviors do so largely with others who behave in a risky manner. Injecting drug users share needles with other IDU. People who have many partners have sex with people who practice like behavior. As a result, STD infection spreads and is sustained within a core group of people who consistently practice risky behaviors.

The pattern of mixing between the core transmitters and the rest of the population determines the speed with which the disease spreads into the general population and the eventual level of prevalence. If those who practice high risk behaviors only associate with other high risk individuals, then the epidemic is largely confined to the group of core transmitters. Conversely, a more widespread epidemic will occur if core transmitters also have sex (or share needles) with those who are uninfected and practice low risk behaviors.

As STD prevalence in a population rises, the relative importance of focusing on core transmitters diminishes but is never erased. Increasing prevalence means that the probability of a core transmitter encountering an uninfected person gradually declines. Hence, a smaller fraction of total new infections emanates from the behavior of core transmitters. Conversely, as prevalence rises the number and proportion of new cases attributable to those who are infected but have only a few partners will increase.

The concept of core transmitters has sometimes been misused as a reason to engage in coercive, discriminatory or abusive conduct against those believed to fall into this category and who are therefore blamed for the spread of HIV or other STD; e.g., abuse of sex workers or gay men. This is both unethical and foolish, serving no public health purpose. Stigmatizing those engaged in risky behaviors or infected with HIV only makes matters worse by driving the problem underground and vitiating efforts to extend educational and health services to populations that are already usually marginalized. Moreover, a focus on those practicing high-risk behaviors should not detract from encouraging and reinforcing wider norms of

TABLE 2-12. Percent Reporting 5+ Sexual Partners Other than Spouse/Regular Partner in Previous 12 Months

Country	Women	Men
Central African Republic	1	2
Cote d'Ivoire	1	10
Guinea-Bissau	0	1
Togo	0	2
Burundi	0	2
Kenya	1	4
Lesotho	0	8
Tanzania	3	5
Lusaka	1	8
Sri Lanka	0	0
Thailand	0	11
Rio de Janeiro	1	10
United States	2	4

responsible sexual behavior. Rather, the core-bridge-general construct is an aid in targeting resources, depending on the stage of the epidemic.

What are the patterns of sexual behavior? Data from multi-country surveys sponsored by the World Health Organization are instructive. Table 2-12 shows the percentage of men and women reporting 5 or more sexual partners over the twelve month period preceding the survey[61].

Though the authors of the study suspect some under-reporting by the women, the general conclusion is clear—only a small proportion of the population in any of the countries studied has a large number of sexual partners and this behavior is far more likely among men than women. The WHO team estimated that the average number of non-regular partners in the African sites studied at about two, which is substantially lower than the number used in earlier models of African sexual behavior.

Though the proportion of the population that has many partners (5 or more) is relatively low in most societies, there is wide variation in the degree of extra-marital sex. Concurrent partnerships—as opposed to sequential partnerships—can play an important role in the transmission of HIV/STD. Concurrent partnerships serve as the bridge between the core transmitters and the general population practicing lower risk behaviors. Concurrent partnership is also linked to having more lifetime partners, thereby increasing the possible number of people infected. In addition, the presence of a concurrent partnership increases the likelihood that sexual contact will occur during a period of high infectiousness. For example, a man contracting HIV from a partner is more likely to transmit the disease immediately after becoming infected (and to be unaware of the infection). If he has other, non-infected partners during this same period there is greater probability of transmission than if the relationships were sequential and the peak viral load passed. Table 2-13 shows the percentage of all adults aged 15–49[62] who had a sexual relationship other than with the spouse or primary partner[63].

The role of commercial sex as a component of non-marital sex varies considerably by society. Using the WHO data[64], the proportion of men reporting commercial sex ranged from one percent in Sri Lanka to just under twenty-five percent in Tanzania, with a median

TABLE 2-13. Percent Reporting a Sexual Relationship with Someone Other than the Spouse/Regular Partner During the Preceding Twelve Months

Country	Men	Women
Central African Republic	13.6	4.7
Cote d'Ivoire	50.7	13.4
Guinea-Bissau	43.5	20.5
Togo	19.5	1.3
Burundi	7.1	1.9
Kenya	30.9	12.2
Lesotho	23.7	19.1
Tanzania	32	14
Lusaka	35.9	9.7
Sri Lanka	4.3	3.1
Thailand	28.2	1.7
Rio de Janeiro	44.3	9.8

of 9.7 percent. The proportion of women who reported giving money or gifts in exchange for sex ranged from virtually zero to just over eleven percent in Tanzania, with a median of 1.3 percent.

There are a number of factors that are associated with extra-marital sex and a high number of sexual partners:

1. Men are much more likely than women to practice extra-marital sex and more likely to have a large number of partners.
2. The number of partners is correlated with age, tending to peak in the early twenties and decline with age.
3. Single people are more likely than the married to have multiple partners.
4. Schooling is also associated with the number of partners in most but not all countries; more years of schooling generally means more partners, though this effect is more pronounced and consistent for men than for women.
5. Non-cohabiting partners are more likely to have other sexual relationships; the economic circumstances that force many men in developing countries to spend long periods away from home in search of wage employment contributes to the spread of STD.
6. Virginity at marriage among women is strongly linked to lack of extra-marital sexuality during marriage, which reflects societies where there are strong social controls on female sexuality. Controls on female sexuality are, however, usually not associated with similarly strong controls on male sexuality.
7. The use of alcohol is also correlated with the number of partners.

Perhaps surprisingly, the WHO survey data do not show a relationship between urban-rural residence and sexual behavior after one controls for other factors, such as education and marital status. Social norms governing sexuality in cities do not appear to be markedly different from those in rural areas.

Using these data, we can cautiously draw a portrait of the population practicing high risk sexual behaviors. They tend to be young men who have more than a primary school education, use alcohol and are single or, if married, are spending a substantial amount of time away from their wives or regular partners. In some, but not all, societies, these men are apt to use commercial sex workers for non-marital sex. The proportion of their non-regular partners who are sex workers ranges from less than twenty percent in Rio de Janeiro and Cote d'Ivoire to more than 75 percent in Tanzania, Central African Republic and Thailand.

There is wide variation in the degree to which this portrait applies to any given setting. But one can see how drawing a profile of the high-risk population would help programmers design and target interventions. Using the profile in the foregoing paragraph, program managers might focus on changing the behavior of men aged 15–25 who are single or separated from their wives and the sex workers who serve them, giving special attention to the locales where alcohol is sold as a place to make condoms and education easily available. Creating a picture of the network of sexual contacts in this manner can help managers apply interventions where they make the most difference.

3

Behavior Change

Recall the definition of reproductive security—*the ability to identify, prevent and manage risks to reproductive health*. Healthy behavior is therefore one essential component of reproductive security. The risk analysis described in Chapter 1 serves to identify the most important reproductive health problems in a given population and the context specific dynamics of the problems. The purpose of behavior change programming is to foster behaviors that help households manage the most important problems identified by the risk analysis.

Behavior change is a complex but not mysterious process. Effective behavior change programs use our increased understanding of the process of behavior change. This chapter draws upon the Transtheoretical Model of behavior change as the basis for fostering healthy reproductive behaviors. This model argues that people go through stages of change as a consequence of specific processes that increase both the net benefits of change and the confidence to undertake new behaviors. We show how the Transtheoretical Model can be used to segment an audience into theoretically meaningful groups that can receive appropriate, targeted interventions.

The second part of the chapter provides practical guidance for translating theory into practice. The uses of audience research, the characteristics of effective communications and some basics on managing behavior change programs are discussed.

Before proceeding, however, we must be clear as to the behaviors that enhance reproductive security. Clear goals are a necessary starting point for any behavior change program. Behavior change goals derive from the context-specific reproductive risk analysis. Hence, a universal statement of behavior change goals would be inappropriate. Nonetheless, we can suggest a general framework drawn from the earlier discussion of the epidemiology of reproductive health. Figure 3-1 provides an illustration of specific goals that might be set by a program manager.

Healthy reproductive behaviors, then, fall into four general domains—achieving household fertility goals, safe pregnancy and childbirth, infection free sex and consensual sex. In the earlier discussions of the epidemiology and technology of reproductive health we identified specific behaviors that foster reproductive security. These include contraception, securing appropriate maternal health care, practicing safe sex and reducing the incidence of FGC and

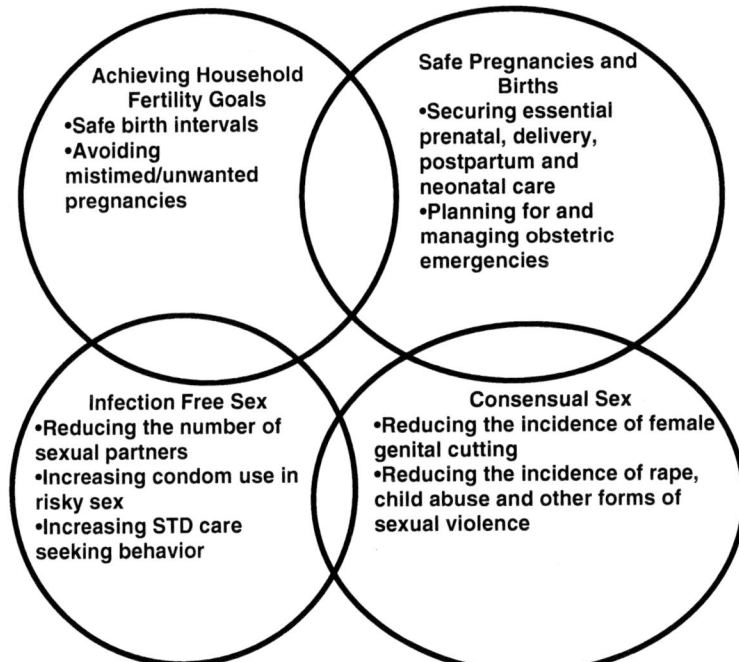

FIGURE 3-1. Goals and domains for reproductive health behavior change.

other forms of sexual violence. Context specific objectives can be stipulated with respect to all of these behaviors. The setting of clear behavioral objectives is a necessary first step in all behavior change programs. If you don't where you are going you can't get there!

The conceptualization of household reproductive behavior presented here suggests that the components of reproductive security are linked. There is reason to think this is true on biomedical and behavioral grounds. As was described earlier, reproductive health risks in one area tend to exacerbate risks in another; e.g., high fertility and STD increase the likelihood of maternal morbidity and mortality. Hence, biomedical risks tend to compound, while many risk reduction behaviors tend to have multiple health benefits. The reproductive security framework also hypothesizes that the ability (or inability) to prevent, identify and manage risks in one arena spills over into related areas. Women who do not access care for maternal health are also less likely to get help for suspected STD or to use contraception as compared to women who seek out proper obstetrical care. People who do not use a condom to protect against STD are also less likely to use contraception to avoid unwanted pregnancy. Conversely, individuals and couples who engage in conscious behavior to manage risk are more apt to do so across several related domains. Hence, the objective of programming for reproductive security is to create a core pattern of behavior that minimizes or mitigates reproductive health risks. Reproductive health providers and managers can help households develop the knowledge, skills, resources and confidence needed to protect their reproductive health.

This chapter emphasizes individual/household level change and therefore largely focuses on psychological approaches to behavior change. Psychological approaches alone, while important, have inherent limitations. As was emphasized in the discussion of the reproductive security framework, households are embedded in particular communities and larger societies. To a greater or lesser degree they are encouraged or constrained in the search for reproductive security by the social and institutional environment. Young men are unlikely to practice safe sex if they are subject to ridicule by their peers and older men. Women cannot protect their reproductive health if they are deprived of access to information, services and choice. In Chapter 4 we take up the issue of community empowerment for health, with the focus on changing norms and organizing for reproductive health. The individual, household and community are linked. Nonetheless, individual and household level behavior change programs are an essential component of promoting reproductive security and can be effective in a wide array of settings.

THEORETICAL BASIS FOR BEHAVIOR CHANGE

If we conduct a simple thought experiment and imagine a household that is practicing healthy reproductive behaviors, we can infer a process that might lie at the origin of appropriate behaviors. Imagine we first encounter our imaginary household during a period of low reproductive security—unwanted pregnancy, unsafe sex and poor maternal health care. Two years later, we return and the family has been consistently practicing healthy reproductive behaviors for over six months. What might have happened? Here is one possible chain of events:

- A process of awareness raising occurred, either through personal experiences or an education campaign. New information created awareness that current behaviors carried significant risks to the welfare of the household. For example, the household members might have learned that a short birth interval could threaten the health of their next child or the death of a neighbor in childbirth may have increased fears about maternal health.
- Household members thought about the risks, discussed them and developed goals and general plans for reducing risk; e.g., avoiding unwanted pregnancies, securing maternal health care, safe sex. They may have discussed their concerns with friends and family, who expressed similar fears and encouraged them to take appropriate action.
- The household members possessed or acquired the skills and resources needed to act on their goals. For example, they may have consulted with the village health worker or visited the local clinic to learn what steps they could to mitigate the risks. They might have pooled resources with neighbors to establish a contingency fund for emergencies.
- The household reasoned that the benefits of new reproductive health behaviors would exceed the perceived financial, psychic and social costs. Implementing the new behaviors involved time, money and some embarrassment in discussing private family matters with a health worker. However, a new government program made it easier to access services, thereby reducing costs. In the end, the family decided that the costs involved were a good investment in protecting its welfare.
- The household members possessed or acquired the confidence to act on their goals. The family was a bit tentative at first, but their initial forays were reinforced through encouragement from a variety of sources. The health worker provided good empathetic counseling and encouraging words came from the religious leader. The local men's dairy cooperative and the Mother's Club, to which the husband and wife belonged, also joined a local campaign to encourage healthier reproductive behaviors.

- The household members pursued reasoned action that furthered their reproductive health goals, such as seeking out the help of a health provider and adopting new behaviors. Good quality of care, including access to essential drugs, facilitated the adoption of new behaviors.
- The household members were able to sustain healthy reproductive behaviors over time and in the face of changed circumstances. For example, a loss of income forced the husband to seek employment in a distant town. During the separation from his wife, he practiced safe sex to avoid contracting an STD. The wife consulted with the health worker to manage contraceptive side effects and switched to a long-term method when the couple opted against having additional children.

The scenario that has just been sketched underlines that behavior change is a *process*, not a one time event. The family went through a series of stages or steps, including developing awareness, thinking through the consequences for household security, preparing and learning, experimenting with new behaviors and sustaining behaviors in the face of changed circumstances. Moving from stage to stage required emotional support, a careful calculation that the benefits outweighed the costs and access to appropriate services.

By thinking about behavior change as a process we can also see that the information and interventions needed changed dramatically over time. Initially, the family needed a "wake-up call". They needed a dose of reality—like the death of a neighbor—to heighten awareness of the potential risks they faced. Later, they needed more precise technical information about reproductive health and the benefits and costs of new behaviors. Emotional and social support were also important at various points in the process. Health workers and managers needed to change what they provided to the family as the process unfolded.

The scenario is an illustration of a theoretical approach to behavior change known as the Transtheoretical Model of behavior change[1], which has been widely applied. The Transtheoretical Model encompasses a number of constructs that are very helpful in designing, implementing and evaluating behavior change programs. For behavior change to occur, people must work through *stages of change* that include: (1) gaining awareness of risks; (2) contemplating change; (3) formulating a plan and experimenting with new behavior; (4) acting on the plan; and, (5) sustaining healthy behaviors. More formally, the stages in the model are known as pre-contemplation, contemplation, preparation, action and maintenance. People can move back and forth across these stages of change. Effective programs adapt their approach to the particular stages manifesting in a target population. The transition from stage to stage results from changes in the *decisional balance*—the perceived net benefits relative to the costs of change. The likelihood of behavior change increases as perceived benefits rise relative to the costs of change. The shift in decisional balance involves a number of *processes of change* that heighten benefits and reduce costs. These change processes include increasing knowledge and skills, changing perceptions of oneself and the behavior(s) at issue, recognizing the impact of one's behavior on others, receiving support or incentives from others and changing one's environment to avoid cues to risky behavior. More generally, the presence of supportive people who can answer questions, provide emotional encouragement and motivate progress is very useful in stimulating and sustaining stage change[2]. The change processes also serve to bring about increased *self-efficacy*, which is the confidence to carry out new behaviors. These four constructs—stages of change, decisional balance, processes of change and self-efficacy—are crucial to developing effective behavior change programs.

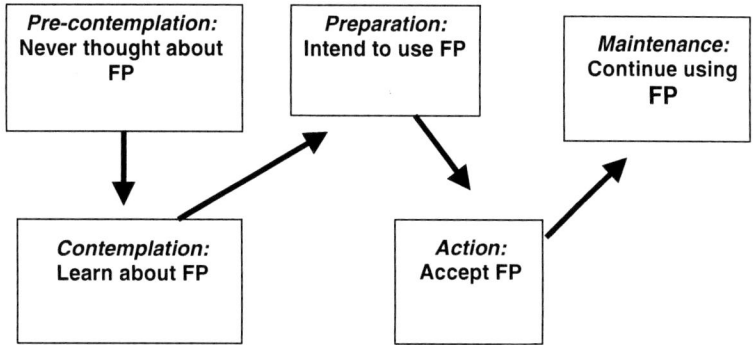

FIGURE 3-2. Applying stage theory to family planning.

Figure 3-2 provides an illustration of how people might move through stages of change in adopting family planning.

The importance of using a theoretically grounded approach to behavior change cannot be overstated[3]. A great deal has been learned about the conditions that foster healthy behaviors. The Transtheoretical Model encompasses many of the key constructs from this body of knowledge, including the notion that behavior change is a staged process rather than a singular event, the weighting of pros and cons in decision-making, the role of self-efficacy, and the combination of cognitive and emotional processes that underlie the manifestation of new behaviors. As a matter of practice, many programs are not grounded in a meaningful model of behavior change. As a consequence, they often yield poor results. There is ample evidence that behavior change programs can make an important difference, but to be successful they must reflect our increasingly sophisticated understanding of how behavior change occurs. We therefore turn our attention to applying the Transtheoretical Model in practice.

Working with Pre-Contemplators: Fostering the Saliency of Health Reproductive Behaviors

In situations where large segments of the population exhibit little knowledge about reproductive risks and/or evince little current interest in adopting new behaviors, program managers may choose to focus on shifting people from the pre-contemplation to contemplation and preparation stages. In these situations program managers should focus on three strategies: (1) ensuring that the target population has accurate, comprehensible and appropriate information about the consequences of healthy and unhealthy behaviors; (2) heightening the emotional distress associated with unhealthy behavior; and, (3) increasing understanding of the impact of unhealthy behavior on others.

People who are unaware of a reproductive risk, misunderstand the degree of risk or do not know about methods for managing risk need additional information. Examples of messages that increase the awareness of risk include:

- The health and financial benefits of family planning;
- Accurate information about the risks and benefits of contraceptive methods;
- The risks associated with pregnancy and labor;

- The importance of birth planning and use of a trained attendant to safeguard maternal health;
- The modes of transmission of HIV/STD;
- The importance of seeking STD care;
- The dangers of female genital cutting;
- The risks of sexual violence.

Increasing knowledge of reproductive risks is a necessary but not sufficient condition for bringing reproductive health issues to the forefront of household discussion and reflection. Effective programs support change by incorporating strong emotional content along with the dissemination of accurate information. The costs of unhealthy behavior to oneself must be brought into stark relief, just as the happiness associated with new, healthy behaviors must be vividly depicted. A wide variety of techniques have been applied to this end, including radio and television spots, soap operas involving reproductive themes, print materials, drama, street theater, billboards, puppet shows, song, testimonials, village and neighborhood meetings and dance. In Thailand, dramatic or humorous messages painted on the sides of elephants have served as mobile billboards promoting family planning and AIDS prevention. All of these programs are designed to associate positive emotions with healthy behaviors and negative emotions with unhealthy behaviors. A poster from Uganda featuring a skull and crossbones and the slogan "I wish I had said no to AIDS", provides a dramatic illustration of eliciting negative emotions in association with unhealthy behavior.

Along with providing information and evoking emotion, effective programs for pre-contemplators induce a heightened awareness of the impact of personal behavior on others in the environment. Family planning is often promoted by appealing to parents' desire to protect the health and welfare of their children. In Kenya, for example, fathers have responsibility for paying school fees. Family planning has been promoted to fathers as a means for ensuring that all of their children will have access to schooling. A poster from Kenya shows a coiled serpent poised to strike an infant, above which is the inscription," If you're not afraid of what AIDS can do to you, think of what it can do to your baby."

The three key processes—increasing knowledge, associating negative emotions with unhealthy behaviors and heightening understanding of the impact on others—are intended to increase the perceived benefits of behavior change. Here we return to the key construct of *decisional balance*. To move people from pre-contemplation to preparation the emphasis must be placed on increasing the perceived benefits of change. The type of benefit communicated must be geared to the specific audience. The benefits may be in the form of better health ("birth spacing means healthier children"), increased income ("fewer children means lower school fees"), increased sex appeal ("real men wear Panther condoms") or other context appropriate messages. Deciding which benefit to emphasize is very much a function of understanding local concerns and priorities.

From Contemplation to Preparation: Paving the Path to Action

The challenge of the contemplation stage is moving people from a rather vague, long-term intention to short-term objectives and testing of new behaviors. Many of the techniques used during the pre-contemplation stage will remain useful as a way of reinforcing the inclination to action. However, there is a distinct shift in focus to re-shaping personal identity to accommodate the new behavior(s).

Healthy reproductive behaviors embody a number of important self-images. A person who practices healthy behaviors is, in effect, saying, "I am a person who has the desire and ability to control my fertility. I can and will secure essential maternal care. I will practice safe sex. I will participate only in consensual, enjoyable sex. Practicing these behaviors us a meaningful expression of who I am and what I want." These are actually fairly profound statements about one's sense of self and, in many contexts, not easily achieved.

Reproductive health programs can help men and women integrate these concepts into their identities. There are at least two practical techniques that can be used to help foster the integration of healthier reproductive behaviors into client self-image. The first is using interpersonal and small group counseling as a vehicle for values clarification. In the Philippines, a guide for health workers in comic book format was developed ("The Stories of Esmeralda") that provided simple guidance on effective counseling. A poster developed for Peru bruited, "We are smart, savvy women. We will help you plan your family", while one in Uganda proclaimed, "Take control of your life. Get HIV counseling and testing." The Planned Parenthood Association of Ghana, in collaboration with the Johns Hopkins University Population Information Program and the Academy for Educational Development, developed a training manual for counselors working with adolescents. The manual covers a wide range of issues, including sexuality, abstinence, negotiation skills, contraception, harmful traditional practices, STD/HIV/AIDS and abortion. All of these are efforts to attract clients to counseling and to provide health workers and counselors with the requisite skills.

At the contemplation stage, there are four key elements to effective counseling[4]:

1. Recapitulation—have the client articulate the reproductive health problem, his or her motivation for seeking help, the perceived benefits, and obstacles to change. This recapitulation is elicited through a series of open-ended questions, such as, "I understand you have some concerns about the possibility of becoming pregnant (or about this pregnancy or about contracting HIV). Can you please tell me about those? What would you like to see change? How do you think the change might help you (and your family)? Is there anything that might make it difficult for you to make the changes you described?
2. Information and advice—the technical expertise of the counselor and health worker now plays a crucial role by providing the client with specific options. This might be in the form of contraceptive alternatives, a maternal health care schedule, strategies for safer sex or culturally acceptable alternatives to female genital cutting.
3. Negotiating a plan—the health provider and the client develop specific objectives and a calendar of actions that will bring about change. This might cover, for example, agreeing on a schedule of prenatal care or developing a birth plan. Another example might be an agreement to purchase and use condoms or simply to bring the spouse for a subsequent counseling session. It is important to ask the client to summarize the plan and be sure there is a common understanding.
4. Eliciting commitment—counseling should incorporate one or two simple questions reaffirming the client's desire to undertake the changes. For example, the counselor might conclude with, "So what I understand is that you will come back in two months for a prenatal check-up. Is this correct?" Where appropriate and feasible, clients should be encouraged to share their plans with household members or other significant individuals, as this tends to reinforce commitment to change.

A second major strategy during the contemplation phase is use of role models. One of the key tenets of social learning theory is that people learn by watching others and then incorporating new behaviors into their own lives[5]. Elevating and encouraging role models can therefore strengthen the transition from contemplation to preparation and action; contemplators will have additional license to adopt new behaviors. Use of role models is an important adjunct to counseling and the two can sometimes be combined. In some instances, celebrities drawn from sports, entertainment or the arts are used as advocates for reproductive health. In Lesotho, for example, the national soccer team was used to promote HIV/AIDS prevention. In Mexico, two singers very popular with adolescents (Tatiana y Johnny) released a song promoting abstinence; Lea Salonga and Menudo in the Philippines released a similar song. Two famous Nigerian singers, Onyeka Onwenu and King Sunny Ade, did a song promoting family planning. These efforts associate healthy reproductive behaviors with popular and respected figures. Consequently, the behaviors gain additional social legitimacy. One must be careful, however, to select role models whose reputation and conduct creates positive associations. There have been instances of unwise choices of celebrities that did not help advance reproductive health.

A complement to the use of celebrity role models is the "satisfied user" or "personal testimonial" approach. In this approach, individuals who have adopted the desired behaviors serve as advocates in their community for better reproductive health, strengthening the argument by explanation of their own experience. Family planning programs have used this approach for years, deploying satisfied contraceptive users as speakers, educators, counselors and distributors of contraceptives. AIDS organizations have used HIV infected persons as speakers and educators who can provide powerful personal testimonials, as well as to help alleviate the stigma associated with the disease. A powerful and tragic tale from West Africa recounts how a village chief became an opponent of female genital cutting following the death of his daughter from bleeding and infection; this led to a precipitous decline in the practice in the surrounding area[6]. Neighbors, family, friends and peers who live in similar circumstances can help re-mold expectations and encourage the adoption of new behaviors. Training and support may be needed by these advocates to be sure that what is said is technically accurate and that they have access to needed materials and transport.

From Preparation to Action: Following through on Commitment

During this stage the emphasis shifts to gaining the requisite skills and self-confidence to act. Skill training can be a very important part of behavior change. An individual may know about the importance of a condom to disease prevention yet lack the skills to use one correctly or negotiate its use with a partner. In the earlier discussions of the epidemiology and technology of reproductive health it became clear that an array of *competencies* are needed at the household level. These includes using contraceptives correctly and managing side effects, crafting and implementing a birth plan, practicing safe sex, couple communication, conflict resolution and so on. Skill building takes time, effort and practice. Identifying skill gaps and helping households gain the requisite skills is part of the change process.

Concomitant with skill building is mounting self-efficacy. The ability to undertake new behaviors requires a strong dose of confidence, including the ability to avoid placing oneself in risky situations. Confidence, like skill, is built by helping the client practice new behaviors in small increments with multiple repetitions. Role-plays can be repeated to practice condom negotiations. Clients can practice putting a condom on a penis model.

The evacuation of an obstetric emergency can be rehearsed. Women in a CARE project in Haiti learned the danger signs of pregnancy through repeating a song that was accompanied by a dance illustrating the manifestations of an obstetrical emergency. The key to building self-efficacy is breaking down a big problem (e.g., managing an obstetrical emergency) into a series of small, manageable tasks that can be mastered through repetition.

The shift from preparation to action also requires that the perceived costs of behavior change decline. As the client gears up for action the barriers and costs become increasingly salient. The cost of reducing reproductive risk can come in many forms – money for services and drugs, travel time, time spent at health facilities, time spent learning and adopting new behaviors, disrespectful or poor quality treatment from providers, embarrassment, restricting the number of sexual partners, and/or disapproval from family and neighbors. Audience research is essential to identify the perceived costs, while alleviating the costs is critical to promoting change. Program managers can help address the costs by facilitating access to services, improving the quality of care, and working with communities to increase the desirability of new norms and behaviors. For example, an important secondary audience for behavior change is community leaders. Cultivating the support of local leaders can help address the social and psychic costs of new reproductive behaviors.

Action and Maintenance: Sustaining New Behaviors over the Long Term

Reproductive risk management is not a one-time event. Most people do not simply adopt a risk management strategy—e.g., contraception or using condoms—and then sustain that strategy indefinitely. The perceived benefits and costs of a strategy change, as do the salient reproductive risks. Hence, creating a supportive environment for long term risk management is important to achieving sustained gains in reproductive health. For example, many family planning programs often devote enormous energy to recruiting new users, while giving inadequate attention to reducing the drop-out rate or encouraging former users to restart. Reducing attrition from healthy behaviors is often more cost-effective than recruiting new participants.

There are a variety of tactics that can be used to help sustain behavior change over time:

- **Problem solving:** As people implement new behaviors they are likely to encounter practical problems that can be dispiriting and prompt a return to unhealthy behaviors. For example, contraceptive side effects are often a major cause of attrition from family planning use. Women are often given no or poor information at the time that they adopt a contraceptive method as to potential side effects and how to manage them. In addition, health providers are often distant so quick consultation about managing the side effects is precluded. As a result, women become discouraged or frightened and abandon the method. Proper counseling as to side effects at the time of contraceptive adoption and easy access to a trained provider in the event of side effects would increase continuation rates. Similar scenarios could be drawn of problems confronting those attempting to implement new behaviors in the arenas of maternal health, HIV/STD and female genital cutting. Good programs sustain feedback from communities and clients to ensure that problems are communicated and addressed.
- **Support groups:** Positive reinforcement from peers and friends can be very helpful in sustaining new behaviors. Mothers clubs, men's groups, agricultural cooperatives, youth groups, savings and loans societies and religious organizations have all served as naturally occurring sites for mutual support. In Bangladesh, an association of commercial sex workers banded

together and supported their collective demand that clients use condoms. In Nepal, a village women's group formed in protest of alcohol abuse and gambling, both of which led to domestic violence. (They eventually succeeded in banning both from the village!) The support groups provide a forum in which members can share problems, receive advice on problems and emotional support in sustaining healthy behaviors.

- **Avoiding risky circumstances**: both unwanted pregnancy and HIV/STD can result where judgment is impaired. In the earlier discussion of HIV/AIDS it was pointed out that risky sexual behavior is often associated with alcohol use and locations in which alcohol is served. In some parts of the world, injecting drug use is a major contributor to the spread of HIV. Accordingly, another useful tactic is helping clients avoid places and circumstances where they are more likely to be tempted to engage in high-risk behavior. Counseling can help clients think through alternatives to locales and associates that are likely to induce risky behavior.

Summing Up: Applying Behavior Change Concepts

One of the most common and critical failures of behavior change programs is the phenomenon of "messaging". In many programs a key message is chosen and then systematically beamed at an audience over and over. Space your children! Use condoms! Seek prenatal care! The problem with this approach is that it ignores the diversity of the population. Stage theory teaches us that a population will be distributed in terms of its readiness to change. Demanding action from people in the pre-contemplation or contemplation stage is fruitless. Those at a more advanced stage of readiness will, conversely, be bored or offended by communications aimed at heightening awareness. I had this experience in India where a group of women quite bluntly told us, "We're bored already. We get it. We are supposed to use family planning. Don't you have anything else to say to us?"

This brief introduction to behavior change theory has underlined the importance of several key constructs—stages of change, decisional balance, self-efficacy and processes of change. Each of these has very clear, practical application to the design, implementation and evaluation of behavior change programs. Most importantly, behavior change theory demands segmenting the audience and then adapting content, medium and processes to the needs of different segments. This is more challenging then a monotone approach, but the only one likely to achieve significant impact.

TRANSLATING THEORY INTO PRACTICE: COMMUNICATION FOR BEHAVIOR CHANGE[7]

The remainder of this chapter is devoted to the practical application of behavior change theory, giving special attention to the uses of audience research, setting objectives and guidelines for effective communications.

Analyzing the Population

Effective behavior change programming is always based on a good, theoretically based understanding of the target population. The Transtheoretical Model provides a framework for analyzing the needs of the target population in terms of their distribution across the stages of change and their readiness to engage in a change process. Behavior change programs segment the over-all audience into meaningful groups reflecting their different needs. The following are some key questions that might be asked in designing a behavior change program:

1. Is there a good understanding of the risks associated with specific reproductive behaviors; i.e., high fertility/short birth intervals, pregnancy and multiple partners? How does the depth of this understanding vary among different subgroups—men, women, youth, socioeconomic class, ethnic group or other contextually appropriate variable?
2. Do households view the risks as salient to their own lives? Do they view themselves as personally at risk? Have they expressed a desire for change? How does this vary by subgroup?
3. Do households exhibit a good understanding of the steps they can take to protect their reproductive health? Do they have an accurate knowledge of contraceptive methods, including sources of supply, benefits and risks? Do they know the danger signs of pregnancy? Have they ever prepared a birth plan? Do they know the signs and symptoms of STD? Do they know how to use a condom properly and to negotiate its use? How do these competencies vary by population subgroup?
4. To what extent do households exhibit personal confidence in their ability to manifest desired new behaviors? How does this vary by subgroup?
5. What are the perceived benefits to new reproductive behaviors among the targeted households? Do these benefits appear to be highly valued? What are the costs and constraints to new behaviors? How do the responses vary by subgroup?
6. To what degree are households currently practicing healthy reproductive behaviors; e.g., contraceptive prevalence, use of trained birth attendants, safe sex, appropriate conflict resolution? How does current behavior vary by subgroup? Are those practicing healthy behaviors likely role models or peer educators?
7. What forms of social support exist to help households sustain healthy behaviors over time? Among those currently practicing healthy behaviors, what has been the duration? What factors are reported as facilitating and inhibiting healthy behaviors? How do these vary by subgroup?

A variety of data collection methods can be used, including surveys, focus groups, in-depth individual interviews and observation of naturally occurring events, such as village and neighborhood meetings, and group education sessions at health facilities. Reviews of previous research are also an important part of building an understanding of behavior change needs.

The most important functions of the data analysis are to (a) segment the population into theoretically meaningful groups and (b) select specific targets for behavior change. Audience segmentation is vital to crafting an effective program. The earlier discussion showed that people are arrayed along a continuum in terms of their readiness to adopt new behaviors. Interventions that are appropriate for people at an early point in the change process are not useful for those at a later point and conversely. The review of the Transtheoretical Model implies that a population might be divided into five meaningful groups, such as those illustrated by Table 3-1.

This sort of analysis is enormously helpful in crafting appropriate interventions. To use the extremes, people who are unaware of risk or who have no intention of managing risk need a very different kind of intervention than people who have been practicing risk management. Consciousness-raising is needed among the former, with the focus on creating a sense of personal risk and urgent need for action. The latter group will require social support and good information to manage contingencies, such as contraceptive side effects.

TABLE 3-1. Illustrative Audience Segmentation for Behavior Change

Stage	Family planning	Maternal health	HIV/STD
Pre-contemplation	Low knowledge of contraception and/or not intending to use contraception	Low knowledge of maternal health risks and/or no plan to reduce risks (i.e., developing a birth plan and/or using a trained birth attendant)	Practices unsafe sex, does not intend to seek STD care and has no intention to practice safer sex
Contemplation	Wants to space or stop childbearing and would like to start contraception	Wants to develop a birth plan and use a trained attendant during the next pregnancy	Is aware of practicing risky behavior and expresses interest in avoiding HIV/STD
Preparation	Would like to start contraception within the next 30 days and may have discussed this with a health worker.	Wants to develop a birth plan and use a trained attendant during the current pregnancy and may have discussed this with health worker	Plans to reduce number of partners, seek STD care and/or adopt regular condom use within next 30 days and may have discussed this with health worker
Action	Has started contracepting within the last 6 months	Has developed a birth plan and has identified a trained birth attendant	Has shifted to safer sex behaviors (fewer partners, condom use) within last six months
Maintenance	Has been contracepting for at least 6 months	Seeks postpartum and neonatal care	Has been practicing safer sex for at least six months

Audience segmentation along lines dictated by behavior change theory is often more helpful than segmentation using conventional demographic variables such as age, gender, income and residence. Women, men and adolescents are not homogeneous groups; each group in a population will exhibit diversity in their current behaviors and readiness for change. Men and women at the preparation stage will be more alike in their needs than a group of women representing all five stages in the change process. It is often useful, however, to combine theoretically relevant variables, such as stage of change, with demographic variables, in order to precisely target populations. Adolescents, for example, may need to be approached as a separate group using peer educators or in adolescent friendly settings. Understanding and responding to the diversity of needs among adolescents can greatly strengthen a behavior change program. Similarly, men and women in some cultures may feel great discomfort in discussing reproductive health issues together and separate settings may be needed. But the programs addressing these groups should not be uniform; they must be differentiated to reflect the diversity within each group.

The analysis also helps define the focus of behavior change efforts and the objectives. Given that a population is distributed along the entire continuum in the change process, a manager may decide to focus on only one theoretically meaningful subgroup. For example, assume that the population analysis shows that a significant portion of the population is at the contemplation stage with regard to family planning—their knowledge levels are high, they understand some of the potential benefits but have no immediate plans to act. This is a fairly common situation. In our discussion of the epidemiology of family planning we pointed to the high level of unmet need—women who want to postpone or end childbearing but are not contracepting. Many of these women can name at least one modern contraceptive method, though they may over-estimate the costs and risks and under-estimate the benefits in increased health and family income. A reasonable posture for a health manager might be to focus his or her behavior change resources on moving those at the contemplation or preparation stage to action. Hence, the behavior change programs would focus on increasing the perceived benefits and decreasing the costs. Relatively little attention would be paid to increasing knowledge among the pre-contemplation group since the greatest efficiency would lie in converting the "contemplators". One could easily imagine alternate scenarios based on the population analysis that might direct resources at sustaining health reproductive behaviors or providing basic information where knowledge levels are low.

Careful, theoretically based analysis of the target population is essential to effective behavior change programming. By arraying the population in terms of their readiness to change, managers can allocate resources effectively and target their campaigns to the needs of different audience segments.

Communications campaigns will typically have to distinguish between primary, secondary and tertiary audiences. The primary audience consists of those people whose behavior is expected to change. In matters of reproductive health, this typically consists of reproductive age women and sexually active men. The secondary audience consists of individuals whose social position or role enables them to influence the primary audience; religious leaders, mothers-in-law and village chiefs are good examples of secondary audiences. The tertiary audience usually consists of policy makers and political leaders who can create a favorable political climate for change. Each audience will then need to be segmented in terms of their stage in order to craft appropriate message content and communication methods.

The data in Table 3-2 on female genital cutting (FGC) from Yemen provide an interesting example of how audience research can shape a communications campaign[8]. One could draw some immediate conclusions from this example:

- FGC is localized in the Coastal region, where two-thirds of the women approve continuing the practice;
- Approval of FGC by the mother (66 percent) and practice (63 percent of daughters circumcised) are highly correlated, as are disapproval by the mother and abandonment of the practice;
- The principal reasons for support are tradition, religion and "cleanliness" (the meaning of which is unclear);
- FGC is carried out by women on girls, largely by traditional birth attendants;
- The medical complications of FGC are not perceived as a major negative even by those who believe the practice should be discontinued.

Interestingly, only a minority of women (32 percent) says their husbands believe the practice should continue, while 45 percent say they do not know their husband's opinion.

Based on these data, one might draw the following conclusions in designing a program:

- The primary audience consists of reproductive age women and traditional birth attendants in the Coastal region.
- The secondary audience consists of religious leaders in the Coastal region since tradition and religion are cited as principal rationales for continuation of the practice.
- The tertiary audience cannot yet be defined based on the available data.

TABLE 3-2. Female Circumcision in Yemen Knowledge, Attitudes, Practices

	Coastal region	Mountain region	Plateau & desert region
% knowing of FGC	91	38	40
% adult women circumcised	69	15	5
% daughters circumcised	63	15	2
% women believing FGC should be continued	66	42	13
Benefits of FGC cited by women approving of FGC		Upholds tradition—48% Follows religion—33 Cleanliness—46 Better marriage—3 Preserves virginity—6 Other/don't know—3	
Negatives of FGC cited by women disapproving of FGC		Bad tradition—68% Against religion—32 Medical complications—12 Painful experience—3 Against dignity of women—10 Other/don't know—5	
Person performing circumcision		Traditional birth attendant—68% Grandmother/relative—19% Barber—5% Nurse/midwife—6% Physician—2% Other—1%	

Setting Objectives

Audience research helps managers set a clear objective by clarifying the audience, their needs and the specific behavior change at issue. Any communications campaign must be limited to one SMART objective. SMART is a term from the management literature that stands for:

- **Specific:** a precise change in behavior
- **Measurable:** a quantitative assessment of behavior change towards the objective must be possible, usually as a percentage change;
- **Appropriate:** responsive to the nature of the problem and the local context;
- **Realistic:** ambitious but clearly achievable;
- **Time bound:** a specific number of months or years for accomplishment of the change is given.

Drawing on the above example, a SMART objective would be "To reduce the practice of FGC among newborn girls in the Coastal region from 63 percent to 50 percent over a five year period." By establishing a clear objective managers and staff can focus their efforts and routinely assess their progress. All program activities can then be tested against the criterion of contribution to the objective.

Focusing on an objective also means saying no to other worthwhile uses of time and resources. Because reproductive health problems and the settings in which they occur are complex and multifaceted, one of the greatest challenges to managers is to focus energy, attention and resources on a clear objective and a specific audience. There are often powerful centrifugal forces that tend to draw attention to other audiences and problems. Sometimes the pressure is to over-promise in the search of political and financial support. However, this usually leads to disillusionment when results inevitably fall short.

Guidelines for Communication

Once the audience analysis has been completed and the objective set, managers must still determine the specific content of the communications to be shared with the audience and the methods by which communication will occur. The following are some practical guidelines that can help managers craft effective communications programs.

Use the Audience Research and the Objective as the Basis for Developing Key Messages

Drawing upon the Yemeni data on FGC will help illustrate the point. The data suggest that:

- The audience is largely at the pre-contemplation stage since they approve of FGC by a margin of two-thirds and are unaware of the medical consequences. Accordingly, the communications strategy should focus on increasing knowledge about FGC; fostering a negative emotional response to FGC; encouraging a positive response to its abandonment; and, emphasizing the long term impact on daughters and their families.
- Message content should focus largely on the commonly cited rationales of tradition, religion and cleanliness, subject to further research on the meaning of these three concepts in the local context. For example, statements from Islamic leaders might help refute the perception that FGC is required by the religion. The health consequences of FGC also need to be dramatically highlighted for the primary and secondary audiences.

This is a very simple illustration using a "bare-bones" data set, but helps illuminate how good data can help focus the target and content of a communication campaign. In practice a much richer data set would be needed to set content.

Good Communication Means a Respectful, Honest Dialogue with the Audience, not a One Way Beaming of Messages

The initial audience research is a way of understanding the needs and concerns of the population to be served. This process of understanding the perceptions, concerns and views never ends in a well-run program. There is an inherent tension in many efforts at behavior change. Public health managers want to respond to the expressed needs of the population to be served while at the same time wanting to introduce new information that will change behavior. Sometimes this tension is easily resolved, as when the objective is to address an expressed unmet need for family planning. In other instances, such as FGC, the public health manager may be trying to change longstanding and highly valued traditions. Constant feedback from the population is essential to understand why current behaviors are practiced and the concerns about adopting new behaviors. Listening to the audience and involving them in a realistic, meaningful way in shaping the communications campaign must consume as much time and energy as transmitting communications. Chapter 4 will describe in detail the many participatory techniques that can be used to involve the beneficiary population.

Be Dramatic

Reproductive health communications are competing with all the other events, messages and "noise" in the life of the audience. They must therefore manifest significant creativity if they are to draw in the desired listeners and watchers. Both sad and humorous forms have been used to good effect. A well-known restaurant in Bangkok uses "condom bouquets" rather than flowers as centerpieces to promote AIDS prevention. A wonderful television commercial developed in Brazil with the assistance of the Johns Hopkins University Population Information Program showed dancing, sexually excited hearts as part of a family planning campaign. A poster developed by the Caribbean Family Planning Association makes a vivid, attention-grabbing statement by showing a forlorn, heavily pregnant young woman saying, "I've lost so much...". Effective communications are both inventive and culturally appropriate.

Communicate a Benefit While Addressing Costs

This guideline is derived from the concept of decisional balance. Movement from stage to stage is a function of the changes in the perceived ratio of benefits to costs in adopting new behaviors. Like all aspects of a good communications campaign, the presentation of benefits and costs must be firmly anchored in the reality that will be experienced by the concerned population. False or misleading claims as to benefits will undermine the credibility of the program. Moreover, the real costs incurred by individuals and households must be addressed on the programmatic side as a necessary adjunct to the communications campaign. The choice of benefits to communicate depends very much on what audience research indicates is of greatest salience to the audience. The following are examples of slogans that have been used to communicate benefits:

- Happy families are planned families (Burkina Faso)
- Birth spacing means better health for your family (Chad)
- A helpful husband makes a happy family (Ghana – promoting condom use)
- Plan your family for prosperity, have children you can afford to feed, clothe and educate (Kenya)
- I'm Juana Segura! Do you want to enjoy me? Then use a condom! (Bolivia)
- Masti lubricated condoms for improved pleasure and complete protection. AIDS equals death but rubbers are protection. (India)

Evoke Emotion While Transferring Knowledge

Behavior change has both cognitive and affective dimensions. Accordingly, a successful communications campaign is very careful to present accurate information in a manner that resonates emotionally with the audience. Many media and techniques can be used to evoke a strong emotional response. The power of the message is limited only by the creativity of the designer; some examples of emotionally powerful messages were presented earlier. But at the core must be perfectly accurate information. After the initial emotional reaction has passed, the remaining kernel of information that is retained must be unimpeachable.

Call for a Specific Action

Effective messages guide the recipient along the change process by encouraging specific actions. It does no good to evoke a strong reaction without providing clear guidance as to what the client should do next. The specific behaviors proposed depend very much upon the nature of the problem and the client's stage. Those in the early stages of change may be called upon to seek out additional information. A poster from Tunisia is a good example of this kind of appeal; the Arabic text calls upon readers to, "Learn before marriage about the benefits of family planning." It is directed at a very specific audience segment—engaged couples with low levels of knowledge about family planning. It does not ask them to adopt family planning, it only suggests they consult a health workers to learn about contraception.

For those in the late contemplation, preparation and action stages, different kinds of behaviors should be encouraged. Clients might be encouraged to develop a specific plan (such as a birth plan), shift from preparation to action (e.g., purchase and use condoms) or join a support group.

Use Attractive and Credible Sources

An effective message delivers appropriate content from a credible source through an appropriate medium. The importance of role models in behavior change was discussed earlier, including the use of both celebrities and peers. *Who* delivers the message is as important as *what* is said. In the United States, the announcement by the basketball star Earvin "Magic" Johnson that he was HIV positive had a huge impact in legitimizing discussion of the issue. Political leaders can play an extremely important role in providing social sanction for new behaviors. President Yoweri Museveni of Uganda has been widely credited with providing a supportive atmosphere for behavior change through his public pronouncements on AIDS. During the mid-1980's, President Seyni Kountche of Niger encouraged health workers to make contraceptive services available through his open support of family planning. Carefully choosing and pre-testing advocates for behavior change is an important component of a communications strategy.

Select an Appropriate Mix of Communication Media and Methods Based on Audience Research

Audience research should include an analysis of how people garner information. In developing country settings, where literacy and access to mass media vary widely, a context specific understanding of the most commonly used communications channels is critical to strategy design. All of the possible modes of communication should be considered, including print, radio, television, film, person-to-person, group and organizational meetings, modern and traditional drama, music, puppet shows and dance. Depending on the local culture and context, any one or combination of these may be the most appropriate for a given message and audience segment. Typically, one communication channel will be selected as the lead modes based on the extant pattern of information gathering. For example, if most people in the targeted audience segment report having a radio in the household and that it is a primary vehicle for getting news, then this might be the principal vehicle for short spots, discussion sessions and a soap opera addressing the behavior change objective. The lead communication channel must, however, be buttressed through some investment in other communication channels to reinforce the key message. No one medium will reach all of the intended audience. Moreover, consistent messages coming from different sources of information can strengthen knowledge and positive perceptions. Radio might be selected as the lead medium, but posters, pamphlets, billboards and group meetings might be used to reach those members of the audience segment who do not rely on radio and/or to reinforce the radio messages. A unifying logo or slogan is usually used to tie together the messages emanating from different sources.

Thoroughly Pretest Messages and Methods and Revise as Needed

No matter how careful a communications professional is in designing a message, there is no way to know what it looks like, sounds like or feels like to the intended audience without careful pre-testing. Submitting draft materials to the review of representatives of the intended audience is extremely important to an effective campaign. Piotrow, et. al., have proposed eight basic questions that pre-testing should answer[9]:

- Is the message clear to the intended audiences? How does the understanding vary among different subgroups (men, women, rural, urban, etc.)?
- Is the message trustworthy and believable? Does it credibly promise a benefit?
- Does the audience like the materials?
- Are the images culturally appropriate?
- Are there too many messages? Must some information be sacrificed for better focus?
- Is there anything offensive in the material?
- Would people talk to their friends and relatives about the message?
- Does it make the audience want to take appropriate action?

Pre-testing typically involves presenting the material(s) to focus groups drawn from the intended audience and then eliciting their reaction, through guided discussion, to the foregoing questions. Suggestions and advice from the focus group as to how to improve the materials are actively solicited and, as appropriate, incorporated into revised versions of the materials. Pre-testing can pick up on a wide range of blatant and subtle deficiencies that may not be apparent to the professional staff. The choice of words, intonations, facial expressions, the type of shoes worn by characters, even the patterns on clothing can create a negative or positive reaction. Slogans may not be understood as intended. Jewelry or clothing on a character depicted in the materials may imply a difference in social class that is off-putting to the intended audience. Focus groups are often extremely helpful in suggesting modifications that make the materials and messages more acceptable. Pre-testing offers the only way to detect flaws from the perspective of the audience and to take corrective action before large-scale distribution.

Political screening of materials is also often required. Reproductive health programs inherently invite controversy. Political and religious leaders are often quite sensitive to the portrayal of reproductive health and sexual issues. Failure to obtain the necessary political support can quickly kill off a communications campaign. Hence, involving representatives of political leaders early in the program design process to set parameters for the communications campaign is essential.

Organize, Staff, and Budget Appropriately for Program Implementation

While many people can contribute to behavior change, individuals with appropriate training and experience must hold key managerial and technical positions. Designing, implementing and evaluating a behavior change program requires specialized expertise. Accordingly, communications professionals must be given the resources and authority to manage the behavior change campaign, while being held accountable for results and rewarded accordingly. Unless they have specialized training, physicians, nurses and other clinicians are generally poorly equipped to manage a behavior change program. There is, however, an important role for health professionals in ensuring that the technical content of communications is accurate. Communication staff can sometimes be carried away with developing persuasive materials that are not necessarily completely grounded in science. Hence, review of all materials for accuracy should be built into the design process and be expected by all involved staff. In addition, both health and communications professionals require supervision to ensure that all messages and materials stay focused on the intended audience and the behavioral objective.

Financing of behavior change programs also requires careful planning. Under budgeting of communications campaigns is a common and cardinal sin. Adequate investment is needed in both the design process and materials acquisition and distribution. One to two years of effort and investment is usually required to carry out the audience analysis and then design, test, revise and mass produce materials. Costs can sometimes be shared among agencies with similar objectives, but this is not always feasible.

Distribution and use of communications materials must also be carefully planned, managed and monitored. Materials are often under-utilized, poorly placed or improperly applied by staff lacking the requisite training. A logistics system for disseminating the materials must be in place. A schedule for broadcasts and placement of materials must be developed and followed. A regular system of feedback must be in place to be sure that materials reach the end user. In one West African country, for example, thousands of dollars were spent on acquiring family planning flipcharts, only to have them hoarded in district warehouses, without ever being placed in the hands of health providers or used to educate potential clients. These system failures are common in many developing countries and examples of programs that failed to deliver carefully developed products are legion. Meticulous planning as to the distribution and use of materials, followed by careful monitoring of the mechanics of a communications campaign is essential. For example, if a radio program has been developed, there must be a clear, appropriate broadcast schedule that has received the necessary approvals. The manager must then monitor that the broadcasts actually take place on the days and at the times planned. Similarly, the delivery, placement and use of flipcharts, posters, pamphlets, billboards, group meetings, street theater and all the myriad forms of communication must also be scrupulously monitored.

Monitor Program Implementation Regularly and Assess Behavior Change

The following is a list of indicators, developed as part of The Evaluation Project, which can be tracked to monitor the implementation of a behavior change program:[10]

- Number of communications produced by type during a reference period;
- Number of communications disseminated by type during a reference period;
- Percentage of a target audience exposed to program messages based on respondent recall;
- Percentage of target audience who correctly comprehend a given message;
- Percentage of target audience who acquire the skill to complete a certain task as a result of exposure to a specific communication;
- Percentage of target audience exposed to a specific message who report liking it;
- Number/percentage of target audience who discuss message(s) with others by type of person;
- Percentage of target population who report advocating healthy reproductive behaviors.

This is a fairly comprehensive list and it is very unlikely that any one program could or should attempt to monitor all these indicators. Attempting to collect too much data that will never be processed or used is worse than no monitoring system at all. Hence, managers should select a few indicators that will help them keep track of progress and that can be readily translated into management decisions. In addition, these indicators do not reflect behavior change *per se*; they largely indicate only whether a message was disseminated or received. This is very useful for on-going management purposes, but should not be confused with an assessment of impact on behavior.

ASSESSING BEHAVIOR CHANGE

In the opening to this chapter we suggested four general domains of behavior change – achieving household fertility goals; safe pregnancy and childbirth, infection-free sex and consensual sex—that foster reproductive security. Specific, measurable behavioral objectives are the starting point for all good behavior change programs. Accordingly, specific, appropriate indicators must be selected by which to measure the behaviors of the population at program inception and assess change over time. Table 3-3 provides a matrix of key behavioral indicators for assessing reproductive security[11].

Other behavioral indicators exist and plausible alternative choices might certainly be made. Given the difficulty in collecting, processing and using data, the challenge to managers is to define a minimum number of indicators that would allow one to determine whether meaningful change in key reproductive behaviors has occurred. These indicators have been chosen because they are directly linked to an essential behavior identified in earlier chapters. Clarifying the specific behavioral objectives to be achieved allows managers to select appropriate indicators of impact.

BEHAVIOR CHANGE

TABLE 3-3. Matrix of Behavioral Indicators for Reproductive Security

Reproductive security domain	Indicators
Achieving Household Fertility Goals	• Contraceptive prevalence • Median length of birth intervals • Unwanted total fertility rate
Safe pregnancy and childbirth	• Mean number of prenatal care visits • % of households with a pregnant woman that have a birth plan • Percentage of births attended by trained health personnel • Percentage of women receiving 2 visits during the first 5 days after birth
Infection free sex	• Percentage of adults practicing low risk behavior for HIV/STD • Percentage of sexually active adults who report current, consistent use of condoms • Percentage of adults practicing care-seeking behaviors that reduce HIV/STD infection
Consensual sex	• Gender specific attitudes towards use of violence in household relations (e.g., approval of wife beating) • Gender specific reports of various forms of sexual violence: psychological abuse, forced sex, other forms of sexual abuse, physical abuse • Help seeking behavior by abused women and reasons for not seeking help • Prevalence of child sexual abuse • Incidence of sexual violence recorded by health providers and law enforcement

The definitions of the indicators are as follows:

- *Contraceptive prevalence* is the percentage of women aged 15–49 who are using a contraceptive method; sometimes restricted to *modern method contraceptive prevalence*, which excludes traditional methods.
- *Median length of birth interval* is the median number of months between a specified reference date, typically the date of the survey, and the last birth among women with one or more births (referred to as open interval) OR the median number of months separating successive births among women with two or more births (closed interval).
- *Unwanted total fertility rate* is the average number of unwanted births per woman where an unwanted birth is one that causes family size to exceed the maximum desired by the mother.
- *Median number of prenatal care visits* assesses the number of visits to a physician, nurse, midwife or other trained health provider by women experiencing a pregnancy during a reference period.
- *Proportion of births attended by trained health personnel* includes births attended by trained health professionals but excludes traditional birth attendants. It is typically calculated as:

    # of births attended by trained personnel / (number of live births × 1.15) with the multiplier of 1.15 used to account for deliveries not resulting in a live birth.
- *Percentage of women securing two post-partum visits during the first 5 days after birth* by a trained attendant as assessed by self-report. This is an indicator of adherence to the recommended ACNM schedule of post-partum visits discussed in Chapter 7.
- *Percentage of adults practicing low risk behavior for STD/HIV*, which includes abstaining completely from sex over the last 12 months OR only one sexual partner over the last 12 months

OR consistent use of condoms with all partners over the last 3 months as measured by responses to survey questions.

- *Percentage of sexually active adults who report current, consistent use of condoms*, which means condoms are used at every sexual act with all partners over the last three months.
- *Percentage of adults practicing care-seeking behaviors that reduce HIV/STD infection* may be measured in terms of any of the following: median interval between onset of symptoms and seeking care; percent of high risk individuals self-referring for care; percent complying with prescribed therapy, and/or percent referring a partner for testing and care.

4

Community Empowerment

HOW COMMUNITY VARIABLES INFLUENCE REPRODUCTIVE HEALTH

The call for community participation in health programming appears in the European public health literature no later than the last half of the nineteenth century[1]. By the 1920s the concept of community participation for health had infiltrated the thinking of British colonial administrators in India and, somewhat later, in Africa. Throughout the 1960s and 1970s there was a growing sense among health programmers that the failure to involve target populations in the formulation and implementation of programs was undermining efficacy. The critique of "top-down" programming reached its zenith in the Alma-Alta Declaration of 1978 in which the World Health Organization endorsed the concept of primary health care as the fundamental strategy for developing countries. The primary health care doctrine encompassed community participation as one of its basic pillars, as exemplified by the following quote from the Alma Alta declaration:

> "Primary health care is the essential health care based on practical, scientifically sound and socially acceptable methods and technology made universally acceptable to individuals and families in the community *through their full participation and at a cost the community can afford to maintain at every stage of their development in the spirit of self-reliance and self-determination.*" (emphasis added)

The concept of community participation for reproductive health has a powerful intuitive appeal. In recent years, there have been urgent appeals for greater community participation in programs addressing family planning[2], safe motherhood[3] and HIV/AIDS[4]. Here are some of the ways that community participation can affect the reproductive health of individuals and households:

1. Community participation in *needs assessment* can help ensure that health professionals focus on issues of high priority to households and/or better understand the context-specific dynamics of reproductive health.
2. Community *norms* can work for or against reproductive health. Positive and negative reinforcement from peers, neighbors, friends and family influence sexual and reproductive behavior.

3. Community participation can develop *leadership support* for reproductive health. Community leaders, such as village chiefs and religious leaders, play a critical role in setting the agenda for collective action, function as role models and can support or oppose healthy reproductive norms.
4. Community participation can help *mobilize resources for collective action.* Given the severe and chronic under-funding of health systems in most developing countries, households can pool resources to secure essential goods and services.
5. Community participation can help extend services to *marginalized and under-served groups* within the wider community.
6. Community participation can help position community representatives to *negotiate effectively with external agencies.*

Working with and through communities is one of the essential responsibilities of health managers. Every community has a social and political structure that mediates its contact with the rest of the world. The quality of the transaction between the health system and the community is one of the key determinants of the success of health programs, including reproductive health programs. Programs that fail to meaningfully involve the community in defining the problem, crafting the response and implementing the program usually fail. The health field is rife with examples of well-intended programs in which an outsider defined for a community its problems and the "right" solution. These efforts almost invariably end in disaster. Even when results are achieved in the short run, the long-term sustainability of programs that are not solidly anchored in a base of community support is seriously imperiled.

THE MEANING OF COMMUNITY

There is no widely shared definition of community in the public health or social science literature—one intrepid sociologist uncovered no fewer than 94 separate definitions.[5,6] Most of the definitions look for a set of common characteristics that bind people together in some way. These characteristics may include living in the same location and/or shared values, culture, interests or problems. A review of the health literature found that community is used to denote "a locality-bound aggregation of people who share economic, socio-cultural and political characteristics, as well as problems and needs".[7]

One very useful example is provided by Indu Aluwalia and Thomas Schmid[8], who have suggested that, "A community is a locale or domain that is characterized by the following elements:

1) Membership—a sense of identity and belonging
2) Common symbol systems—similar language, rituals and ceremonies
3) Shared values and norms
4) Mutual influence—community members have influence and are influenced by each other
5) Shared needs and commitment to meeting them
6) Shared emotional connections—members share common history, experiences and mutual support

This definition would encompass people sharing a place of residence, such as a village or neighborhood, who also share the other characteristics. However, any grouping that exhibits the characteristics defined by Ahuwalia and Schmid also constitutes a community that may be a useful vehicle for promoting reproductive health. Other naturally forming associations, such as those composed of youth, women, members of a religion, ethnic group, caste or category of workers (e.g., transport workers) may form a community. They create a social infrastructure that can be profitably used to improve the health of their members.

The potential drawback to the "shared characteristics" approach to defining a community is that it usually relies on an external observer to infer that a group of people constitutes a community. A case of failed community mobilization will help illustrate the pitfall. An attempt was made to mobilize commercial sex workers (CSW) in Madras, India[9]. The program managers initially presumed the CSW shared many of the same characteristics – living in close proximity, similar profession, the same elevated risk of STD and HIV, and like histories of stigma and exploitation. However, the program was unsuccessful in large part due to the heterogeneity among the CSW. CSW in Madras fall into different groups (street workers, brothel workers, housewives, call girls, male prostitutes and a group of castrated, feminized men known as 'ali'). The sub-groups regard themselves as quite distinct and, in fact, experience sex work in very different ways. These sub-groups also tend to be drawn from different ethnic populations; e.g., many of the brothel workers come from Andhra Pradesh and speak a different language than those native to Madras and the surrounding area. Most importantly, the CSW do not *identify themselves* as belonging to a community of CSW – there is little sense of shared identity or interests. The structural barriers imposed by pimps, brothel owners and police exacerbates the atomization of the CSW. As a result, efforts to promote collective action, such as peer education, proved very difficult. Management inadequacies and a police crackdown that eventually doomed the program compounded these problems.

Communities are often, indeed usually, heterogeneous. Divisions occur along ethnic, caste, gender, age, class and income lines. These divisions can (but need not) inhibit collective action in response to reproductive health problems. They can also play an important role in determining health status, including reproductive health. Groups within a community that are poorer or less powerful are likely to exhibit a higher prevalence of unhealthy behaviors and less access to services. As shall be discussed further below, one of the challenges to community empowerment is integrating marginzalized groups into the decision-making process and ensuring that they capture benefits from reproductive health programs. A health manager cannot simply presume that a village, neighborhood, work group or other collective constitutes a meaningful "community". People may or may not perceive themselves as having a commonality of interests despite living in close proximity or "objectively" sharing similar problems and characteristics. The attempt by an outsider to define or discover the membership of a community must be approached cautiously lest one run afoul of the potential divisions within an erstwhile community.

Moreover, the characteristics proposed by Ahuwalia and Schmid are sometimes the *outcome* of a successful community mobilization process rather than the starting point. Community mobilization helps people uncover shared interests and concerns from which springs a sense of common identity. Mutual influence and shared emotional connection derive from the process of solving problems together. New, shared norms governing sexuality and reproductive health evolve in response to dialogue and discovery. While some level of shared characteristics may be a necessary precondition to collective action, the members' perception of community identity can also be influenced by community mobilization.

Some commentators have simply abandoned the effort to define community in terms of a set of shared characteristics[10]. Rather they have argued that community is a shifting social construct that reflects people's sense of relationships. Community, in this view, must be understood as a mental image that people have about others who play a role in their lives.

A community is represented not by shared characteristics but by the pattern of communication, feeling and influence that people articulate about others in their lives. An outsider cannot observe a community on the basis of "objective" characteristics. He or she can only inquire as to the pattern of meaningful relationships as experienced by individuals.

Specifying the community to be served is one of the first tasks that must be undertaken by the manager. Managers may attempt to observe shared characteristics that define a community. A complementary or alternative approach to defining a community is to look for the pattern of relationships that people identify as particularly meaningful. Using this approach, the analyst simply asks people to define the salient network of contacts and leaders. People who define each other as sources of communication and influence constitute a community. Relatively straightforward questions about the pattern of communication and the degree of influence accorded individuals can help in constructing a "community" for the purposes of health programming.

An interesting example of this approach comes from Bangladesh.[11] All women in a village were asked to identify their contacts and opinion leaders. A visual map of the network of social contacts was then drawn. A circle represented each individual and lines represented contact among individuals. The size of the circle representing the individual is proportional to the number of contacts; the bigger the circle the larger the social network of a given individual. In this way the actual community of women who interact and influence each other was defined. This network became the "target community" for the manager of the family planning program. Women with the largest number of social contacts were identified as nodes for community mobilization; i.e., they were trained and supported to organize community meetings and provide family planning education for their friends and acquaintances.

THE CONFUSING LANGUAGE OF COMMUNITY PARTICIPATION

The professional jargon implying a role for the community includes the phrases *community empowerment*, *community participation* and *community mobilization*. Program managers will speak of seeking community input or consulting with the community before making decisions. The array of terms reveals the multiple roles that a community might play relative to a reproductive health program, including:

- implementing tasks designed by health professionals;
- providing information and opinion to professional program staff;
- contributing labor, money or other resources to initiate or sustain the program;
- establishing a continuing physical or organizational infrastructure, such as community based distribution of contraceptives or transport for obstetrical emergencies, that will sustain the program after external assistance is withdrawn;
- supporting healthier reproductive behaviors through various forms of communal encouragement or sanction;
- providing leadership support for the reproductive health program in the form of public advocacy to constituencies inside and outside the community;
- participating in program decision-making along with health professionals;
- assuming complete control of the program, along with concomitant responsibility for decisions and resource mobilization.

COMMUNITY EMPOWERMENT

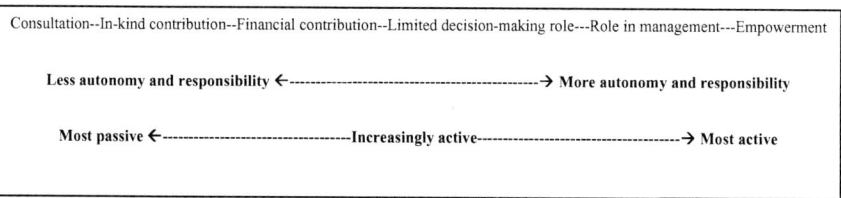

FIGURE 4-1. Spectrum of community participation.

All of these may be legitimate and reasonable expectations of or by the community. There is, however, a clear hierarchy implicit in both the jargon of community participation and the range of roles for communities. Rifkin stipulated five levels of community participation: participation in (1) benefits, (2) activities, (3) program implementation, (4) monitoring and evaluation, and (5) program planning.[12] Kambou suggests a spectrum of community participation depicted in Figure 4-1[13].

A somewhat more cynical view is embedded in the work of Choguill, who suggests the following "ladder of community participation":[14]

- Self-management—the community is left to its own resources without help from the government
- Conspiracy—the community is manipulated by authorities for the benefit of officials
- Informing—the community receives a one-way flow of information without feedback or negotiation
- Diplomacy—authorities seek community "input" without meaningfully affecting the programs (if any) that are eventually implemented;
- Dissimulation—the forms of participation, such as committees and advisory boards, exist, but they are expected to act as a "rubber stamp" for government decisions;
- Conciliation—government authorities are well-intentioned but basically use the structures of community participation (committees, advisory boards) to implement externally conceived programs;
- Partnership—members of the community and outside decision-makers share planning and decision-making through agreed upon structures;
- Empowerment—community members exercise control over planning and decision-making.

These and other similar typologies suggest that the role of the community hinges largely on decisions about the locus of control. All the typologies depict a continuum with regard to the locus of control over health programs as between external agencies and community structures. At one end of the continuum the community is an entity to be changed as a consequence of decisions made elsewhere. Managers might "consult" with the community or seek community "input". However, decisions, resources and control are vested in an agency (whether private or public) external to the community. At the other end of the continuum, usually denoted by the term empowerment, is the transfer of authority, resources and responsibility to community structures.

The typologies also suggest that managers need to develop clear, shared expectations about the role of the community, which can obviously take many different forms. The specific type of community participation appropriate to a given context reflects the philosophy/ideology of the managers, the capacity of the community and the tenor of the general political system. Communities that are highly atomized may not be prepared for an empowerment approach, whereas the opposite conclusion might be drawn for a community that has highly developed structures for negotiating with the health system. An authoritarian political regime may preclude relinquishing decision-making to community structures. There is no one "right" role for all communities under all circumstances. The role of the health manager is to be aware of the alternatives and optimize community participation given the local context.

COMMUNITY EMPOWERMENT FOR REPRODUCTIVE HEALTH

Many definitions of community empowerment have been advanced. Beeker, et. al. define community empowerment as "effect(ing) community-wide change in health related behaviors by organizing communities to define their health problems, to identify the determinants of those problems and to engage in effective individual and collective action to change those determinants."[15] Minkler and Wallerstein define community empowerment as "a social action process through which individuals, communities and organizations gain mastery over their lives in the context of changing their social and political environment to improve equity and the quality of life."[16] Ahuwalia and Schmid define an empowered community as "one in which individuals and organizations apply their skills and resources in a collective effort to meet their respective needs.[17]"

Embedded in these and other definitions of community empowerment are three key ideas. First, community empowerment, much like behavior change, constitutes a *process* rather a singular event. Communities gradually redefine extant conditions, such as high fertility, as problems that need solving or new problems, such as AIDS, emerge. Over time, norms are adjusted and resources mobilized to address the problem. Leaders become advocates for new norms. Communities uncover their own resources and capacity to take effective action in support of reproductive health. Existing organizations, such as health committees or women's associations, take on the responsibility of promoting reproductive health. Alternatively, new organizations, such as an AIDS support group, are formed. Community representatives learn to be effective negotiators with external authorities and resources.

Secondly, community empowerment implies *collective action*. Askew makes the point that community participation only makes sense when the nature of the problem or the task requires collective action.[18] His research found that community participation in family planning programs was often quite low because couples had no particular reason to invest scarce resources to support the government program. If a problem can be resolved at the individual or household level there is little incentive to invest the time and energy needed for collective action. Hence, a necessary element of effective community empowerment is identifying the collective actions essential to reproductive security. The following are examples of collective actions that are likely to foster reproductive health:

- Assessing community reproductive health needs, setting priorities and crafting an appropriate strategy.
- Fostering norms that support reproductive health and mechanisms for encouraging adherence to those norms. These norms might include informed and responsible choice as to family size,

safe birth intervals, utilization of essential maternal health care, safe sex, sympathetic support to people living with AIDS and the absence of violence or coercion in sexual relations.
- Developing leadership support for actions and norms that foster reproductive health.
- Creating or strengthening an organizational infrastructure for identifying and implementing collective actions needed to support reproductive health. These actions might include community based distribution of contraceptives, condom distribution, rapid transport of obstetrical emergencies, blood donation, access to essential drugs, supporting community health workers, support to people living with AIDS, community health education, emergency loan funds, and refurbishing and equipping local health facilities.
- Identifying and mobilizing the resources needed for essential reproductive services.
- Extending reproductive health care to under-served groups in the community.
- Negotiating effectively with government, donors and other actors external to the community with regard to reproductive health resources and services.

The third core concept embedded in the definitions of community empowerment is that of *outcomes*. Community empowerment is more than a process; it must lead to a discernable change in people's lives. One type of outcome is *increased capacity*. All of the collective actions listed above require gains in knowledge, skills and resources. Community empowerment means that people are less vulnerable to the vagaries of their environment and have greater control over their own lives. Communities become less dependent on the will and whims of health professionals, government authorities and other external agents to secure essential reproductive health care and improve their reproductive health status. A second type of outcome is a change in the *quality of life*. Community empowerment should lead to better reproductive health—fewer unintended pregnancies, lower maternal mortality and morbidity, lower incidence of STD/HIV and less sexual violence.

With these core concepts in mind—process, collective action and outcomes—community empowerment for reproductive health is defined as a process by which a community acquires and exercises the capacity for collective actions that foster household reproductive security.

It must be recognized that there is an inherent tension, indeed contradiction between an emphasis on community empowerment and a focus on specific health outcomes, such as improved reproductive health. As a consequence of a genuinely participatory process, a community may determine that reproductive health issues are not a priority or too difficult or controversial to address. The community's first priority may be water supply or improved income, rather than reproductive health.

The dilemma is real and there are no easy solutions, though three general guidelines can help alleviate the tension:

1. The health staff and the community need to engage in candid dialogue from the moment of first contact to set boundaries. It is a disservice to the community to begin an unfettered exploration of needs to which the health professionals cannot respond. By clearly delineating the arena of action, managers can avoid creating unrealistic expectations and the consequent potential for conflict and disappointment.
2. Focus on building skills and capacities that are transferable. Many of the skills needed for collective action for reproductive health, such as participatory research, organizational development, resource mobilization and negotiation, are applicable to other arenas. Training and experience gained in one area can foster a more general community capacity at collective action.

3. Look for linkages to other partners and resources. Health professionals can serve as good faith conduits to resources in other arenas. Organizational and funding constraints may demand that health professionals focus on reproductive health. This does not preclude helping the community gain access to organizations and resources in other fields.

THE COMMUNITY EMPOWERMENT CYCLE

Defining community empowerment as a specific process of collective actions leading to better reproductive health creates a roadmap for the health professional as a facilitator of community empowerment. Community empowerment is not amorphous; it can be focused in concrete ways—defining the community to be served, needs assessment, resource identification and mobilization, organization building, leadership development, and implementation of specific collective actions that foster reproductive health. The intervention strategy must be adapted to the point in the process at which a community finds itself at any point in time. Awareness raising may be needed early in the process, but will be useless if the community is struggling with organizational development or resource mobilization. The health professional must descend from his or her perch as an "expert" and engage with the community as a genuine partner. The task becomes one of working with the community in its own efforts to identify problems, craft appropriate solutions and mobilize resources.

Figure 4-2 provides a graphic representation of the process of community empowerment.

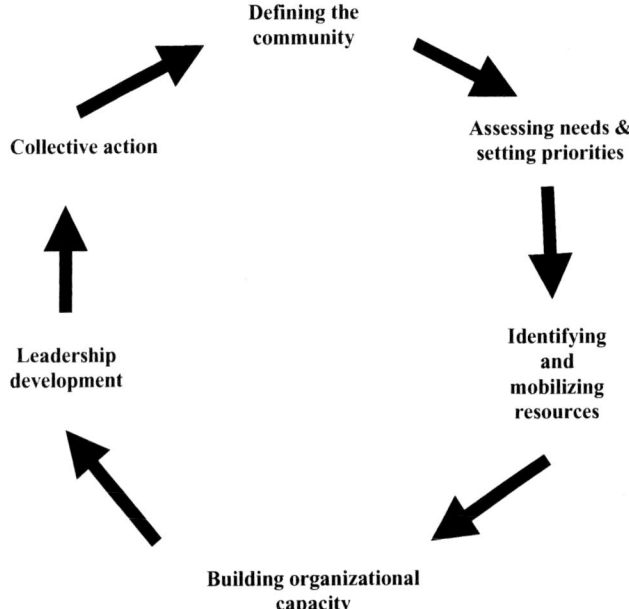

FIGURE 4-2. The community empowerment cycle.

COMMUNITY EMPOWERMENT REQUIRES PARTICIPATORY APPROACHES

The rest of this chapter is devoted to practical techniques for working with communities to achieve greater reproductive security. The emphasis is on participatory approaches. There is a role for "outsiders" as providers of capital, technical expertise and access to external resources. But sustaining collective action for reproductive health requires a strong sense of community commitment and ownership. Cleland identified seven conditions for optimal community participation in his study of four countries[19]:

1. The activity was perceived as high priority within the community;
2. Most community members benefited;
3. There was little or no controversy;
4. Community resources were available and committed;
5. Modest external technical resources were made available;
6. Straightforward management; and
7. External authorities and sponsors were willing to adapt to local needs.

What ties together these seven conditions is relying on the community to identify its problems, craft solutions and mobilize resources, with external authorities playing a modest supportive role.

Conversely, collective action is impeded when:[20,21,22]

- Health officials adopt an authoritarian approach to the community;
- Health officials perceive "participation" as community implementation of government defined services and priorities;
- Health systems are internally authoritarian and therefore cannot model participatory approaches;
- The community structure is rigidly hierarchical or authoritarian;
- There are few or weak community organizations with which to mobilize collective action.

What follows is a menu of participatory techniques that can help elicit collective action. Deciding which techniques to use and in what order is a matter of judgment based on the community's position relative to the community empowerment cycle. Different techniques are needed at each point in the cycle; some techniques are best suited to problem identification, while others are better used for resource mobilization. Selecting techniques depends very much on how far the community has progressed in mobilizing for collective action and on the nature of the problem to be resolved.

Usually, multiple techniques will need to be employed over time, which serves two purposes. Most participatory techniques are actually *learning processes* by which the community discovers ways to further its collective interests. Each successive technique can be used to complement, confirm or call into question findings from earlier exercises. Triangulation from different exercises is an important part of the process of learning to solve problems. Properly applied, using multiple techniques can also expand the circle of participation. Each successive application of a participatory technique provides an opportunity for soliciting information and action from community members who may have been missed by earlier exercises.

Most importantly, participation for empowerment is a long-term, on-going process. Participatory techniques originally gained currency for their use in program appraisal. A range of approaches—participatory rural appraisal, rapid rural appraisal, rapid assessment procedures—were championed as a complement or alternative to more conventional social science research. These are short-term exercises that use many of the same techniques described below for the purpose of gaining insights that are incorporated into program design. Participation for empowerment is very different, stretching out over months or years. Community empowerment is an iterative, incremental process of defining needs, mobilizing assets and building capacity. The techniques described below are tools to which a community can turn again and again for problem solving.

DEVELOPING A FACILITATION TEAM

Community empowerment is *work*. It requires significant investment of time and energy. Health managers must be willing to devote staff time to facilitating the process. This requires an understanding that community mobilization is just as important to health outcomes as the delivery of clinical services.

Health managers need to assemble a *facilitation team* to plan and implement participatory exercises and support collective action by a wide range of individuals and groups. The village or neighborhood health committee can be the starting point for the facilitation team. The facilitation team should include health professionals, community leaders and other interested community representatives; a good gender balance will also be needed. Issues of ethnicity, language, caste and class may also need to be taken into account in assembling the team. A non-governmental organization can often play a helpful role in organizing, staffing and supporting the facilitation team.

DEFINING AND DESCRIBING THE TARGET COMMUNITY[23]

A necessary first step in community empowerment is defining the community to be served and describing its salient characteristics. The key to this process is employing participatory methods that unveil the knowledge people already have about their locale and the web of relationships in which they function. Here are some simple techniques that can be used with small groups to help define and describe a community:

Social Mapping: A social map is a visual presentation of a residential area. The work group, using locally available materials, draws or depicts the physical boundaries of the community on a large piece of paper or on the ground. Using symbols, all the residences and other salient features of the community are depicted, including health facilities, water supply, roads, schools, and places of worship. The object is for the group to prepare a detailed visual representation of the community and its features. If the map is initially depicted on the ground using objects (which is often more practical), then it should be transferred to paper to keep a permanent record. Where a community is large and complex, it may be necessary to create maps of zones within the community that are later combined. This process is almost always surprising to users in terms of the richness of information revealed about resources and diversity within the community.

Census Mapping: Once all the residences have been identified on the social map, basic demographic data is recorded about each household, including number of adults, number of children by sex and age, school attendance and literacy. Census data can be recorded in one of two ways. The information can be recorded directly on the map. Alternatively, a card can be prepared for each household with the relevant information. Important health information about each household can also be recorded. A CARE family planning project in Bangladesh used this approach to record contraceptive use via colored dots associated with each household on the map. This allowed very precise tracking of changes in contraceptive prevalence as well as targeting of education efforts.

Transect Walk: A transect walk is basically a structured walk through a community. It is used to verify and supplement information on the social map. It may be carried out with specific objectives in mind, such as identifying places where people congregate or optimal sites for education and services.

Wealth and Well-being Ranking: The purpose of this exercise is to identify those households with the least resources that can eventually be targeted for special emphasis in programming. However, the wealth and well-being ranking must be carried out very carefully and sensitively, as it tends to arouse suspicion about its misuse. Dialogue with community members, leaders, and local authorities is important to clarify the reason for the exercise. The group carrying out the exercise should determine criteria for wealth and well-being, such as the quality of housing, ownership of livestock or goods, farm holdings, school attendance, health and/or access to food. The group then creates categories of well-being, such as poorest, poor, better-off, best-off. The group then assigns each household to a category. This technique was used by a CARE adolescent reproductive health project in an urban neighborhood in Zambia to designate the well-being of households. Adolescent boys and girls used their knowledge of their neighborhoods to assign each household to a well-being category. This ultimately provided very useful insights into social divisions within the community and barriers to service delivery access among sub-groups.

Social Network Analysis: In discussing the definition of community, it was pointed out that the network of social relations may be a "truer" representation of a community than a group living in the same place that shares a set of demographic characteristics. The two approaches are complementary rather than opposed. Social network analysis allows for an understanding of patterns of mutual influence within a larger grouping. This influence manifests as exchange of assistance, information, companionship and emotional support. The object of the analysis is to map the pattern of regular exchange among subsets of community members.[24] The basic technique is to survey respondents as to the identity of others who have an influence on their lives. In general, the questions ask the respondent to identify four kinds of people: (1) those with whom they exchange assistance in time of need; (2) those with whom they exchange information; (3) those with whom they exchange companionship; and (4) those with whom they exchange emotional support.[25] Network analysis can also be used to identify sexual partners. An interesting example of the use of network analysis comes from Thailand, where urban adolescents were contacted in school dormitories, shopping centers and entertainment spots.[26] Each adolescent was asked to name "people you like to spend free time with" and "boy/girlfriends, sex partners and lovers". This provided rich information on the network of relations, locations where adolescents congregate, risk behaviors, gender relations and negotiation that could be used to design interventions.

The combination of social mapping, census mapping, wealth and well-being ranking and social network mapping can provide the community and the manager a detailed understanding of the boundaries and members of a community, diversity within the community and the pattern of influence.

ASSESSING NEEDS THROUGH PARTICIPATORY APPRAISAL

Participatory needs assessment is a complement to the health service statistics, surveys and other conventional forms of community health analysis that rely on epidemiological and demographic techniques.[27] They are not a substitute for conventional health assessments. They are, nonetheless, a very important and valuable part of crafting an appropriate reproductive health program. They elicit a richness of detail about reproductive health problems as perceived and explained by the community that cannot otherwise be secured. As importantly, participatory appraisal, properly applied, contributes to the empowerment process. Participatory research provides a mechanism by which the community uncovers and articulates its own problems, enhancing the sense of ownership in an eventual problem-solving strategy.

Free Listing and Pile Sorting: The purpose of this exercise is to elicit community members' perceptions of reproductive health problems that they experience. Community members are asked to assemble in small groups. Each member is asked to individually name reproductive health problems that exist in the community. For example, a group might be asked to, "Name health problems or illnesses that women have from being wives and mothers." Each reported illness is recorded on a card, using symbols when groups are illiterate. Only one "illness" is placed on each card. Community members will typically report symptoms, such as vaginal discharge or postpartum bleeding, as health problems. An appraisal in India that asked women to identify their health problems generated the following list:[28]

- vaginal discharge
- backache
- excessive menstruation
- fever
- headache
- weakness
- pain in hands and legs
- scanty menstruation
- stomach ache
- malaria
- irregular menstruation
- body ache
- cough
- problems during menstruation
- cold

Each group is then asked to sort the cards into piles of problems that tend to occur together. Problems associated with childbirth, for example, will commonly form a cluster. Vaginal discharge, itching and pain will form another. Free listing serves a number of useful purposes. It elicits terminology used by the community to describe reproductive health problems; e.g., in a Somali community the CARE team found that "waist pain" was used to signal reproductive tract infections, while "kidney pain" was used to identify urinary tract infections. It provides the health professional with insight into the health problems perceived by the community and those left unstated. It helps crystallize for the community portraits or clusters of health problems surrounding life events commonly shared in the community. This can be helped if the clusters are depicted using visual aids and clear symbols.

Ranking and Scoring: Ranking and scoring is used to help the community set priorities among reproductive health problems. Small groups are asked to order the previously identified health problems in terms of importance. An alternative procedure is to assign each participant a fixed number of points that he or she can allocate among the problems. For example, a participant might be allocated ten points. Some or all of the points can be allocated to any health problem or problem cluster generated through the free list. The problems allocated the highest number of points are priorities for the group. Community priorities can be inferred as the results from multiple groups are reviewed.

An alternate use of ranking and scoring is to identify at risk populations. Sub-groups within the community may be known or can be identified using focus groups, interviews or Venn diagrams (see below). Ranking and scoring can then be used to rank the perceived vulnerability of different groups to reproductive health problems. A CARE project in Zambia, for example, found that adolescent boys in an urban area were grouped into various cliques, clubs and gangs[29]. The boys carried out a ranking of which groups were most likely to contract an STD. The boys used their knowledge of the sexual behavior of the different categories to develop the ranking.

Flow Diagrams: Flow diagrams are charts drawn by groups of community members to describe both the causes and impacts of the problems identified through listing and ranking exercises. A literate community member or facilitator is needed for this exercise. The problem is placed in a circle in the middle of a large piece of paper. The participants are then asked to identify causes of the problem. Each individual cause is placed in a separate circle on the page with an arrow drawn from the cause to the problem. In some instances a second level of underlying causes may be identified. For example, female genital cutting (FGC) may not be named as a problem but the exercise may lead to FGC being identified as an immediate or underlying cause of reproductive health problems experienced by women.

Once the causes have been identified, a similar exercise is carried out to identify the impacts of the problem. Each participant identifies one or more impacts. Each impact is placed in a circle with an arrow drawn from the problem to the impact.

The relative importance of the various causes and impacts can be imputed through a ranking or scoring exercise. Participants in the exercise each have a fixed number of points that they can allocate among the causes. The cause receiving the highest number of points is deemed the most important and the one needing immediate attention. Figure 4-3 provides an example of a flow diagram developed by Zambian adolescent girls[30]. The numbers inside the circles represent a *severity* score out of a fixed maximum of 100, while the numbers outside the circles represent a *frequency* score out of a maximum of 100.

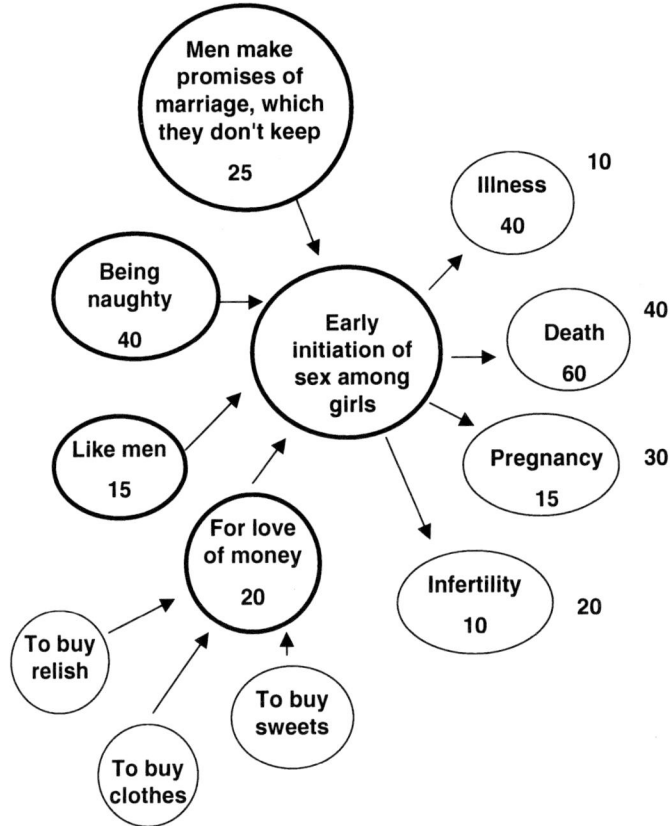

FIGURE 4-3. Causes and impacts of early initiation of sex among girls Lusaka, Zambia.

Body Maps: Small group participants are asked to draw pictures of the male and female bodies, including the reproductive organs. The drawings are made on large pieces of paper or on the ground using chalk. Men and women are usually segregated for this exercise. The participants are then asked to describe the bodies. This is a very useful exercise to gain insight into participants' understanding of basic reproductive functioning and of misinformation circulating in a community. This exercise has been applied frequently by CARE with adolescents.

Participatory Sex Census: This technique is designed to gain information about patterns of sexual behavior in a community. Two to three facilitators are needed for this technique. The technique has been used successfully with both segregated and mixed-gender groups. Each participant in a group receives a stack of slips of paper and a pencil. The group is advised that sensitive questions about sexual behavior will be asked. People may decline to participate altogether or refuse to answer any given question. Participants are instructed not to include their names in responding to the questions. As each question is asked the participants write down their answers on the pieces of paper. The responses are placed in a basket passed through the group. One facilitator tallies the responses, while the leader moves on to the next question. Every slip of paper is destroyed in front of the group after each question is tallied. It is often useful to repeat the same question in various ways over the course of the exercise as confidence grows that the responses will not be shared. If gender specific information is desired in a mixed-gender group, each respondent can indicate his or her sex with a symbol on the response and the results are tallied separately.

The results are displayed on a prepared matrix, such as that displayed in Table 4-1. The response categories in Table 4-1 are purely arbitrary. Facilitators may use the actual responses received to create response categories for age at intercourse, number of partners and other variables. The questions presented in Table 4-1 are illustrative. Many other questions could be asked. The specific questions to be raised depend on the facilitators understanding of the local circumstances and sexual behavior questions that will be most useful in designing interventions, as well as raising community awareness. Exercises of this type carried out with adolescents by CARE in Zambia and Haiti were very helpful in alerting parents to the extent of teen sexuality and mobilizing a community response.

Cartooning and Story Telling: In this exercise participants are asked to draw a cartoon sequence or write down a story around a particular theme. Themes might include a day in the life of a woman, what happens between teenage boys and girls, seeking health care, relations between husbands and wives, becoming pregnant or giving birth. These can be very powerful exercises when respondents tell common stories. The sharing of life experiences through the vehicle of pictures and stories can help identify felt needs and the depth of emotion surrounding those needs. The cartoons and stories provide insight for the facilitators of the needs assessment, as well as providing impetus for community action as common experiences are uncovered. In a CARE project in Zambia 36 adolescent girls were asked to draw a cartoon of daily life. Thirty-five of the 36 responded by drawing pictures that involved fending off sexual advances from boys!

Focus Groups: Focus groups are structured, facilitated discussions around a particular topic or theme. Focus groups often precede and follow other participatory techniques. They are used to elicit a preliminary set of concerns or issues that can be subjected to more detailed scrutiny or to react to findings from other sources. Key questions for discussion are prepared in advance by the facilitator. For example, a group of parents might be asked to discuss their concerns about the sexual behavior of teens in the community. Alternatively, they might be asked to respond to the findings of a flow diagram or sex census. Focus groups can be used to obtain community views on perceived reproductive health needs in the community, patterns of sexual behavior, attitudes towards sexual and reproductive behavior, the accessibility and quality of reproductive health services, understanding of reproductive health issues and sources of information about reproductive health.

Focus groups typically consist of groups of 8–12 individuals drawn as convenience samples from sub-populations of the community. For example, separate focus groups might be run for adult women, adult men, adolescent boys, adolescent girls and/or other sub-groups relevant to a particular context. The facilitator presents the central question or topic and

TABLE 4-1. Matrix for Tallying Sex Census Responses

Question	Responses
Have you ever had sex?	Yes – No –
Age at first sex?	6–9 – 10–12 – 13–15 – 16–18 – 19–21 – Over 21 –
With whom did you first have sex?	Neighbor – Friend – Sex worker – Cousin – Other family member – Other –
Did you ever give or receive money or gifts for sex?	Yes – No –
How many people have you had sex with during your life?	0 1 2–3 4–5 6–8 9–11 12–14 15 or more
How many people have you had sex with during the last three months?	0 1 2–3 4–6 8–10 11–14 15 or more
How many times have you had sex during the last 30 days?	0 1–4 5–8 9–12 13 or more
Did you use a condom the last time you had sex?	Yes – No –
Have you ever had sex with a family member (father, mother, daughter, son, brother, sister, grandmother, grandfather, cousin, uncle, aunt)?	Yes – No –

then encourages response from all members of the group. The facilitator tries to ensure equitable participation so that the views of all members are aired. The facilitator tries to remain unobtrusive to avoid impeding the flow of the conversation or signaling "correct" responses. As needed, the facilitator will ask additional probing questions to generate more information and keep the conversation going. In addition to the facilitator, each focus group should have a recorder who captures themes and different perspectives in responding to the key questions. A report should be prepared as soon as possible after each focus group using the notes of the recorder.

Synthesizing the Findings

The findings from the various needs assessment techniques must be synthesized into a report that defines *problems requiring collective action*. The needs assessment must generate an agenda for action. The findings must be carefully recorded in the field as the participatory exercises unfold. The report should then address the following topics:

- Reproductive health problems identified by the community and their relative priority;
- Causes and impacts of the problems as perceived by the participants;
- Knowledge, attitudes, norms and behaviors that influence reproductive health;
- Recommendations for collective action needed to address reproductive health problems.

Participatory Appraisal in Southern Sudan

A participatory appraisal of reproductive health needs in southern Sudan used a variety of participatory methods—freelisting, ranking, story telling, focus group discussions and interviews. The appraisal covered two towns and nine surrounding villages. The participatory techniques were complemented with a review of secondary data. The major findings were:

1. Reproductive health needs are among the leading health concerns in the community. The top ten health concerns include HIV and other STD, miscarriages and childbirth. HIV/STD ranked in the top 3 perceived causes of illness and death. Sexual violence also emerged as an issue though there was reluctance to engage in public discussion of this topic.
2. There was a mismatch between health needs identified by the community and those identified by the health providers; e.g., health providers denied that abortion was occurring, which was refuted by community members.
3. There were differences in perceived need by age and gender, as well as between refugee and displaced populations. For example, young women gave much higher priority to pregnancy and childbirth as health problems than did men.

Source: Palmer, Cecilia "Rapid appraisal of need in reproductive health care in southern Sudan: qualitative study" *British Medical Journal* Vol. 319 (7272) 18 Sep 1999 pp. 743–748

MAPPING AND MOBILIZING COMMUNITY RESOURCES

Identifying problems and needs is only the beginning of community empowerment. Needs assessments can, in fact, be counter-productive if not quickly followed by a process of crafting solutions and mobilizing resources. Appraisal processes that lead nowhere can exasperate communities and block later efforts at community organization. Attention must quickly turn to identifying and mobilizing resources to solve problems.

Here is a suggested five-step process for resource mobilization that is an adaptation of a process developed by Kretzmann and McKnight:[31]

1. Identify the assets and skills of *organizations and associations*;
2. Identify the skills and capacities of *individuals* in the community;
3. *Build relations* among the individuals and organizations with assets;
4. *Mobilize cash resources* within the community;
5. *Seek external resources*.

The fundamental premise of this process is that every community has assets that can be brought to bear for collective action and problem-solving. Most communities have indigenous organizations and all communities have individuals who can bring skills and/or influence to bear. Asset mapping is the systematic process of identifying community resources and encouraging collaboration among community resources to solve problems. Kretzmann and McKnigt argue that asset mapping should actually supplant needs assessment. In their view, community empowerment springs from building onto the positive assets that a community already has in place, rather than "meeting needs". They argue that needs assessment often dispirits community members by focusing energy and attention on community deficits and pathologies. Asset mapping draws attention to what the community already has accomplished over the course of its history. Community empowerment then becomes the much more manageable task of incrementally adding to the extent capacity for collective action. The rather vague and daunting challenge of "organizing for reproductive health" becomes a series of small changes, such as helping the existing women's club maintain a supply of contraceptives or organize transport for obstetrical emergencies.

Mapping Assets: Associations and Organizations

The social map, as modified by the transect walk, is a good starting point for developing a list of community assets. A good social map will show many of the physical assets and institutions within the boundaries of a community. These should include social and political institutions (school, health facility, community building, church, mosque or temple, police or military post, government facilities), businesses and hubs of economic activity (such as markets), and places where people congregate (wells, bars, squares, crossroads, transportation hubs). Using the social map, two lists should be developed: a list of physical assets and a list of community institutions.

The list of community institutions from the social map should then be supplemented with a list of associations and organizations that do not have physical facilities that appear on the map. Small groups of community members and community leaders should take responsibility for developing this list. In some places, local authorities maintain an organizational registry. In urban areas, the names of local organizations will appear in newspapers. This list might include the village council, ethnic/family clans, mothers' clubs, youth groups, savings and loan groups, health committees, farming cooperatives, burial societies, labor cooperatives, water and sanitation committee, literacy club or any of the myriad possible political, economic or social organizations that might be found in a community. Look for *informal associations*; these are small groups of people who provide mutual assistance but are not necessarily organized into an association with a name and a structure. The social network analysis can help identify these informal associations. All the formal and informal associations are potential assets in mobilizing for collective action. An exhaustive list is not necessary. A good "first cut" list of organizations will suffice to begin resource mobilization; others can be added over time.

COMMUNITY EMPOWERMENT

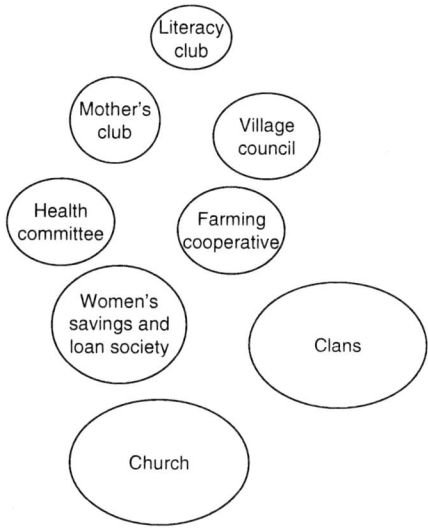

FIGURE 4-4. Map of community assets.

Once the list has been developed, the facilitation team can begin a dialogue with the organizations. The purpose of the dialogue is to communicate the findings of the needs assessment and identify organizational assets that might help with collective action. An organization's assets might include skills, labor, space, materials, cash, vehicles, prestige, influence, legitimacy and advocacy. Once an initial round of dialogue has been completed the facilitation team can use the *Venn diagram* technique to identify those that appear to be of greatest potential help in terms of assets and interest. On a piece of paper or chalkboard place the name of each organization inside the circle. Vary the size of the circle in accordance with the organization's perceived ability to contribute to collective action around a specific problem. Figure 4-4 gives an example of a map of organizational assets and their potential contribution to maternal health care.

In this example, the clans and the church would be the primary sources of source for collective action to reduce maternal mortality and morbidity. In Ekpoma, Nigeria, a maternal mortality prevention project began by holding focus group discussions that identified lack of emergency transport as a major obstacle to maternal mortality reduction.[32] The most important associations in the town are the 13 clans, each with a head and grouped under a traditional leader, the *Onogie*. Each clan agreed to create a loan fund for women needing obstetrical care. Clan meetings were used to solicit contributions to create the funds. Twelve of the thirteen clans succeeded in creating a loan fund. Over the first year of operation, 380 women received loans, with 97 percent of the loan funds recovered.

Mapping Assets: Individuals

The facilitation team can use a very similar process to map individuals who are potential assets to the reproductive health program. In this instance the objective is to identify individuals in the community who possess skills or resources that might be used to support

TABLE 4-2. Skills and Capacity Matrix

Skill area	Individuals
Health care	
Construction/facility repair	
Vehicle ownership/access/use	
Artistic/communication skills	
Literacy/writing skills	
Community organizing	
Sales	
Money management	
Teaching/education skills	

the reproductive health program. Individual assets should also be catalogued through a *skills and capacity matrix*. The facilitation team should draw up a list of skills and assets that might be needed. Small group work can be used to draw up lists of individuals who have relevant assets. This list can be complemented through consultation with community leaders and the facilitation team's own knowledge of the community. Table 4-2 provides an illustration of the skills and capacity matrix.

The skills suggested in Table 4-2 are all applicable to fostering better reproductive health care. The potential contribution of modern and traditional health care providers is the most obvious. However, many other people can contribute. Construction and repair skills are needed to build and refurbish health facilities. Vehicle access is essential to obstetrical emergency transport. Skills at drawing, painting, song, dance, music and public speaking can all be deployed in behavior change programs. Those who are literate in a community can play many roles in program development, management and record-keeping. Almost every community has people who are experienced at organizing friends and neighbors for tasks. Those who can sell are good candidates for social marketing of contraceptives and essential drugs. People who are trusted to manage community funds will be needed for maintaining revolving funds for essential drugs and obstetrical emergencies. Teachers are often respected figures in the community who can play a vital role in training and community education. This list is not exhaustive. Rather, it serves to illustrate that every community has a reservoir of skilled people who are assets for the reproductive health program. A CARE program in Haiti, for example, depended upon troupes of community women skilled in song and dance who put on dramatic performances vividly demonstrating the pregnancy danger signs and the importance of rapid care for obstetrical emergencies. A maternal health program in Nigeria developed a list of vehicle owners who agreed to provide emergency transport on a 24-hour/7-day basis at pre-established fees.[33] Building on the skills and resources of people in the community helps sustain reproductive health programs over the long term.

Building Relations among Organizations and Individuals

After identifying needs and assets the next major challenge is to build relations among associations, institutions and individuals. The asset maps are a good way to begin this exercise. Place any one of the associations in the middle of the map. Now array other associations and

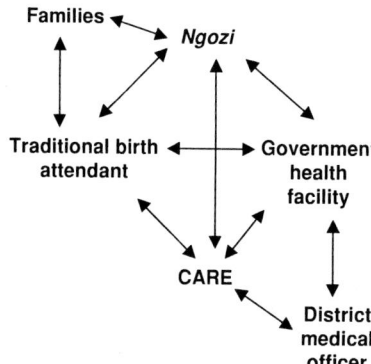

FIGURE 4-5. Relationship web for managing obstetrical emergencies (Uganda).

individuals in a circle around the organization in the middle. Encourage dialogue around a simple question: "How can any combination of individuals and institutions work together to solve a clearly defined reproductive health problem?" In a CARE project in Uganda, dialogue between the health facility and a traditional self-help group known as the *ngozi* helped address obstetrical emergencies. The *ngozi* members agreed to serve as stretcher-bearers. The traditional birth attendant, with support from the CARE office, was trained by the government health facility to recognize obstetrical emergencies. In the event of an emergency the birth attendant would contact the *ngozi* leader, who would organize a stretcher team to bring the woman to the health facility. Figure 4-5 provides an illustration of the web of relationships that was cultivated in support of managing obstetrical emergencies.

In small, tightly knit communities the process of relationship building is fairly straightforward. The parties know each other and have established relations. The task is simply one of extending extant relations to solve new problems. The Uganda case is an example of building on existing assets and relationships. All of the associations and institutions were in place and the individuals had longstanding, even lifelong relations. Small infusions of training, facilitation and capital sufficed to address a critical reproductive health problem.

In some instances, building relations requires breaking down barriers of suspicion and hostility. Divisions along class, caste, gender, age, ethnic and other lines can make it very difficult for dialogue to take place, let alone collective action to solve problems. Even where there is no overt hostility, tradition may make it difficult for different segments of the community to communicate effectively. In many cultures it is very difficult for women to speak out in the presence of men. Person from lower castes or classes may be similarly inhibited from engaging in dialogue. These divisions within a community require special effort to break down barriers and encourage dialogue.

A CARE project in Bolivia aimed at preventing sexually transmitted disease provides a case in point. The project was located in Tarija, a town near the border with Argentina. Tarija is a trading center through which a major highway passes. Commercial sex workers (CSW) serve the truckers and transport workers along the highway. The town also has a significant gay community. Both the sex workers and the gay community were subject to harassment, violence and extortion from the police. The sex workers and the gay community were internally disorganized and highly suspicious of outsiders, such as CARE HIV/STD prevention educators, who were suspected of being agents of the police, government or church. HIV/STD prevention was initially very difficult in these high-risk populations due to the levels of suspicion and police harassment. Over time, CARE workers in Tarija were able to broker relations among the communities. CARE provided a small building that served as a safe haven for the gay community at night and for sex workers and their children during the day. These groups worked with CARE to develop rules of conduct governing appropriate use of the building. A core of activists developed within each community. CARE engaged the police and other local authorities in extended discussion that greatly reduced harassment of the CSW and gays, which made prevention activities feasible. CARE trained leaders among the CSW and gays to serve as peer educators and condom distributors. These leaders in turn reached out to their peers to promote safer sex and healthier lifestyles. At least five different parties had to be brought together in a productive relationship: CSW, gays, police, municipal authorities and the local CARE office. By focusing on a problem of mutual concern—the spread of HIV/STD along the highway and through the town—mutual suspicion and hostility were suspended in an effort to find a productive solution.

Over time, relationship building can be transformed into regular consultation for identifying and solving problems. Entry into most communities will require consultation with and the support of official and traditional leaders. Participatory appraisal builds a shared understanding of community problems among many segments of the community. Asset mapping illuminates resources and draws additional people and associations into the process. Problem focused dialogue helps build trust among individuals and associations. Shared problem solving will help increase confidence and community capacity. The facilitation team can encourage many partners in the web of relationships to meet on a regular or as needed basis to solve problems and develop plans for continuing improvement.

Mobilizing Cash

Poor people always pay for health care, though the absolute level of expenditure is often very low. In many developing countries out-of-pocket expenditures constitute a high percentage of total expenditures on health, far outweighing public expenditures. Table 4-3 presents data on out-of-pocket expenditures for a set of countries in sub-Saharan Africa[34]. The amount the poor pay is often high relative to meager incomes and frequently misdirected at measures that may not yield optimal improvements in health. The challenge to health managers is helping people direct their scarce health resources to expenditures that will have the greatest impact on health. Participatory appraisal and asset mapping can help communities make choices about where to direct slim cash resources.

Here are some ideas for mobilizing cash at the community level for goods and services that cannot be secured using other assets:[35]

- *User fees* set at a reasonable level (e.g., 1 percent of income assuming two patient contacts per year) that help defray the cost of basic reproductive health services. The fee level should be negotiated between the community and the health providers.
- *Pre-payment plans* in which people pool their risk by contributing to a health fund on a regular basis. Those participating in the fund are then entitled to services and/or essential drugs. These prepayment schemes have been used in countries as diverse as Benin, India, Philippines, Indonesia and Bangladesh.

TABLE 4-3. Out-of-pocket Expenditures

Country	Out-of-pocket expenditures as a % of total health expenditures	Out-of-pocket expenditure at official exchange rate (U.S. $)
Angola	40.4	NA
Benin	52.8	6
Botswana	36.4	48
Burkina Faso	69.1	6
Burundi	64.4	4
Cameroon	79.9	24
Cape Verde	36.2	12
Central African Republic	31.1	3
Chad	20.7	1
Congo	63.4	37
Cote d'Ivoire	61.6	14
Democratic Republic of Congo	90.1	NA
Eritrea	44.3	3
Ethiopia	63.8	3
Gabon	33.5	46
Ghana	53	6
Guinea	42.8	8
Guinea-Bissau	24.4	3
Kenya	35.9	6
Lesotho	27.4	8
Madagascar	46.2	2
Malawi	36.7	5
Mali	48.7	5
Mozambique	19.6	1
Namibia	48.3	74
Niger	53.4	3
Nigeria	71.8	22
Rwanda	49.9	7
Senegal	44.3	10
Sierra Leone	90.3	10
South Africa	46.3	124
Sudan	79.1	10
Swaziland	27.7	13
Togo	57.2	5
Uganda	48.2	9
Tanzania	39.3	5
Zambia	42.4	11
Zimbabwe	38.2	24

- *Production based pre-payment schemes* capitalize on existing economic cooperation organizations, such as farming or marketing cooperatives. In India, for example, some dairy cooperatives add a small surcharge to each liter of milk that pays for health care for members.
- *Drug sales* that generate income for sustaining an essential drug supply. An initial per capita assessment may be needed to secure the initial stock of drugs. The size of the initial drug supply depends on judgment about the difficulties of re-supply. Typically, a three to six month supply of drugs is needed, which is replenished periodically as drugs are sold.

- *Loan funds* that are capitalized through community contributions and lent for specified purposes with sufficient interest to sustain the fund. An example from Nigeria was described earlier.
- *Fund raising events* such as festivals and raffles have been used to raise money for health activities, equipment and facilities. This is not a regular source of income, but can be used for special projects

Procedures governing use of cash resources must be appropriate and clearly specified. The procedures should safeguard the monies and ensure that they are used for the intended purposes. The rule should govern how money is collected, how it is stored, how and when it is disbursed and record-keeping. Accountability for cash resources should be clear, so specific individuals are held responsible for stewardship of community resources. The community may choose to waive fees and charges under exceptional circumstances. However, the rules governing such exemptions should be transparent and agreed to through a participatory process.

Given the low absolute level of income and health expenditures in many communities, cash contributions will often be low. However, when combined with other assets, the mobilization of cash resources can contribute significantly to making essential reproductive health services accessible.

Seeking External Resources

I have put seeking external resources as the last resource mobilization strategy because it should follow rather than precede building on community assets. The process of participatory appraisal, setting objectives that reflect community defined priorities and mobilizing internal resources strengthens the community's ability to negotiate effectively with external sources of money. Internal resources will rarely suffice in securing essential reproductive health services. External donors will almost always have an agenda of pre-existing priorities. Donor concerns and strategies may or may not match community needs. Moreover, there is always the danger that the relationship with donors breeds dependence. The community and its representatives will be better positioned to direct external resources properly if donor support comes after, rather than before, a process of community mobilization. The community should carefully define its needs prior to engaging the donor in a dialogue and focus its request on securing resources that *cannot* be acquired through community assets.

Here are some practical suggestions for communities trying to work with external sources of resources:

1. Map the potential sources of funds in the local environment – national government, local government, domestic and international non-governmental organizations, bilateral aid agencies, foundations, and corporations. Learn about the interests and priorities of these sources and the mechanisms they use to disburse funds.
2. Funds flow to organizations that can be held accountable, so the community must designate a credible organization to receive the funds and authorize representatives to speak on behalf of the community and the organization.
3. The relationship between the community and the external resource should be treated as a partnership between equals seeking to solve a shared problem or achieve a common objective.
4. The community should prepare a succinct statement of its needs that includes a statement of the contribution it is making through mobilizing community assets.

COMMUNITY EMPOWERMENT

5. It will sometimes help communities to pool their requests or work through an intermediary organization. The administrative burden of responding to many small requests is often a barrier for potential donors. Donors may prefer to make one larger grant to a single entity that will be held accountable; this intermediary can then disburse the funds to multiple communities.
6. Communities and their organizational representatives should be prepared to show how they will keep track of funds and report on progress.
7. Maintain regular contact with a donor over the life of the grant and keep the donor informed of both positive and negative developments. They will want to know about successes and should be apprised of problems early to avoid embarrassment. The support of the donor should be publicly acknowledged.
8. Seek multiple sources of funding. Communities and community-based organizations that depend over-much on a single source of external resources are extremely vulnerable. External resources should always be subsidiary to locally available assets.
9. Plan for the end of external support. Contributions from external resources invariably end. The community must build in a strategy for sustaining services after external resources are withdrawn. The plan for sustaining services after external resources are withdrawn should be built into the agreement with the donor.

BUILDING ORGANIZATIONAL CAPACITY

Community organizations and associations may lack basic management skills that are essential to sustaining collective action. Health managers can foster community capacity by providing appropriate training, counseling and technical assistance. The specific skills needed by a community association will vary and participatory techniques can be used within associations to identify capacity building needs.

Employing the techniques of participatory appraisal and participatory asset mobilization described above is part of the capacity building process. In using these techniques the community associations gain skills that can be used in many contexts, as well as confidence in their ability to undertake collective action.

Here is a checklist of basic management skills that may be needed by community associations:[36]

- Developing and following a work plan
- Coordinating activity within and between organizations
- Managing staff
- Managing community health workers
- Collecting and using information for decision-making
- Managing the supply of drugs, contraceptives and other expendable supplies
- Managing equipment and facilities
- Budgeting and cash management
- Negotiating with donors and external authorities

Capacity building will be discussed in greater detail in Chapter 5. Health managers can use many of the same techniques discussed earlier, such as freelisting, ranking and scoring, to work with organizational leaders to define capacity building needs and set priorities. There are also tools and methods for assessing the management capacity of community organizations, such as the Management Capacity Assessment Tool developed by CARE or the situation analysis methodology pioneered by the Population Council[37]. These tools define a set of core competencies that are needed for organizations to flourish and procedures for assessing the status of the organization relative to the core competencies. A sustained program of management development for community based organization is part of the process of community empowerment.

LEADERSHIP DEVELOPMENT

Certain individuals in any community possess relatively high levels of power, influence and prestige. Their support or opposition can play a critical role in the success of a reproductive health program. In some instances these individuals hold "official" positions in the community—chief, clan leader, religious leader, mayor, council president and so forth. In other instances the authority is informal and clings to the person rather than the position. However, the attitude of these informal leaders can also be very important.

The "mapping" techniques discussed earlier can be used to discern the structure of community leadership. The facilitation team should ask small groups from the community to free list people who are influential and whose support is needed or potentially helpful. The groups should be asked to pictorially represent the relative influence, authority and potential support of the community leaders using a Venn diagram exercise. The size of the circle should be proportional to the degree of influence and authority perceived by the group. Repeating this exercise with groups drawn from different segments of the community will create a map of leaders.

The individuals identified through the mapping exercise should be invited to participate in a program of leadership development for reproductive health. The elements of leadership development might include the following:

- Including leaders in the appraisal process so they feel a sense of ownership of the needs and priorities defined by the facilitation team.
- Providing leaders with appropriate, non-formal adult education in key aspects of reproductive health as they affect the community.
- Supporting visits by leaders to other communities that are engaged in successful reproductive health programs for dialogue with peers.
- Supporting attendance by community leaders at sub-national or national meetings at which reproductive health issues are discussed. This is particularly useful in working with community religious leaders. Meetings on reproductive health issues featuring prominent religious leaders can help allay concerns about transgressing core values.
- Providing leaders with examples or models of actions that supported improved reproductive health in comparable communities.
- Providing organizational leaders with management training or other specialized training that would help build capacity for collective action. The Center for Population and Development Activities (CEDPA) based in Washington, D.C. has done a marvelous job training thousands of women community leaders in a wide range of skills relevant to reproductive health.
- Soliciting specific support from sympathetic leaders, especially public advocacy that would legitimize community action and allocation of resources.

COMMUNITY EMPOWERMENT

TABLE 4-4. Illustrative Matrix for Assessing Community Empowerment

Dimensions of community empowerment	Key questions for assessment
Defining and describing the community	Has the community to be served been clearly defined? Is there a good understanding of the community's boundaries, members and physical attributes? Are social networks within the community understood?
Participatory appraisal	Has a participatory appraisal of reproductive health needs been carried out? Were all segments of the community reached through the appraisal? What were the findings? How have the findings been used? Is the process on-going?
Resource mobilization	Have organizational and individual resources been mapped? What has been the contribution of organizations and individuals in time, labor, facilities, materials, skills, cash and advocacy? Is there continuing communication between the involved people and organizations? Is there a system for collecting cash to support RH services? How much is collected on a monthly or yearly basis? How have the funds been used? Has support been received from external sources? How much and what is the relationship with external sources of support?
Organizational capacity building	Which are the organizations engaged in supporting reproductive security? What are the specific tasks in which they are engaged? Do they have the technical and managerial ability to undertake the intended actions? What are the strengths and weaknesses? What specific actions have been taken to build capacity?
Leadership development	Who are the community leaders? Are they supportive of collective action for reproductive health? What has been done to develop supportive leaders? What specific actions have the leaders taken, especially in advocacy and resource allocation?
Collective action	Which of the following actions are being carried out: community based distribution of contraceptives, condom distribution, rapid transport of obstetrical emergencies, blood donation, access to essential drugs, supporting community health workers, community health education, emergency loan funds, support to people living with AIDS, and refurbishing and equipping local health facilities.

ASSESSING COMMUNITY EMPOWERMENT

The community empowerment cycle implies a framework for assessing community empowerment. A community empowered to protect its reproductive security will have:

- Carried out a participatory appraisal of its reproductive health needs that is updated regularly as part of an on-going learning process;
- Mapped and mobilized locally available organizational and individual resources and negotiated successfully with external sources of resources;
- Strengthened the managerial and technical capacity of community organizations;

- Developed a cadre of leaders supportive of reproductive health; and,
- Undertaken specific, relevant collective actions that foster reproductive health.

Table 4-4 provides an illustrative matrix for assessing community empowerment. The questions proposed in the table are not definitive or exhaustive. Assessment should also be a participatory process. Small group work can be used to define criteria that are particularly relevant to a community and many of the techniques used for appraising needs can also be applied in monitoring change.

5

Building Institutional Capacity

Reproductive security demands the delivery and utilization of essential reproductive health services. Behavior change and community empowerment, while fundamental to improving reproductive security, must be accompanied by high quality services. Reproductive security demands contraception, obstetric care, management of sexually transmitted diseases, care for victims of sexual violence, and other services appropriate to the local context. Reproductive health mangers have four fundamental responsibilities in delivering services:

1. Optimizing the mix of technical interventions so as to improve reproductive security. A limited set of interventions can have a dramatic effect on reproductive morbidity and mortality—contraception to prevent unintended and high risk pregnancies, birth planning and emergency obstetrical care, STD case detection and management, prevention and treatment of sexual violence. The specific mix of services that is appropriate to a given context depends on the findings of the reproductive risk analysis. Since resources are always very scarce it is important that managers focus on the services that will have the greatest impact.
2. Maximizing access to essential services by clients. Health facilities and health providers are often at considerable physical distance from clients. Hours of travel on foot may be required to access care. The cost of care may exceed the economic resources of households. Social barriers also serve to inhibit care; e.g., women may be reluctant or unable to visit male health providers or differences in caste and class may serve as a barrier between the provider and the client. Mangers must select a mix of service delivery strategies and service providers that facilitate access to essential services by the communities they serve. As will be discussed below, effective programs combine clinical, community based and commercial approaches to maximize access.
3. Ensuring that the quality of care is adequate. Clients are entitled to technically competent providers, access to essential drugs and supplies, accurate and comprehensible information, follow-up, and respectful treatment from providers. Poor quality care can vitiate efforts to extend access and alienate clients from services. Managers must have clear standards of quality and processes for encouraging quality improvement.
4. Implementing effective management systems. Service delivery is partially a function of the ability of health institutions to carry out the basic management functions of planning, managing people, controlling resources and using information. These systems are often weak in

developing country health institutions. Managers must therefore be clear about the basic management functions required for service delivery and strengthen management systems where necessary.

A capable health institution will therefore be marked by four characteristics: (1) an appropriate mix of interventions; (2) easy client access to services; (3) high quality care; and (4) effective management systems. Virtually all health institutions fall short of this ideal. Many health managers in developing countries work in institutions that are quite weak relative to these standards. Hence, the fundamental task of all managers is strengthening institutional capacity. The remainder of this chapter is devoted to further refining our understanding of these four key characteristics and to strategies and methods for strengthening institutional capacity.

ESSENTIAL SERVICES FOR REPRODUCTIVE HEALTH

One of the recurring themes of this book is that reproductive security encompasses a constellation of inter-linked issues and concomitant services. The choice of contraceptive method is affected by the risk of sexually transmitted disease. Family planning and STD have an impact on maternal health outcomes. Sexual violence influences contraception, the risk of STD and maternal health outcomes. Moreover, the often difficult and arduous trek by a client to access care for one purpose, such as family planning, provides the opportunity to raise and address other reproductive health concerns. Given the difficulty and infrequency of contact between the health system and the poor, especially poor women, the most efficient possible use should be made of this encounter. This implies designing client interview protocols to surface related concerns, responding to multiple concerns during a single visit rather than requiring return visits, and rapid referral to additional services where necessary. Good quality care implies the integration of *essential* services, with the definition of essential services depending on the outcome of the reproductive risk analysis.

Family planning, maternal health care and HIV/STD management are included in the minimum package of health services defined by the World Bank. They are generally considered to be highly cost-effective public health interventions in terms of the disease burden alleviated relative to costs[1]. In most low and middle income countries these three interventions will form the core of a reproductive health package. Preventing and treating sexual violence should be included in the set of core reproductive health services. Sexual violence and the threat of sexual violence contribute to other reproductive health problems, including unwanted fertility, poor maternal health outcomes and the spread of STD[2]. Additional interventions may be included as a consequence of the reproductive risk analysis, which identifies the most salient reproductive health problems in a given population.

The accumulated body of knowledge about effective reproductive health care must also be incorporated into the choice of interventions. We know, for example, that family planning programs must offer the widest feasible array of methods to be effective. Maternal health programs must give priority to emergency obstetrical care if maternal deaths are to be reduced. HIV/STD case detection and management must be part of an STD control program. Support groups for women are needed to reduce sexual violence. Every health manager should develop a taxonomy of essential reproductive health services that reflects the local context and the global body of knowledge.

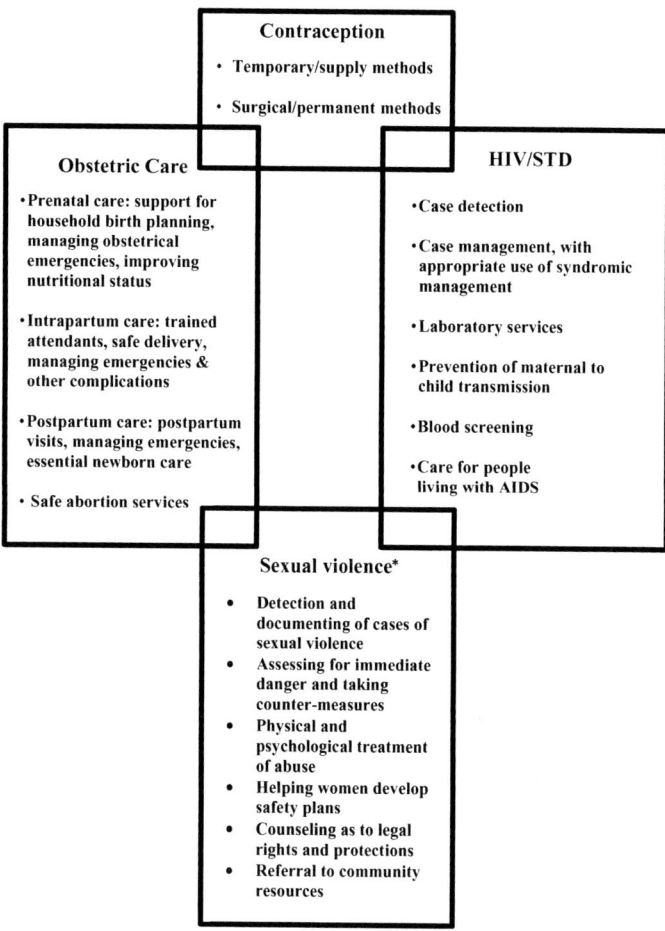

FIGURE 5-1. Essential services for reproductive security.

Figure 5-1 provides an illustration of the essential interventions needed to advance reproductive security. A detailed discussion of the interventions is provided in the chapters on Contraception, Maternal Health, and HIV/AIDS and Other Sexually Transmitted Diseases. While context specific adaptation is always needed, these interventions are known to have a major impact on reproductive morbidity and mortality. Within the framework suggested by Figure 5-1, managers may be required to make choices in light of resource constraints. These may be choices as between the four major domains and/or within each domain. The decision as to which interventions to support should be guided by the criteria discussed earlier: *frequency, severity of health impact, household impact* and *feasibility*. Moreover, managers should avail themselves of the participatory approaches that have been discussed at length in making choices. This both shifts the burden from the manager of making the choices and

---

*Interventions adapted from Heise, L., Ellsberg, M., and Goetemoeller M. "Ending Violence Against Women" Population Reports Series L., No. 11. Baltimore: Johns Hopkins University School of Public Health, Population Information Program, December 1999.

provides the concerned communities with the opportunity to exercise greater control over the decisions that affect their lives.

In defining the package of essential services it is very important to be sure that the population has been defined correctly and adequately. Reproductive health programs have been conventionally focused on married women of reproductive age living in relatively stable settings. As a consequence, refugees, the displaced, youth, single women, men and older women have often been left out. Marginalized groups also tend to be left out in the assessment of reproductive health needs. The consequence has been to significantly reduce the potential impact of reproductive health programs. A glaring example has been the almost complete omission, until recently, of refugee and displaced populations. With the exception of emergency care (including assistance at childbirth), refugees and the displaced have been neglected by health programs, especially in the area of reproductive health. However, refugee and displaced settings are especially vulnerable to reproductive health problems of all kinds, including unwanted pregnancy, poor maternal health care, sexually transmitted diseases, rape and violence. Re-defining the audience to include refugees and the displaced has had a very important impact on the package of essential services.

There is a potentially dangerous flip side to integrated reproductive health care that must be recognized and addressed. The laudable desire to screen for and address multiple problems can be misused. Integrated care may mean, in practice, that nothing is done well as providers try to do too much with too little. Managers and providers must still make choices and set priorities in the face of limited resources. Integrated care can lead to medical barriers to care. Clients may be subjected to long, inconvenient, unnecessary or expensive diagnostic procedures in the effort to ferret out problems. Care in one domain is sometimes withheld without reasonable cause pending delivery of services in another domain; e.g., in Bolivia, IUD insertion was not, until recently, permitted unless a cervical cancer screening was completed. Providing an appropriate constellation of services should increase and not limit access to care.

MAXIMIZING ACCESS TO SERVICES

Mapping the Network of Health Providers

As used in this book, the term "health institution" applies to the entire array of health providers who can contribute to improved reproductive health. This includes public, private, for-profit, not-for-profit, professionally trained, and traditional health care providers. Most populations are served by an array of providers, including physicians, nurses, trained midwives, medical assistants, pharmacists, drug sellers, traditional birth attendants and traditional healers. Depending on the country, many types or categories of health providers may be found. Managers need to think in terms of a network or system of health providers drawn from many sectors. The identity, skills, role and contribution of the relevant providers must be considered in building a delivery system that extends high quality services to the entire population of concern.

One useful technique is mapping the location and identity of providers serving a target population. The provider map is very much akin to the social map described in the discussion of community empowerment. It provides a readily grasped picture of where

BUILDING INSTITUTIONAL CAPACITY

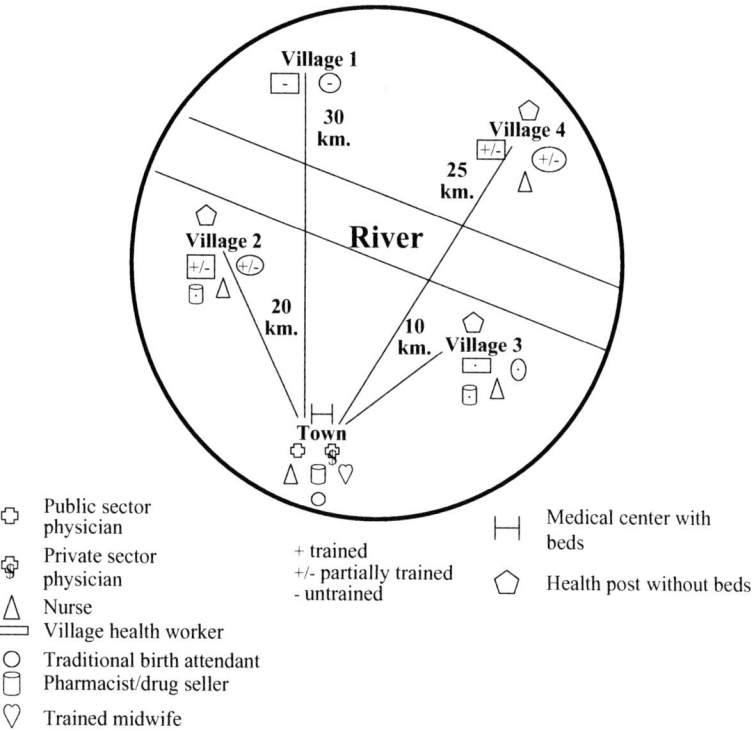

FIGURE 5-2. Mapping service providers.

providers are located and the types of providers available to each community. A visual representation of the network of service providers can serve several useful purposes. First, it provides a roster of providers whose support for reproductive health can be solicited, encouraged and developed. Second, a map provides a portrait of physical access to care and can be used to help deploy resources and personnel appropriately. Third, coding of providers in terms of skills allows managers to target training appropriately and visually gauge changes in the availability of trained personnel. Fourth, a network map can be used to optimize technical support and supervision visits. Figure 5-2 provides an example of a health provider map. In this example, which is fairly typical of developing country situations, health facilities and trained staff are concentrated in the town. The further a community is removed from an urban area, the less the facilities and trained staff, a condition often exacerbated by natural barriers such as rivers, mountains and monsoons. Village 1 lacks any facility and has no trained staff. Village 4 is somewhat better off with access to a health post staffed by a nurse and village health worker and traditional birth attendant who have received some training in reproductive health care. Villages 1 and 4 are also far away from the medical center in town and residents must traverse a river to reach town in the event of an emergency. Village 2 is somewhat better off, though providers need additional training. Village 3 is relatively well off with a health post and trained providers, which probably reflects its proximity to town. The town has a diverse range of trained providers, including a pharmacy. Even this very simple example provides immediate clues as to how a capacity building effort might be targeted. Over time, increasingly sophisticated information could be incorporated, without rendering the map too complex to read easily.

Matching Providers to Services

The map of providers should be integrated with the taxonomy of essential services. The object of this exercise is to expand access to services by using the widest feasible array of providers who can deliver safe and effective services. There is no universal prescription for the effort to match providers to services. A physician oriented health care delivery system is out of the question in many contexts because they are simply unavailable. Other categories of health professionals—nurses, nurse-midwives, midwives, medical assistants, pharmacists—may bear primary responsibility for health care delivery. Paraprofessionals, community health workers and traditional providers play a critical role in many contexts. Moreover, the health-seeking behavior of the population plays an important role in matching services to providers. In most of the developing world, large proportions of the population rely on traditional healers and traditional birth attendants (TBA) as their first and primary recourse for health care. India, for example, has an elaborate formal health care system and an equally elaborate traditional system. The formal system is composed of public and private health professionals (physicians, nurses, midwives, pharmacists, etc.) trained in Western medicine, while the traditional system includes Rural Medical Practitioners, quacks (a recognized category), ayurvedic healers, drug sellers, traditional birth attendants and traditional healers. All of these providers can be found serving the same population, with the majority of clients obtaining their health care from the traditional system. Attempts to divert clients away from these preferred providers are likely to prove futile, whereas a strategy of collaboration between the formal and informal health care sectors is more apt to expand access to appropriate care. This collaboration should be based on strengthening the ability of community health workers and traditional healers to provide a basic level of care while encouraging referral to better trained providers for more sophisticated services.

The general trend in primary health care has been to expand the range of services offered by health providers with less formal training. For example, community health workers were once largely restricted to distributing barrier methods of contraception (condoms and spermicides), but it is now commonplace for them to distribute oral contraceptives and even, in countries such as Peru, contraceptive injections.

The role of the health manager is to optimize the contribution of each category of provider to reproductive health care. The specific distribution of interventions, as between levels and types of providers, must be context specific. Choices are generally driven by the availability of trained staff to deliver essential services. In a country like Mozambique, where physicians are extremely scarce because of years of civil war, greater reliance has been placed on training and equipping nurses and midwives to handle obstetrical emergencies. In Bangladesh, the Ministry of Health has established "satellite clinics", which are homes or community buildings at the village level that are made available on a monthly basis for an itinerant family planning worker who can provide all contraceptives save implants, ligations and vasectomies. The worker also provides a variety of other reproductive health services, such as antenatal screening and tetanus toxoid injections.

In allocating responsibilities among types of providers the manger should consider the following criteria:

1. *Whether the evidence supports safe and effective delivery of a specific service by a category of provider.* For example, it is clear that community health workers can be trained to offer a range of contraceptives and that nurses and midwives can carry out IUD insertions. Traditional birth attendants can be trained to assist effectively with normal deliveries but must have clinical back-up in the event of complications. Community health workers can help promote STD prevention, case detection and referral, but treatment will usually require access to clinical staff. Local experimentation is important in accumulating relevant evidence. Much of the progress in extending access to care has come about as a result of carefully documented efforts to use providers in new and unconventional ways.

2. *The barriers faced by the population in accessing care.* Managers must make best use of the health providers that the target population can actually reach. Physical, economic or social barriers may effectively constrain the real choices people have about the health provider they will use. The allocation of responsibility for health interventions must reflect this reality, with the objective of minimizing the barriers to essential reproductive health services. One might argue, for example, that every birth should be attended by a trained health professional. However desirable this objective, it will be many years in most developing countries before this option is available because of the dearth of trained staff. Hence, best use must be made of traditional birth attendants, while recognizing and managing the inherent limitations in their ability to manage emergencies.

3. *The existing pattern of reproductive health care seeking behavior.* People may seek care from any of a wide array of health providers. One of the tasks of the manager is to understand the pattern of health seeking behavior and optimize the quality of care by all types of providers. In many instances health professionals are not the first choice; rather, first recourse is to traditional providers or drug sellers. District health managers have three options that are not mutually exclusive: (1) try to change the pattern of care seeking behavior; (2) improve the quality of care provided by the extant array of providers; and, (3) build linkages and referral systems between categories of providers. Traditional birth attendants (TBA) again provide a good example. Women in the developing world overwhelming use a TBA or have no assistance at birth. Many years will elapse before using trained health professionals will become the norm. One might attempt to discourage women from using TBAs, but this would almost certainly fail and drive a wedge between the formal health system and the traditional provider. A more useful approach might be to optimize the potential contribution of TBAs to maternal health, while building productive relations that facilitate prompt referral of women experiencing problems that are beyond the capacity of the TBA to manage. Similarly , in many cultures the traditional healer and the local purveyor of drugs are the first choice for treating STD. Responding creatively and effectively to the reality of health care seeking behavior is one the principal tasks of the manager.

4. *The ability of the manager to elicit the cooperation of the providers and of the health care system to provide training, support, drugs and supplies.* Formal regulatory authority is rarely a useful tool for public health managers in developing countries. Rather, they must rely on participatory approaches, persuasion and the judicious allocation of scarce resources to induce providers to adopt new or modified practices. The decision to support the reproductive health care role of a provider implies a decision to provide training, regular technical assistance visits, and access to essential drugs and supplies.

A tool that can be used by managers in conceptualizing the allocation of responsibilities is a Provider/Services Matrix that matches providers to services. Table 5-1 provides an example

TABLE 5-1. Illustrative Provider/Services Matrix

Level	Family planning	Obstetric care	HIV/STD	Sexual violence*
Community	• Behavior change promotion • Condoms, spermicides, pills, (injectables?)	• Behavior change promotion • Birth planning • Nutrition counseling • Safe normal delivery • Obstetric first aid • Emergency transport • Postpartum visits • Newborn care	• Behavior change promotion • Condom distribution • Referral for care & testing • Access to antibiotics • Prophylactic treatment of newborns for opthalmia neonatorum • Social support to people living with AIDS (PLWA)	• Behavior change promotion • Support groups • Safe houses • Reporting of violence
Rural dispensary	• Behavior change promotion • Condoms, spermicides, pills, injectables, (IUD?)	• Support community interventions • All community services • Life saving skills – vacuum extraction; IV antibiotics, sedatives, rehydration; manual removal of placenta & retained products	• Support community interventions • All community services • Syndromic case management • Care for infected newborns • Case detection/Contact tracing • Palliative care for PLWA • Referral to care & testing	• Support community interventions • All community services • Case detection • Treatment of victims • Counseling • Referral to community resources
Medical center	• Behavior change promotion • Condoms, spermicides, pills, injectables, IUD, (implants?, ligation?, vasectomy?)	• Support dispensary services • All dispensary services • Surgical interventions if properly equipped and trained • Manual vacuum aspiration	• Support dispensary services • All dispensary services • Prevention of maternal to child transmission • Simple lab tests	• Support dispensary services • All dispensary services • Documentation and consciousness raising
Hospital	• Behavior change promotion • Condoms, spermicides, pills, injectables, IUD, implants, ligation, vasectomy	• Support medical center services • All center services • Cesarean section • Blood replacement	• All medical center services • Blood screening • All lab tests	• Support dispensary services • All medical center services • Promote policy change

* Adapted from Heise, L., Ellsberg, M., and Goetemoeller M. "Ending Violence Against Women" *Population Reports* Series L., No. 11. Baltimore: Johns Hopkins University School of Public Health, Population Information Program, December 1999, pp. 30–34.

of Provider/Services matrix for reproductive health care. This matrix is illustrative and must be adapted to the health care system of each country. This example is drawn from west Africa. The typical health district has four levels of health providers:

1. The community, which includes village health workers, traditional birth attendants, and traditional healers;
2. Rural health dispensaries, staffed by a nurse, that oversee and support community level providers;
3. Medical centers staffed by a physician, a nurse and/or midwife, and a medical technician, and equipped with a small laboratory; the centers oversee the rural health dispensaries;
4. The hospital located in the district capital, which oversees the medical centers.

Reproductive health programs are aided by dense provision of services from multiple sources. Clients differ in their needs and tastes. They will enter the health care system at many different points, both formal and informal. Successful service delivery strategies offer the client many opportunities to access reproductive health care because the barriers to care are multiple and diverse. Women confined to the home or village by *purdah* in south Asia need a different kind of provider and service delivery strategy than men who are free to visit a clinic, but embarrassed to do so. The health care system should be diverse enough to accommodate this diversity of needs. Strengthening the competence of an array of providers and building links among providers heightens the probability of overcoming the barriers to care.

One of the great advances of the reproductive health movement has been a steady diversification of the range of service delivery strategies and providers. Over the years, it has been demonstrated that safe, effective services can be provided by a wide range of providers using different service delivery strategies. Three major modes of service delivery can be distinguished: clinical services, community-based distribution and commercial distribution. The following sections discuss how managers can support increased access to reproductive health services through these different strategies.

Strengthening Clinical Services

Clinical services are offered by health professionals at medical facilities, though there are examples of mobile clinics housed in trucks and recreational vehicles. Clinics potentially offer the best trained staff and the widest array of services. Clinics serve as the lynchpin for virtually any service delivery strategy. In addition to service provision, they also usually serve as a point of training, supervision and re-supply for community and commercial strategies. Because clinics are typically multi-purpose, they can attract reproductive health clients coming for other services or, conversely, help reproductive health clients who need other forms of medical care.

There are different types and levels of clinics. The process suggested above of matching services to providers sets the type and quantity of services to be delivered by each clinic. Using the African example, the manager would have clarified which reproductive health services are to be offered by health posts, medical centers and the hospital. Specifying the quantity and type of services to be provided logically requires defining the resources that must be available at each clinic and the standard of care that must be achieved. Clarity about the minimum requisite resources and the standard of care allows managers to assess the capacity of clinics and target capacity building interventions.

The Situation Analysis Methodology developed by the Population Council[1] and the COPE Self-Assessment Procedure[2] pioneered by EngenderHealth have helped define the general areas of concern that must be addressed by clinic managers. Clinic performance can be assessed along the following dimensions:

1. The number, type, training and experience of the staff relative to the norms set by public health authorities and/or to the reproductive health services the clinic is expected to deliver.
2. The availability of drugs and other essential commodities for reproductive health care (e.g., contraceptives, antibiotics, anticonvulsives, rehydration fluids) concomitant with the role of the clinic.
3. The adequacy of the physical facilities and clinic relative to established standards and/or the services to be provided.
4. The quality and use of record keeping.
5. The frequency and type of supervision or technical support provided from outside the clinic.
6. The frequency and type of reproductive health education offered by clinic staff to clients, including the availability and use of educational materials.
7. The efficiency of patient flow through the clinic.
8. The quality of care during the provider-client transaction (see below for a more extended discussion of quality of care issues).
9. Client satisfaction with the services provided and client recommendations for improvement as assessed by client interviews.
10. Health provider satisfaction with the support functions provided by the clinic. Many clinics have "extra-mural" responsibilities that involve training, supervising and supplying providers at lower levels in the health pyramid. Interviews of these dependent providers can also be used to assess clinic performance.

Both Situation Analysis and COPE rely on defining a standard of performance along multiple dimensions and then assessing actual performance relative to the standard. Training, technical support and material resources can then be targeted at performance deficiencies in an orderly sequence of capacity building activities. Both methods use a variety of data gathering approaches, including interviews, observation, focus groups and review of records. The Situation Analysis methodology tends to give greater weight to using external analysts to develop findings and a capacity building plan, whereas the COPE Procedure relies more heavily on clinic staff participation. A common finding from multiple applications of both methods is that many lapses in clinic performance are remediable by staff and management at little or no cost. They often involve changes in procedure or the use of available resources in a more effective manner. The participatory approach to assessment lends itself to this kind of change by helping staff identify problems and solutions.

Unfortunately, clinics alone are not a solution to the problem of limited access to reproductive health services. For one thing, the absolute number of health professionals is often quite low relative to population size, especially in the rural areas. Scores of millions of potential and actual clients face severe obstacles to access. Clinics are often physically remote (more than 10 kilometers distance), requiring long, difficult and expensive commutes. Social barriers in many cultures make it difficult for women to travel outside the immediate environs of their homes or villages, further inhibiting contact with clinical providers. Lost productivity and childcare impose hidden costs on accessing services, to which must be added charges for services and commodities. As a consequence, clinical services must be complemented by community based services that rely on lay health workers.

Supporting Community Health Workers

Community based reproductive health care is a service delivery strategy that uses lay community members as service providers. Table 5-1 suggested some of the functions that can be carried out by community based health workers (CHW). CHW serve as distributors of contraceptives and condoms, birth attendants, health educators, community organizers, and sellers of essential commodities, including drugs. In many settings they are the first source of health information and health care for the majority of the population. Properly trained, supplied and supported CHW have been shown to deliver a wide array of services safely and effectively.

Traditional healers and community health workers can also undermine reproductive security by providing inaccurate information and poor quality care. Most notably, TBA mishandling of obstetrical emergencies and mistreatment of STD by traditional healers and drug sellers contribute significantly to poor reproductive health outcomes. In a study in western Kenya, for example, traditional healers, non-credentialed practitioners and chemists were found to be the preferred source of treatment for STD[3]. The use of traditional medicines was found to be widespread, partner notification was nonexistent and some traditional healers recommended unprotected intercourse as part of the therapeutic regime. Integrating community-based workers in a productive manner into the health care system could help optimize their contribution and minimize harm.

There are a number of important determinants of the effectiveness of CHW:

1. **Recruitment and selection:** The community must perceive the CHW as a credible, effective source of reproductive health care if the CHW is to be effective. Many different criteria have been proposed for selecting CHW, including age, gender, marital status, number of children, social status and reproductive health practice (e.g., use of contraceptives). There is little evidence that these criteria per se are good predictors of CHW effectiveness. Rather, the personal credibility and acceptability of the agent to the population being served is key. Therefore, involving the client population in selecting the agent is usually very helpful in increasing community acceptance of the CHW.
2. **Training:** CHW are often illiterate and typically have very little formal education. CHW are usually volunteers or receive very small emoluments in the form of receipt from sale of drugs, compensation from community funds or rewards from external sponsors. Hence, the bulk of their time must be devoted to other forms of productive employment. Training must be adapted to these realities. CHW training should consist of multiple short, practice-oriented, mutually reinforcing sessions, rather than long training programs. Adult education methods, which emphasize experiential learning, observation and practice, should be emphasized, with a minimum of lecturing. Typically, a training session for CHW will last a few days to a week, after which they are encouraged to practice their new skills. Refresher training and/or acquisition of new skills should be provided on a regular basis. Child care during training is often needed as many CHW are women.
3. **Supervision:** Regular, supportive supervision is critical to the effectiveness of CHW. CHW must receive periodic visits from skilled staff who can answer questions, provide on-the-job training, observe performance and resolve problems. The investment in training and supplying CHW can be easily wasted if CHW do not receive reinforcement of newly acquired skills. Supervisors should serve as coaches, answer questions, reinforce training, monitor progress and re-supply CHW with drugs and other essential supplies. Supervision is often a serious lacuna in programs that rely on CHW. CHW supervision is usually entrusted to

clinic staff who also have patient care and clinic management responsibilities; e.g., the nurse at the rural health post is expected to visit the CHW in the surrounding villages. Unless adequate provision has been made, clinic staff will not have the time, means or incentive to make regular field visits. Such field visits as do occur are often mishandled because clinic staff lack supervisory skills. The supervisor is critical rather than supportive and arrives without supplies to replenish community stocks. Effective supervision requires dedicating staff time to this role, training in supervision and a budget to support the costs of travel. Because of the constraints on the ability of clinic staff to travel, an alternative strategy is to have the CHW assemble on a periodic basis for discussions with clinic staff. This also provides the opportunity for reviewing progress, answering questions, solving problems and providing additional training. Conversely, requiring travel of the CHW can prove impractical in many settings unless CHW are reimbursed for their travel costs and time.

4. **Range of tasks:** A critical management responsibility is defining a reasonable range of tasks that responds to priority needs but does not over-burden the CHW. Because of the multiple dimensions of reproductive health, CHW are often asked by Ministries of Health, sponsoring non-governmental organizations and/or communities to take on multiple tasks, including family planning, maternal health care and STD prevention. Reproductive health is, in fact, often only one dimension of the ostensible responsibilities of a CHW, which may range over the whole of primary health care and include distribution of a wide range of drugs. This may result in placing unrealistic expectation on the CHW, who is usually an uncompensated volunteer. As a practical matter, the CHW who is asked to do too much will often end up focusing on a very few tasks or abandoning the role. There is no formula for determining the appropriate range of tasks other than genuine dialogue involving the CHW, the community and the manager. Responsibilities may be allocated across several CHW. New tasks should be added gradually to the responsibilities if the public health system can provide adequate training, supervision and supplies.

5. **Range of drugs and commodities distributed by the CHW:** CHW can play a critical role in storing and supplying essential drugs and commodities at the community level. However, there is disagreement as to the ability of CHW to distribute drugs safely and effectively and wide variation in practice. Countries vary as to the range of contraceptive methods they permit CHW to distribute; in some CHW are only permitted to distribute barrier methods (condoms and spermicides), while others authorize CHW distribution of hormonal methods (pills and injectables). Making a greater variety of methods easily available in response to diverse fertility desires and contraceptive preferences among clients enhances contraceptive prevalence. Most countries encourage TBAs to adopt use of a safe birth kit, but only a few authorize CHW use of oxytocics or antibiotics. This may help prevent misuse but may also limit access among women in need of obstetric first aid. There is very little experience with training CHW to provide antibiotics for STD treatment, despite the prominent role of traditional healers and drug sellers in STD care. There is compelling evidence to support CHW distribution of barrier and hormonal contraceptives, less dispositive evidence with regard to the use of obstetric care drugs at the community level, and very little experience or evidence with regard to training CHW in prescribing drugs for STD.

6. **Modality of service delivery:** The potential role of the CHW range along a continuum from very assertive to passive. At the assertive end of the continuum the CBD uses the social map of the community to define reproductive behavior in each household. Each household is coded with regarded to contraceptive use, pregnancy, birth planning, and so forth. The CHW maintains a regular pattern of household visitation where behavior change is encouraged and commodities are distributed. The CHW can also play a more or less assertive role in organizing collective action for reproductive health. The assertive CHW is needed in the early stages of a reproductive health program or when there are cultural constraints that inhibit women from

leaving their homes. However, it is a time consuming and expensive strategy. Alternatively, CHW may hold regular "public" sessions for education, counseling and care. The social map is used to identify places where potential clients congregate, such as marketplaces, crossroads and bus depots. These sites are visited by the CHW in accordance with a publicized schedule. The CHW sets up a table, booth or simply a large square of cloth on the ground. These sessions are then used as an opportunity for public education, small group counseling and distribution of commodities. Arrangement can be made with clients who desire private consultation. In Nigeria, Togo and Ghana, for example, CHW sell contraceptives at tables in the marketplace. At the passive end of the continuum CHW is largely responsive rather than pro-active. In this approach the trained CHW stores commodities in his or her dwelling and responds to requests for assistance from clients who come to the home. This is often accompanied by periodic public education on reproductive health by the CHW, who has been provided with educational materials. This approach is most useful when demand for reproductive health services has already been generated and the time of the CHW is best spent responding to that demand plus targeted educational efforts. Good judgment by the CHW, the manager and the community is needed to determine the CHW service delivery approach best adapted to the local context.

7. **Record keeping:** CHW must keep records to track the status of clients and monitor the disbursement of drugs and supplies. However, record keeping forms must be adapted to the needs of illiterate or low literacy providers. Pictograms are often used, wherein CHW can simply make marks against a symbol to indicate the number of clients served, the type of service provided and the amount of supplies distributed. The most important use of this record is as an element of the dialogue with the supervisor. Trends in service utilization and commodity distribution can be displayed visually in a form meaningful to the CHW and then discussed as to their significance. For example, the CHW might look at trends in contraceptive use and use of maternal health services. Factors underlying the trends can then be discussed with an eye to rewarding positive outcomes and resolving problems when trends are negative or static. The data are also used to determine the amount of new commodities supplied to the CHW by the supervisor. Contact with the supervisor can also be used to transfer information for purposes of aggregation and comparison across communities.

8. **Client access to clinical services:** CHW must be linked to clinics and be able to ease client use of clinical services. Family planning clients must be able to opt for clinical methods. Pregnant women must be able to secure clinical care in the event of an emergency. STD care requires clinical intervention for diagnosis and treatment. The very important contribution of CHW has limits and the services of trained clinicians must be available. The process of consultation, training, supervision and re-supply is very important to building the relationship between the CHW and the local clinic. Part of the process is arriving at a mutual understanding of the services that the CHW can perform and those that require a clinician. For example, a critical element in training TBA is enhancing prompt recognition of obstetrical emergencies and a protocol for eliciting rapid response from clinical staff. More generally, effective programs establish a method for referring clients for clinical care. In the Dominican Republic, for example, CARE developed a relationship with the family planning association whereby clients desiring a ligation or vasectomy were given a referral slip that generated prompt, subsidized care. In Bolivia, some communities have acquired two-way radios that are used to alert the local clinic of medical emergencies.

9. **Incentives and retention:** Retention is a constant challenge to programs that use CHW. The public health system in most countries cannot afford to pay for a national network of CHW. Where payment is provided, CHW wages can quickly become a major burden to the health system as the program expands. Alternative strategies have therefore evolved. One option is allowing CHW to sell publicly supplied commodities and retain all or part of the

proceeds. In some programs the agent is provided with a bicycle, horse or donkey that can be used to visit remote dwellings, but is also available for personal use. Other programs reward the agent with gifts, such as a uniform or shirt that adds to a meager wardrobe and confers status. Other options include awarding tools or free access to medical care at the clinic in exchange for service. Many programs motivate continued service by offering CHW medals, plaques and ribbons in honor of their service. However, the reality is that significant attrition is a regular feature of CHW programs that rely on volunteers. Acknowledging this fact can help communities and managers plan for turnover. There should be a regular process by which CHW opt out of continued service, which prompts a new cycle of recruiting and training.

Using the Commercial Sector Effectively

The commercial sector can make an important contribution to reproductive health services in two ways. In some contexts, private, for-profit health care providers serve a significant portion of the population. Building skills and incentives in the for-profit sector to deliver reproductive health services can increase access to services by current or potential clients. Optimizing the use of for-profit providers has a number of advantages. In countries such as the Philippines, Dominican Republic, Indonesia and India, for-profit providers already provide a significant percentage of reproductive health services and commodities. Improving the reach, scope and quality of care offered by for-profit providers would benefit their clients at relatively low cost to the public health system. Limited public sector resources can then be more effectively targeted at those unable to pay for private care. In addition, the application of commercial marketing approaches can increase the demand for and distribution of reproductive health services and products.

The social mapping and provider mapping suggested at the beginning of this chapter can be used to define the array of for-profit providers that could increase access to services and products by the population of concern. These commercial providers can be grouped into the following general categories:

- Physicians;
- Nurses and midwives;
- Pharmacists, chemists and other sellers of drugs;
- Employers who provide health care for employees and their families; this is typical of large employers such as factories, mines and plantations;
- Health insurance providers;
- Retail sales outlets not specifically directed at health care that include or could include the sale of contraceptives, birth kits, micronutrients and other reproductive health commodities.

Here are some key issues and considerations in working with the commercial sector[4,5]:

1. **Proportion of the population is served by for-profit providers:** In many developing countries for-profit providers serve less than five percent of the population and this tends to be in the larger urban areas. However, there are important exceptions and each situation must be appraised individually. In Indonesia, for example, midwives in private practice play an important role in the delivery of reproductive health care. The current market share of the for-profit sector is an important determinant in deciding whether to invest in this sector.
2. **Ability of clients to pay:** The for-profit sector will respond to customers who can pay. A realistic assessment of the ability to pay for services and products must be made. Household

income; household expenditures on health care; the degree to which households direct their expenditures to the private sector; and, the market price of reproductive services and goods must be taken into account. Private sector services may not be possible where household income and health expenditures are very low. It is often helpful to compare the projected price of reproductive health goods and services with household expenditures on other commonly purchased items (food, soap, beer) to judge projected demand.

3. **Demand generation:** There is no incentive for individual providers to expend time and money on generating demand for reproductive health services when they may not capture the benefit. Hence, the burden of demand generation usually rests on the public sector. It is usually pointless to increase the supply of trained and equipped for-profit providers unless there is a systematic effort to generate increased demand. The growth of the supply system and the behavior change program must be meshed. Social marketing programs have often relied on commercial advertising firms to promote the need for care and the availability of private sector services.

4. **Regulatory and political environment:** Government attitude towards private health care ranges from supportive to hostile. Written and unwritten rules can serve to block for-profit service delivery. These rules may govern the type of service allowed, the permissibility of selling drugs or other commodities, advertising, pricing, importation, taxation and record-keeping. Private providers may also fear they will incur the hostility of community leaders or important constituencies by offering specific services, such as family planning. Any or all of these may serve as disincentives to private providers. Understanding the policy and political environment can help guide the development of the for-profit sector.

5. **Training:** For-profit providers will often need training in reproductive health care, for which they may not be prepared by earlier experience or schooling. Private providers usually have specific needs with regard to training that differ from those of public sector providers. Training schedules must be adjusted to accommodate normal working hours; weekend or evening training is therefore often preferred. Moreover, business and technical subjects must often be integrated to foster the sustainability of private sector services.

6. **Access to capital:** For-profit providers may be unable to provide services unless they are able to procure necessary facilities, equipment and supplies. This will require access to loans that can then be re-paid. Creative arrangements are often needed involving the provider, the public health system, donors and local financial institutions to generate the necessary capital. It is usually too time consuming and expensive for financial institutions to make loans to individual providers. Therefore, the use or creation of associations that can serve as intermediaries is often a prerequisite to securing capital. For example, CARE helped launch a midwives association in Tanzania that could then serve as the conduit for training, technical assistance and capital.

7. **Competition from the public sector:** One of the major reasons for working with the for-profit sector is to alleviate the financial burden on the public sector. However, this objective can be vitiated if the public sector provides free goods and services that undermine the private sector. This has been a frequent obstacle to the commercialization of contraceptives, which are often distributed free by public sector family planning programs. Clients may be willing to pay for private services and goods because the real costs of public care, including lost time, poor quality care and inconvenience, may exceed the prices charged by the private sector. Some clients may have a strong personal preference for private providers that overcomes the difference in price. Nonetheless, a strategy designed to maximize access by encouraging private sector services must try to avoid undermining private providers through indiscriminate use of subsidies in the public sector. For this reason, cost-recovery in the public sector should be harmonized with private sector prices, while reserving free goods to those who cannot pay.

IMPROVING THE QUALITY OF CARE

Defining the package of essential services and easing access to care sets the stage for meeting client needs. The next challenge to the health manager is ensuring that the client receives high quality care wherever she or he enters the system. The experience of clients in their encounter with health providers profoundly affects reproductive health outcomes, as well as the reputation of the program in the wider population. High quality care preserves the investment in building systems and attracting clients. Competently treated clients are more likely to achieve good outcomes and satisfied clients more likely to encourage friends and neighbors to seek needed care.

Quality of care is both a *standard* and a *process*. Quality standards define what is required in the transaction between the client and the health system. Quality processes provide for on-going amelioration of the client-provider transaction, including regular measurement of whether standards are being met.

Quality Standards

Judith Bruce has developed a very useful framework that sets forth the fundamental elements of quality of care in family planning.[6] The WHO has developed quality of care standards for maternal health.[7] The Evaluation Project sponsored by the U.S. Agency for International Development developed a framework for assessing the quality of care in STD programs.[8] Table 5-2 summarizes the standards or elements of quality in each of these domains:

As can be seen from Table 5-2, the essential elements of quality care are similar across reproductive health domains. The WHO definition of quality of care in maternal health is somewhat broader than other approaches since it also encompasses behavior change and

TABLE 5-2. Quality of Care Standards for Reproductive Health

Family planning (Bruce framework)	Maternal health (WHO framework)	Sexually transmitted diseases (Evaluation Project framework)
Choice of methods	Promotion and protection of health	Availability of drugs, condoms an other essential supplies
Information given to clients	Accessibility and availability of services	Informing and counseling clients
Technical competence of providers	Acceptability of services to clients	Technical competence of providers
Interpersonal relations	Technical competence of health care providers	Acceptability of services to clients
Continuity of care and follow-up	Essential supplies and equipment	Continuity of care and follow-up
Appropriate constellation of services	Quality of client-provider interaction	
	Information and counseling for the client	
	Involvement of clients in decision-making	
	Comprehensiveness of care and linkages to other reproductive health services	
	Continuity of care and follow-up	
	Support to health care providers	

access to services, which have been discussed earlier in this text. Both the Bruce and WHO framework call for delivering an appropriate package of reproductive health services, which was the subject of the opening section to this chapter. The approaches summarized in Table 5-2 can then be synthesized into a quality of care framework for reproductive health consisting of the following six essential elements:

1. **Access to essential drugs, supplies and equipment:** Reproductive health care requires that clients have access to an essential set of drugs and supplies. STD care requires access to antibiotics to treat curable STD and drugs for care of AIDS patients. Laboratory supplies and equipment are also needed for STD diagnosis. Obstetrical emergencies demand antibiotics, anti-convulsives, anesthetics and blood products. Routine maternal health care includes tetanus toxoid injection and micronutrient supplementation. Failure to provide essential drugs to STD and maternal health clients will lead to serious illness or death. Family planning clients need access to a wide range of contraceptive methods to accommodate differences in health status and fertility desires. Programs that offer clients a range of methods and help clients make informed choices experience higher rates of contraceptive adoption and continuation. One of the responsibilities of the health manager is to define the commodities (drugs, contraceptives and other supplies) that should be available at every service delivery point. This should follow logically from the Provider/Services Matrix. By specifying the services to be provided by each type and level of provider it should also be possible to identify the commodities needed to provide care.

2. **Information and counseling given to clients:** Clients are entitled to accurate, comprehensible information that empowers them to make informed choices, understand the medical procedures to which they are subject and adopt healthy reproductive behaviors. Family planning clients must be aware of contraceptive options, and the benefits, risks and proper use of each method. Pregnant women must know the danger signs of pregnancy, develop a birth plan and be knowledgeable about essential actions that will help safeguard their health and that of their babies. Clients must know how to recognize, prevent and manage STDs. Women must know how to protect themselves against sexual violence. Both men and women need better information on communicating about sex with one's partner. The encounter between client and provider should be seen as a time for teaching and counseling, as well as proper administration of medical procedures. The teaching and counseling role is not necessarily part of clinical training and requires different skills. Training, monitoring and supporting staff in these functions is part of establishing the norm of high quality care.

3. **Client involvement in decision-making:** Closely related to the information and counseling standard is the standard of genuine client power over reproductive health care choices. Barring absolute medical contraindication, it is the client and not the provider who must choose the most suitable contraceptive method. Women are entitled to make choices about many aspects of pregnancy, labor and delivery, including location, attendant, position and companion. Clients must be able to exercise control over the manner of partner notification in the event of an STD so as to avoid physical and social repercussions. Other examples might be given, but the principle is clear. There are clearly moments and domains where the technical expertise of the provider must hold sway. However, the client is in charge of her body and good quality of care requires respecting the right of the client to make choices.

4. **Technical competence of health care providers:** Technical competence has two dimensions: *capacity* and *implementation*.[9] Capacity refers to the ability of health providers to provide care in accordance with established guidance, including medical care and counseling. This means that providers have received appropriate training, have access to current information, have been given clear guidelines as to standards of practice, and have adequate facilities, equipment, drugs and supplies. Implementation refers to the degree to which skills are

actually applied; i.e., the proportion of clients who actually benefit from the proper use of knowledge and skills. Implementation of technically appropriate care by capable providers is influenced by proper supervision, rewards for meeting quality standards, encouragement and feedback from clients, peers and managers and back-up from other providers who can provide complementary skills and assist over-burdened staff. Technical competence therefore depends on systems that continuously build staff capacity, while encouraging and rewarding the application of high standards of care.

5. **Interpersonal relations:** There is a very important affective component to high quality reproductive health care. Clients are often embarrassed or uncertain in approaching providers for reproductive health care. Especially for women, the decision to seek contraception, STD care, maternal health care or violence prevention may take great courage. The client view of quality is often quite different from that of providers. The latter tend to define quality in terms of the technical competence exhibited and the governing treatment protocols. Clients consider technical skill, but only as one aspect of the interaction with the provider. Clients also look for respect, understanding, access, fairness, accurate information and results.[10] The need for privacy and assurance that conversations and records will be held in confidence are also important to clients. Clients use these criteria in deciding whether to seek care, return for care, pay for care, comply with provider instructions, seek alternative care or recommend a provider to others. Clients are more likely to turn away from providers who are seen as rude, not listening, providing incomplete or inaccurate information, inaccessible and/or altering care in response to the social status of the client. Client satisfaction may not mesh with technical norms. Clients habituated to poor quality care often express satisfaction with incompetent treatment or, conversely, may demand services that are inappropriate. Raising and adjusting client expectations to match the standard of technical competence is part of the client education process. Client dissatisfaction, however, is always a warning sign to managers that intervention is needed to improve the quality of client-provider interaction.

6. **Continuity and follow-up:** The initial contact between the client and the provider is only the beginning of proper care. Reinforcement of behavior change, proper use of contraceptives and drugs, compliance and evolving client needs require continuity of care. For example, contraceptive continuation is very important to the over-all health and fertility impact of family planning programs. Large investments are made in attracting new clients. However, discontinuation rates are often quite high—rates of 50 percent in the first year for oral contraceptive users are common. Follow-up of contraceptive acceptors to identify concerns, assist with compliance and help manage side effects is often a better investment then recruiting new users. Similarly, good maternal health care requires a sequence of linked interactions, including prenatal care, childbirth and postnatal care. Over-investing in prenatal care without adequate provision for the remainder of the pregnancy cycle can vitiate the impact on maternal morbidity and mortality. The end of pregnancy signals the need to start contraception. STD care usually requires follow-up to ensure compliance with the drug regimen, safer sex practices and partner notification. Intervention in cases of sexual violence is almost always a multi-stage effort. Clients may be inhibited from seeking follow-up care for reasons ranging from lack of understanding to fear of physical violence from sexual partners. Good quality care therefore encompasses mechanisms for following up on clients who need additional care.

Quality Processes

Virtually all institutions fall short of the desired standard of care. Health providers and health institutions need systematic processes for assessing their performance and upgrading

BUILDING INSTITUTIONAL CAPACITY

quality. Health programs have borrowed the concepts of *total quality management* and *continuous quality improvement* from the management literature. These concepts emphasize regular measurement of performance relative to quality standards and on-going, incremental changes developed by concerned staff. Quality improvement involves five distinct but related processes: demonstrating leadership commitment, defining quality standards, measuring the quality of care, developing and implementing a quality improvement plan, and sustaining quality improvement over time.

1. **Demonstrating clear leadership commitment to improving the quality of care:** A concern for quality must emanate from the top. Staff are very unlikely to undertake the effort to identify, publicize and correct deficiencies in quality unless there is clear, overt encouragement from organizational leadership. Quality improvement requires staff to actively identify errors in processes and performance. This can only happen if management makes clear that such behavior will be rewarded and not punished.

2. **Engage staff in developing and disseminating quality standards:** The six elements suggested above provide a framework within which context appropriate standards can be developed. Clarity of expectations is essential to measuring and improving quality. Staff cannot be expected to improve quality in the absence of a clear barometer against which to measure performance. In some countries, guidance as to quality standards will be available from the Ministry of Health or other appropriate national institutions. Alternatively, standards developed by the World Health Organization, other countries or professional associations might be used as references. Standards should be set for essential drugs and commodities, counseling methods, client satisfaction, treatment algorithms, client follow-up procedures and the essential package of services. The process by which standards are established is very important, as they must be technically sound but also properly adapted to the context. Hence, a participatory process that involves managers, providers and clients in defining standards can enhance their applicability and acceptance.

3. **Measure the quality of care relative to standards:** In practice, quality assessment often takes place before the formal adoption of quality standards. Standards are implicitly embedded in the assessment instruments. The process of developing, adapting, implementing and using the quality assessment serves as the *de facto* procedure for setting quality standards. Much like the assessment of client needs, the assessment of quality typically involves triangulation of information from multiple sources using different data gathering techniques. Three and possibly four different perspectives are usually needed to assess quality: (1) The perspective of the client must be the starting point. Exit interviews and surveys can be used to determine the degree of client satisfaction and pinpoint areas where clients are particularly troubled by provider performance. Re-orienting staff to understand and respond to client perspectives is usually one of the most important steps in establishing continuous quality improvement. (2) The perspective of staff, broadly defined, is also essential. Staff includes everyone working at a service delivery point from the physician managing a clinic to the sweeper responsible for cleaning the facility. Widespread involvement in quality assessment is important to fostering support for the effort and in generating ideas from as many sources as possible. Group processes and interviews are very useful in eliciting staff concerns about quality. In general, staff are very adept at identifying flaws in work flow and infrastructure that inhibit good quality care, such as the reasons underlying long client waiting times. There is often less ability to identify shortcomings in technical competence and communication with clients. (3) The perspective of managers is also important in assessing quality, though it must not override the perspective of staff and clients. Supervisors are often needed to identify technical problems and lapses in coordination and communication between different units or personnel that are inhibiting

TABLE 5-3. Illustrative List of Quality of Care Indicators

Quality of care domain	Illustrative indicators
Drugs, equipment and commodities	• Approved drugs, contraceptives and medical supplies available • Approved equipment available • Space for private examination and consultation available
Information and counseling	• Service delivery point has clear guidelines governing counseling and information provided to clients • Provider elicits client concern/problem/reason for seeking care • Provider elicits essential information on reproductive health status and history per guidelines • Provider gives information on family planning, maternal health, HIV/STI and sexual violence per guidelines • Provider responds accurately to questions and concerns raised by client • Provider reinforces skills needed by client to address reproductive health concerns; e.g., condom negotiation, contraceptive method use, compliance with drug regimen
Client involvement in decision-making	• Provider describes feasible options in balanced presentation • Client participates actively in discussion and selection of option • Client expresses satisfaction with option selected
Technical competence	• Service delivery point has clear guidelines regarding client assessment and management for core reproductive health services • Staff demonstrate mastery of technical knowledge concomitant with their responsibilities • Staff practice assessment/diagnosis in accordance with guidelines • Staff practice client treatment/management in accordance with guidelines • Staff receive regular technical supervision
Interpersonal relations	• Provider establishes and sustains rapport with client • Client believes transaction will be kept confidential • Client experiences acceptable waiting times • Client expresses satisfaction with provider comportment
Continuity	• Service delivery point has established guidelines for client follow-up • Staff apply follow-up guidelines

good quality care. (4) External consultants can be very helpful in carrying out observation of performance by staff in their interaction with clients. Table 5-3 provides an illustrative list of indicators of quality that might be used at a service delivery point.

Simplicity in collecting, interpreting and using quality of care data is essential. Using data in this manner is usually a new skill for health providers. Staff may initially see little reward or relevance to the exercise. It is always better to begin by collecting data on a very few indicators and inculcate the habit of regular self-examination. One might begin by selecting only one quality of care standard, such as information and counseling, and focus on change in this area for a number of months. Alternatively, a small subset of the indicators suggested in Table 5-3, representing several quality of care standards, might be selected. Over time, additional indicators can be gradually added to develop a richer understanding of the quality of care provided. Collecting, displaying and interpreting data on a few key indicators should become part of the normal work routine. Simple, prominent graphic displays can be very helpful. For example, a reproductive health program in Zambia supported by CARE assembled clinic managers from the Livingstone area on a monthly basis. Each manager would enter the quality of care data from his or her clinic on large paper wall charts. This allowed the managers to track changes over time and compare progress among clinics. The managers would interpret the significance of trends and exchange experience in promoting better quality. Because the data were used immediately to enhance the quality of work, resulting in positive feedback from clients, staff developed a positive attitude towards quality of care assessment. The simple and rapid use of data to improve work performance is essential to sustaining staff support for routine quality monitoring.

4. **Develop and implement a quality improvement plan:** Staff are amazingly creative and innovative in addressing quality problems when provided with a supportive environment. Quality improvement efforts rely on assembling staff teams embodying multiple perspectives without regard to rank or formal role to review the data and devise appropriate responses. Many improvements in quality can be achieved at very low monetary cost and save staff time. In one clinic in Niger, for example, a private area for physical examinations was created at the cost of a piece of cloth and a small rope purchased on the local market. The objective of a quality improvement plan is to achieve progress with regard to all six of the dimensions of quality. However, it is usually advisable to begin by concentrating on a few of the more pressing and soluble issues. Because quality improvement is an on-going process managers should seek constant, small changes that accumulate in their impact over time.

Quality improvement can be sought through changes in standards, work processes, staff capacity, staff incentives and infrastructure:

- **Clarifying standards:** Health providers often lack clear guidance from their institutions as to appropriate client management. Health providers need relevant, comprehensible and explicit guidance on counseling, the information to be provided to clients and patient assessment and care. These guidelines are often available at the national level but are not adequately disseminated or promoted at the local level. Clarifying and communicating standards is therefore an important part of improving quality.
- **Improving work processes:** The analysis and revision of work processes is another common tactic for improving quality. For example, waiting times at clinics are often very long because of poorly designed patient flow procedures. Simple changes can often dramatically reduce waiting times. Patient management is often inadequate because patient records are irretrievable due to a poor or non-existent filing system. The patient's medical history is either ignored or re-created at the time of each visit. Drug shortages are often due to poor inventory management; simply tracking inventory and submitting the required forms on time could help alleviate shortages. Identifying and rectifying these types of flaws in work processes can ultimately make a big difference in the quality of care experienced by clients.

- **Increasing staff capacity:** Training is a very important component of quality improvement. Staff cannot be expected to achieve the desired standard of care if they have not been afforded the opportunity to develop the requisite skills and competencies. Targeted, competency based training that helps providers acquire and practice needed skills will usually be required. The specific objectives of the training should reflect the assessment of staff capacity.
- **Staff incentives:** Health providers in developing countries are generally very poorly compensated. Public sector employees sometimes go months without being paid and supervision is characteristically infrequent. Staff must be recognized and rewarded for quality improvement. These rewards are often non-financial, but nonetheless important. To return to the Zambia example described above, clinic managers who showed significant gains in quality received small prizes and certificates in public ceremonies recognizing their accomplishment.
- **Infrastructure:** Quality of care depends on the availability of facilities, equipment and supplies conforming to the services delivered at each service delivery point. Resource availability is obviously a major constraint to addressing this dimension of quality. Nonetheless, creative partnerships can sometimes be used to address this problem. In eastern Uganda, for example, the United Kingdom Department for International Development provided funding to CARE for infrastructure development. CARE purchased materials and provided needed engineering skills, while each participating community contributed the labor needed to build a new clinic. The strategies for community mobilization discussed in the preceding chapter can often be put to good use in addressing quality of care issues if there is a genuine promise of improved access and quality as a consequence.

5. **Sustaining commitment to quality over time:** Quality improvement programs typically start out with a burst of enthusiasm and activity, often generated by input from a donor or at the behest of senior managers. Intensive data collection is carried out and one round of improvement takes place. However, quality improvement is not institutionalized as a way of doing business. It is a one-time exercise. This basically vitiates the philosophy and purpose of continuous quality improvement. Quality of care tools should be gradually introduced at a reasonable pace that can be absorbed by staff and integrated into work routines. Quality improvement should become part of normal work rather than an exercise in addition to core business. This brings us back to the first step in quality improvement—leadership commitment. Quality improvement can be sustained only if leadership insists on regular, data based assessment of quality and on adjusting incentives to reward those who bring about quality improvements.

STRENGTHENING MANAGEMENT SYSTEMS

The fourth critical dimension of capacity building is strengthening management systems. Both access and quality depend on the proper functioning of basic management systems. Assessing and strengthening management systems is one of the fundamental responsibilities of managers. Management development is very similar to and often overlaps improving the quality of care. Management development involves (1) clearly defining the management systems essential to optimal institutional functioning; (2) assessing the functioning of management systems; and, (3) implementing a management development plan.

Defining Management Systems

Seven management systems are essential to the capacity of health institutions: community liaison, planning, human resources management, information management, financial management, commodity management, and facilities and equipment management. The remainder of this section briefly defines each of these systems.

1. **Community liaison:** Capable institutions have an accurate understanding of and support from the communities they serve. Community liaison serves at least three functions
   - *An investigative function* that identifies reproductive health needs and resources using both participatory techniques and conventional tools of epidemiology and social science, such as service statistics and surveys. The investigative function underpins the reproductive risk analysis and the consequent setting of priorities. The investigative function plays a critical role in defining and segmenting the population served, as well as determining the magnitude and type of services offered. Managers must decide what information is needed, how it will be collected and the frequency of data collection.
   - A *consultative function* that managers use to recognize and seek out key constituencies whose support may be needed for programs to succeed. These include leaders of the formal political structure (village chiefs, municipal leaders, etc.), ethnic and religious leaders, women's groups, civic groups, non-governmental organizations, businesses and business associations. These consultations are held regularly and are used to gain agreement on priorities, address concerns and secure commitments of support and resources. The consultative function is sometimes formalized in the form of an advisory board or committee.
   - A *decision-making function:* The discussion of community empowerment described the levels of community participation that ranged from seeking advice to decision-making. Appropriate structures and processes are needed to share decision-making with the community. Typically this is in the form of a village or community health committee that includes the health manager. Issues that must be considered in crafting the decision-making function are membership (who will make the decisions), the scope of authority (what will be decided) and procedures (how decisions will be made).
2. **Planning:** If there is any basic law of management it is, "If you don't know where you are going, you can't get there." Planning serves to clarify purposes, assign responsibility, allocate resources and create the basis for accountability. A well wrought plan will normally include the following elements:
   - *Internal and external analysis:* A widely used tool in planning is SWOT Analysis, which stands for **S**trenghts, **W**eaknesses, **O**pportunities and **T**hreats. The internal analysis is typically devoted to defining strengths and weaknesses in three areas: management systems, technical capacity and resources. The assessment of technical capacity focuses on the match between the reproductive health needs of the population and the ability of staff to deliver essential services. The assessment of financial resources looks at the correspondence between the demand for services and the available budget. The external assessment looks for opportunities and threats in the external environment. This analysis should look at five issues: the target population, trends in the profession, competitors, constituencies and policy. Planners need to be particularly alert for shifts in the composition and needs of the population that may affect the content or magnitude of service needs. A review of trends in the profession serves

to contrast the existing program of the institution with best practices. Comparisons with other organizations serve to delineate advantages and weaknesses in terms of the type of service offered, the quality of care provided and the cost to clients, governments and donors. The constituency analysis deepens understanding of whether the health institution has the necessary support of social, political and economic groups whose blessing is needed for programs to succeed. The policy analysis defines government laws, rules and regulations that are facilitating or inhibiting the success of the reproductive health program.

- *Long term goals:* As a consequence of the SWOT analysis the organization sets long term goals, typically for a three to five year period. These goals are aimed at capitalizing on strengths and opportunities, while countering weaknesses and threats. A weakness in technical capacity, for example, would be addressed through a goal of increasing the number of trained, experienced staff. A threat of an alienated constituency would be addressed through the goal of re-building relations.
- *Strategy:* Each goal has an associated strategy or strategies. A strategy can be thought as the path or approach that will lead to attainment of the goal. For example, implementing a technical training program and disseminating technical guidelines would be strategies for attaining the goal of increased technical capacity.
- *Short-term objectives:* Every strategy is realized by setting short-term objectives, typically for a one-year period. The objectives, in aggregate, lead to the attainment of the goal. For example, the three year goal may be, "Ensure that all providers demonstrate an adequate level of competence in reproductive health care." The objectives for the first year of the plan might be, "Ensure that 1/3 of all providers demonstrate adequate reproductive health care knowledge and skills by the end of the first year."
- *Activities:* Every objective is achieved by specific activities leading to achievement of the objective. The training objective, for example, would involve defining training objectives, developing curricula, developing training materials and carrying out the training. The magnitude and type of activities should be logically derived from the objective.
- *Allocation of budget and staff:* A budget and staff time must be allocated to every objective and activity. This ensures that resources will be available and that there is clear accountability for executing the plan.

3. **Human resources management:** Human resources management serves to align people with the purposes of the organization. The planning process is the starting point for human resource management. The number and type of staff needed should be evident from the goals, strategies, objectives and activities. To return to our example, building technical capacity in reproductive health requires trainers with a specific set of skills. A goal of achieving a specified level of service delivery would logically lead to an assessment of the number and type of service providers needed. Once hired, staff need a supportive system that optimizes their performance. The minimal elements of a supportive human resource system include:

- Clear job descriptions that let every employee know his/her responsibilities.
- A personnel manual that specifies the rules governing employment and that is binding on both the employer and the employee.
- An orientation program that helps new staff gain an understanding or expectations, rules, procedures, responsibilities and privileges. The manual and orientation program usually cover the same issues.
- Regular, supportive supervision.
- Clear annual performance objectives.
- Periodic training that increases skills
- Regular, written appraisal that links rewards to performance.

BUILDING INSTITUTIONAL CAPACITY

4. **Information management:** The management information system is used to help organizations determine progress relative to the plan and gain information that may indicate needed changes in the plan. A good management information system has the following characteristics:
   - A parsimonious set of indicators covering all the key dimensions of organizational functioning has been defined.
   - The data are reasonably accurate.
   - The data are processed in a timely fashion.
   - The data are presented to managers and concerned staff in a lucid, comprehensible fashion with reasonable frequency.
   - The information from the system is shared widely, especially with staff and managers who need it for effective decision-making.
   - The data are actually used in decision-making.

5. **Commodity management:** Reproductive health demands the availability of drugs, contraceptives and other essential supplies. An effective commodity management system ensures that the right commodities are in the right place at the right time in the right amount. Effective commodity management is characterized by:
   - Appropriate selection of essential commodities.
   - Proper procedures for forecasting commodity needs.
   - Proper procedures for procuring commodities.
   - Proper procedures for inventory control.
   - Appropriate storage of commodities that prevents wastage.
   - Proper procedures for distribution of commodities.
   - Periodic audits of the commodity management system.
   - No stock-outs or over-stocks of essential commodities at any point at any level of the health system.
   - Integration of commodity data into the management system.

6. **Budgeting and financial management:** Scrupulous control of the usually meager cash resources of developing country health institutions is a critical management system. Effective financial management requires:
   - A budget that is consistent with the program of activities in the annual plan in total amount and allocation among functions.
   - Regular expenditure reports that compare disbursements to budget.
   - A balance sheet.
   - Periodic audits.
   - Proper procedures for monitoring income, including a register for recording receipt of cash, checks and other forms of income.
   - Proper procedures for monitoring expenditures, including a register of disbursements.
   - A register of accounts payable.
   - Proper procurement procedures.
   - A schedule of fees that is realistic and appropriate.

7. **Facilities and equipment management:** Like cash, fixed and durable assets must be carefully managed to preserve their utility at the least possible cost. Simple procedures can help, including the following:
   - Developing specifications for the physical appurtenances and appearance of each type of facility.
   - Establishing a list of essential equipment appropriate to the level of the facility.
   - Developing and implementing a facility maintenance schedule, which should be reflected in the budget.

- Projecting the useful life of equipment and planning for replacement.
- Maintaining a fixed asset register.
- Periodic inventories of fixed assets.

Assessing Management Capacity

Clarity as to the dimensions of effective management systems sets the bar against which current performance can be measured. Health institutions in developing countries will usually fall far short of the ideal, which poses a fundamental barrier to service delivery. Weak community liaison, poor planning, inadequate supervision, inability to monitor progress, lapses in access to drugs and other commodities, and inefficient control of scarce resources can all wreak havoc on service delivery. As is the case for quality of care, assessing the most damaging gaps in management performance can set the stage for institutional capacity building. There are a number of tools and methods available to assess management capacity, including the CARE Management Capacity Assessment Tool. A variety of useful instruments can be obtained through Management Sciences for Health, which has posted materials to their web site. Most assessment procedures combine interviews, participatory techniques, observation and review of administrative records to assess management systems. Table 5-4 provides an example of the key questions usually asked in the process of carrying out a management systems assessment.

Designing and Implementing A Management Development Plan

Management development looks much like quality improvement, relying on many of the same methods and tools. Management development and quality improvement are two sides of the same coin and are in practice sometimes indistinguishable. Both are an effort to incrementally modify systems that affect service delivery. Management systems are often determinative of quality. Commodity management systems determine the availability of essential drugs and contraceptives. Human resource management determines the technical competence of staff. Hence, many of the same processes are used to strengthen management, including:

- Reliance on staff participation to identify problems and develop solutions with judicious use of external analysts and consultants.
- Establishing and disseminating appropriate management procedures that clarify how systems are expected to function and the responsibility of each staff for implementing systems.
- Training staff in management systems and procedures.
- Staff incentives that reward systems improvement and discourage disregard for appropriate procedure.
- Aiming for and achieving a series of small successes that improve working conditions and staff performance.

Case Study: Improving Institutional Capacity in Bangladesh[11]

The Non-Governmental Organization Services Project (NGO-SP) was implemented by CARE-Bangladesh during the period 1992–1997. The project was designed to address the problem of inadequate coverage by family planning services in rural areas of Bangladesh. The

TABLE 5-4. Illustrative Questions for Assessing Management Systems

COMMUNITY LIAISON
- Is there a good understanding of reproductive health needs and the social and political environment?
- Is there a process for garnering new information on a regular basis?
- Is there a regular process for consultation with the community?
- How does the community participate in decision-making?

PLANNING
- Is there a systematic planning process?
- Does the planning process involve the right people?
- Does the plan show an understanding of the multiple dimensions of reproductive health?

HUMAN RESOURCES MANAGEMENT
- Does the institution use the basic tools of human resource management, such as job descriptions?
- Are staff provided with clear expectations? Do performance assessment and rewards reflect expectations?
- What is the system for supervising and supplying community health workers?

MANAGEMENT INFORMATION SYSTEM
- Is there a clear set of management indicators that are tracked on a regular basis?
- Is information collected, processed and disseminated on a timely basis?
- Is the information used in decision-making?

COMMODITY MANAGEMENT
- Are essential drugs, contraceptives and supplies in stock?
- Is there a working system for tracking, ordering and receiving drugs, contraceptives and other essential supplies?
- Is the institution able to project commodity needs?
- Are drugs, contraceptives and supplies properly stored?

FINANCIAL MANAGEMENT
- Is there a budget?
- Are there basic accounting procedures and controls?
- Is financial information used for program management?

FACILITIES AND EQUIPMENT MANAGEMENT
- Are the basic facilities and equipment necessary to service delivery present?
- Is there evidence of acceptable clinic management as indicated by the state of record keeping and inventory control?

---

basic strategy adopted was to strengthen the ability of twenty Bangladeshi non-governmental organizations (NGOs) to deliver family planning services. From the outset, the project had two basic goals. The first was a behavioral goal, expressed as an increase in contraceptive use in the populations served by the NGOs. The second was a systems goal, expressed as an increase in the institutional capacity of the NGOs.

A fundamental key to the strategy was the regular use of information on three key variables. Contraceptive use was monitored on a regular basis through the use of service statistics and surveys. Service statistics were used to monitor the number of new acceptors of family planning, family planning users and couple-years of protection[12]. A baseline and post-project survey were used to assess gains in contraceptive prevalence. The CARE Quality of Care Supervision Tool was used to provide a quantitative measure of quality of care as defined by the Judith Bruce framework. This tool can be completed very quickly in the field by supervisors to provide a quality score for each service delivery point. Client satisfaction was also monitored on a regular basis. The CARE Management Capacity Assessment Tool (MCAT) was applied

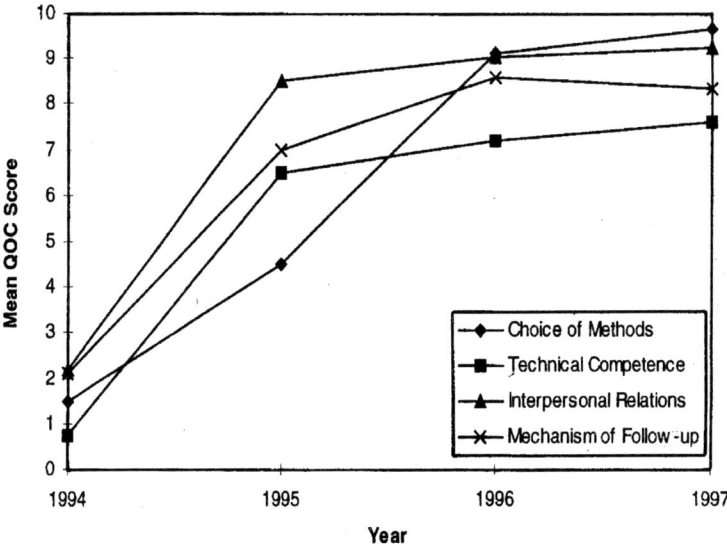

FIGURE 5-3. Quality of care in family planning service delivery CARE-Bangladesh NGO-SP project.

every six months at each NGO to score the functioning of management systems. The MCAT provided a numerical score for each of five key management systems: planning, field program management, logistics, personnel and finance. Managers and staff from the NGO met with CARE-Bangladesh staff on a semi-annual basis (or more frequently if needed) to review the data and plan specific capacity building interventions for the succeeding six month period.

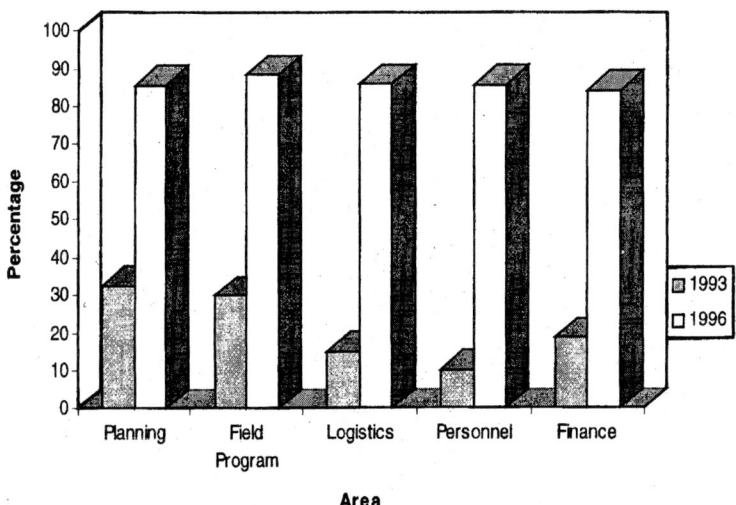

FIGURE 5-4. Aggregate changes in management capacity in 20 NGOs CARE-Bangladesh NGO-SP project.

Linking frequent measurement, participatory review of the findings and targeted capacity building efforts was key to the eventual success of the program.

Institutional strengthening interventions included:

- Cash grants to the NGOs
- Technical and management training of NGO staff
- Placing two CARE staff in each NGO for an extended period to provide technical assistance
- Inculcating the use of participatory processes in NGO managers
- Establishing technical and administrative standards of performance
- Reform of work processes and systems

Contraceptive use increased substantially as the NGOs extended access to under-served populations. The NGOs relied heavily on community health workers with referral of clients needing clinical services to government health clinics. Access to services increased markedly among the target population. The percentage of households visited by a health worker increased substantially, as did the number of women receiving clinical family planning services. The project provided over 446,000 couple-years of protection and served over 525,000 family planning users, including 366,000 new acceptors of family planning. Contraceptive prevalence increased in all four project areas, with gains ranging from 9 percent to 28 percent.

In addition, significant gains in the quality of care and the functioning of management systems were recorded. Figures 5-3 and 5-4 show the changes in quality of care and management capacity.

6

Contraception

THE BIOLOGY OF CONTRACEPTION

Understanding the way contraceptives work requires a basic knowledge of reproductive physiology, especially the menstrual cycle. This section briefly describes the basic physiology of reproduction, which sets the stage for the ensuing discussion of contraceptive methods.

The Menstrual Cycle

The woman's menstrual cycle averages 28 days, although women can have perfectly normal cycles ranging from 23 to 35 days. This discussion assumes a 28 day cycle. The menstrual cycle consists of two phases: the follicular phase and the luteal phase.

Days 1 to 15 constitute the follicular phase. During days 1 to 5, the lining of the uterus—the endometrium—from the previous menstrual cycle sloughs off (menstruation). Estrogen and progesterone levels in blood plasma are low. The low level of estrogen stimulates the release of Gonadotropin Releasing Hormone (GnRH) from the hypothalamus. GnRH triggers the anterior pituitary gland, which releases Luteinizing Hormone (LH) and Follicle Stimulating Hormone (FSH). FSH enters the ovary, stimulating development of several ovarian follicles, which are small sacs containing the unfertilized ova. One of the follicles will become dominant by day 7 and eventually release an oocyte (unfertilized egg). The remaining follicles will regress and die, along with their eggs. FSH and LH work together on the cells of the remaining follicle to promote the production of estrogen. The rising level of estrogen inhibits further release of FSH and LH, stimulates the development of the endometrium and provokes changes in the mucous property and secretion of the cervix, which facilitates sperm transport. The growth of the endometrium prepares the uterus to receive the fertilized ovum.

Estrogen levels continue to rise and peak on day 13. The peak level of estrogen has a *positive* effect on GnRH secretion, which induces additional release of FSH and a large surge of LH, which reaches its maximum level on day 13. Ovulation is triggered on Day 14 approximately eighteen hours after the LH peak and the mature follicle bursts, releasing the oocyte into the fallopian tube.

Days 16–28 constitute the luteal phase. During the luteal phase, LH induces a transformation of the burst follicle, which becomes the corpus luteum. The corpus luteum secretes estrogen and progesterone, which are necessary to the maintenance of the endometrium. Progesterone levels rise and peak on day 21. Body temperature rises in response to the increasing levels of progesterone. The rise in progesterone also changes the properties of the cervix and the mucous, which inhibits sperm transport. Estrogen levels, which decline between day 13 and day 16, rise to a secondary peak on day 22. FSH and LH levels decline steadily during the luteal phase. The endometrium enters the secretory phase, releasing proteins that are essential to implantation of the embryo.

The unfertilized egg has a life span of about 12 hours, while sperm can live in the female reproductive tract for up to five days. Hence, a woman who ovulates on day 14 of her cycle can become pregnant from a deposit of sperm as early as day 9. The oocyte is fertilized in the fallopian tube and is transported to the uterus within 2 to 3 days. Implantation of the conceptus occurs 6 days after fertilization.

In the absence of fertilization, the corpus luteum degenerates, with a consequent decrease in estrogen and progesterone levels. This leads to decreasing blood flow to the endometrium and, consequently, menstruation. Between 20 and 80 ml. of blood is normally lost during menstruation, which lasts 4 to 6 days. Seventy percent of blood loss occurs by the third day and 90 percent by the fourth day. The low level of estrogen triggers the hypothalamus and the cycle is repeated.

The processes underlying the menstrual cycle provide the key to understanding hormonal contraceptives. Manipulation of estrogen and progesterone levels can inhibit pregnancy in the following ways:

- Production of FSH and LH is inhibited and, consequently, growth of the follicles and ovulation are suppressed;
- Transport of the ovum through the fallopian tube is inhibited;
- Growth and maintenance of the endometrium is inhibited, preventing implantation; and,
- Sperm transport is inhibited.

Understanding of the menstrual cycle is also the basis for "natural" methods of family planning, which rely upon the symptoms associated with the different events in the menstrual cycle to time intercourse and abstinence.

Male Reproductive System

The two testes are responsible for production of sperm and testosterone. Within the testes, sperm are formed in the tightly coiled seminiferous tubules. The interstitial cells of Leydig, which lie between the coils of the seminiferous tubules, produce testosterone. The seminiferous tubules flow into the epididymis, which is connected to and rests on the top and posterior surface of the testicle; the role of the epididymis is to store the sperm. The epididymis becomes the vas deferens, a tube which runs into the pelvic cavity behind the urinary bladder. The seminal vesicles, glands lying just below the bladder, empty into the vas deferens. The seminal vesicles extrudes fructose, which serves as an essential nutrient for the sperm. The vas deferens then empties into the urethra. The prostate gland surrounds the upper portion of the urethra. The prostate secretes an alkaline, milky fluid that aids in sperm transport and neutralizes the acidic seminal fluid. Below the prostate is the Cowper's gland, which releases a mucus-like substance that lubricates the distal end of the penis. During ejaculation, the secretions of the epididymis, seminal vesicle, prostate and Cowper's gland all flow into the urethra.

As in the female, an elaborate feedback system controls male reproductive function. Declining levels of testosterone stimulate the hypothalamus to release GnRH, which acts on the pituitary to foster release of LH. Within the seminiferous tubules are the Sertoli cells. Declining testosterone levels also decrease Sertoli cell release of the hormone inhibin, which in turn stimulates release of FSH from the anterior pituitary. Rising levels of LH and FSH leads to spermatogenesis. LH stimulates Leydig cell production of steroids, primarily testosterone. FSH stimulates the Sertoli cells, which, among other functions, use the testosterone for spermatogenesis. As testosterone is used in spermatogenesis or for other functions, testosterone levels drop and the cycle is repeated.

One of the principal barriers to the development of male contraceptives is that the biochemical pathway requires inhibiting testosterone production and, consequently, spermatogenesis. Testosterone has many other functions, including protein synthesis, regulation of bone growth and establishing secondary male sexual characteristics. Hence, the side effects of inhibiting testosterone production have been a major barrier to development of a male hormonal contraceptive.

CONTRACEPTIVE TECHNOLOGY[1]

This section provides a brief guide to all contraceptive methods. In thinking about contraception, clients and health professionals should consider the following questions:

1. What is the mechanism of action? How does the contraceptive actually work? Misconceptions about how contraceptives act can serve as an unnecessary barrier to their use, so accurate information is important.
2. How effective is the contraceptive method? Women who are fecund, engaged in sexual union and not using any form of contraception run an 85 percent probability of becoming pregnant after one year. One key issue for all contraceptives is the degree to which they decrease this probability. Here we must be careful to distinguish between *perfect use*, which assumes the client uses the method exactly as needed to prevent pregnancy, and *typical use*, which looks at actual behavior and the consequences for efficacy. Generally speaking, the contraceptive methods described in this section are very effective when used perfectly, but typical use significantly lowers the efficacy of many methods. A somewhat different facet of effectiveness is *continuation*. While clients must have the option to stop using a contraceptive method, discontinuation is often due to side effects or inconvenience. Hence, the likelihood that clients will discontinue use is one aspect of effectiveness.
3. What are the advantages and disadvantages of the method? Efficacy is only one criterion in choosing a contraceptive method. Health providers and clients must also consider a variety of other factors, including:
    - Health impacts other than contraception; these can be positive or negative;
    - Ease of access;

TABLE 6-1. Risk of Mortality Due to Contraception

Method	Chance of dying in one year
Oral contraceptives (non-smoker, <35)	1 in 200,000
Oral contraceptives (non-smoker, >35)	1 in 28,600
Oral contraceptives (more than 25 cigarettes/day, <35)	1 in 5300
Oral contraceptives (more than 25 cigarettes/day, >35)	1 in 700
Intrauterine device	1 in 10,000,000
Diaphragm, condom or spermicides	None
Fertility awareness methods	None
Tubal ligation	1 in 38,500
Vasectomy	1 in 1,000,000

- Ease of use;
- Reversibility;
- Cost;
- Psychological aspects; e.g., enhancement/detraction of sexual relations

4. What key information must the client have to make an informed choice and use a method effectively? Good counseling and accurate, comprehensible information is essential to appropriate use of contraceptives.

The perfect contraceptive would be easily accessible by all clients, require very little to no effort by the user, have no unwanted side effects, provide some ancillary health benefits (such as protection against STD), be 100 percent effective, instantly reversible and low cost. No such contraceptive exists. The decision to use any method requires careful and informed choice that matches the characteristics of the method to the needs and desires of the client.

One critical point that deserves emphasis is that modern contraceptive methods are very safe and have been subject to extensive study. More than 73,000 studies have been carried out on oral contraceptives alone! Table 6-1, which shows the risk of death associated with each contraceptive method, is a good indication of the safety of contraceptives[2]. In considering this table, it is also very important to remember the significant *increases* in infant and maternal survival that could be achieved through spacing of births and avoidance of unintended pregnancy. By way of example, an African woman who becomes pregnant has a one in twenty chance of dying from complications of pregnancy or childbirth.

The discussion of each method includes a brief description, the mechanism of action, efficacy, benefits and risks, and key points in counseling clients.

Abstinence[3,4,5]

Description

The definition of abstinence varies. For purposes of *contraception*, abstinence means avoiding heterosexual vaginal intercourse. If the objective is *avoiding infection*, then abstinence must include refraining from vaginal, anal and oral–genital intercourse. Abstinence can therefore take many forms: abstaining from any form of sexual expression; avoiding contact with a partner's genitals; or engaging in sexual acts other than vaginal intercourse. The time frame for abstinence can also vary significantly—from as short as one day to many years.

Benefits and Risks

Strict observance of abstinence is 100 percent effective in preventing pregnancy. It is free and easily available. It is instantly reversible for clients who choose pregnancy. It does not require the use of any chemical or mechanical device. Individuals may choose abstinence for religious or ethical reasons. Others will find abstinence conducive to their psychological health and sense of well-being. Abstinence may be chosen to prevent sexually transmitted infections. Certain physical conditions may also induce people to avoid conventional intercourse, including sexually transmitted diseases; recovery from some forms of surgery; pelvic, urinary or vaginal tract infections; painful intercourse; gastrointestinal illnesses; the latter stages of pregnancy; the postpartum or post-abortion period; and recovery from myocardial infarction. Many adolescents choose to either postpone initiating sexual activity or return to abstinence after a period of sexual experimentation.

The potential for sexual frustration, consequent inability to adhere to abstinence and conflict between discordant partners are the main drawbacks to the method. Clients may wish to keep condoms and/or spermicides readily available should they choose to end a period of abstinence, though some may find this impedes rather than helps them remain abstinent.

Guidance to Clients

Like all family planning clients, people who choose abstinence need careful counseling and a plan of action for realizing their objectives. The following guidelines are useful in counseling clients choosing abstinence[6]:

- Ask them to develop, *clearly, soberly and in advance*, a personal definition of abstinence; i.e., what sexual activities they will engage in and which they will not accept;
- Advise them to discuss with the partner *in advance of a sexual encounter* what they will and won't do;
- Teach them how to negotiate effectively with a partner, including how to say no authoritatively;
- Provide essential information about reproductive health and contraception so they can make informed choices; and,
- Suggest they consider having an alternative means of contraception available, especially condoms, in case they change their minds in the "heat of the moment".

Withdrawal[7,8,9]

Description

Withdrawal or *coitus interruptus* is the removal of the penis from the vagina prior to ejaculation. Withdrawal is widely used as a method of contraception. In Turkey, it is the single most widely used method, employed by one out of four couples. Among 22 countries included in the Demographic and Health Surveys, ever-use of withdrawal ranged from less than one percent of women surveyed in Niger to almost 24 percent in Zambia. In eight countries, ever-use exceeded 15 percent. With the notable exception of Turkey, current use rarely exceeds 3 percent, indicating that withdrawal is often a first method before transitioning to other forms of contraception.

Efficacy

Though often presumed to be ineffective, the efficacy of withdrawal is actually comparable to that of barrier methods. Perfect use efficacy is estimated at 96 percent after one year of use, while typical use efficacy is about 81 percent.

Efficacy is largely dependent upon the ability of the man to control the moment of ejaculation, ensuring it takes place outside the vagina. Pre-ejaculate, which consists of lubricating fluid from the Cowper's glands, does not contain sperm. However, sperm from a previous ejaculation may remain in the urethra and become mixed into the secretions of the Cowper's glands. Pre-ejaculate, which goes unnoticed by both the man and the woman during intercourse, may therefore lead to pregnancy.

Benefits and Risks

Withdrawal is free, always available, involves no use of chemical or mechanical methods and has no side effects. The obvious risk is that a man may not withdraw in time, leading to pregnancy. Withdrawal does not provide protection STD, since open lesions or pre-ejaculate may contain infective agents.

Guidance to Clients

Clients should be advised of the importance of consistent and correct use. Withdrawal must be practiced at every act of intercourse and care must be taken that ejaculate does not land on the woman's genitalia. Men should urinate prior to intercourse and wipe off the tip of the penis to remove any sperm that may persist in the urethra from a prior ejaculation.

Fertility Awareness Methods[10,11,12]

Description

As discussed earlier, the menstrual cycle produces observable clues to ovulation and the fertile period. Most women have a discernable pattern of menses; while the cycle is not necessarily 28 days in length, many women can determine the normal length of their menstrual cycles. Body temperature reaches its cyclical low approximately 24 hours before ovulation and then begins to rise, peaking three days after ovulation. Cervical mucus during the period when fertilization can occur is generally thin, clear, sticky and of high volume.

There are four fertility awareness methods:

- *Calendar method* relies on calculating the days of the cycle during which fertilization is possible.
- *Basal body temperature method* uses shifts in body temperature to determine when ovulation has passed and intercourse is safe.
- *Cervical mucus method* requires the woman to feel for changes in the properties of mucus in the vagina to judge the period when intercourse is safe.
- *Symptothermal method* combines the other three approaches to provide multiple signs of the fertile and infertile periods.

CONTRACEPTION

Mechanism of Action

Conception can occur only if intercourse occurs during the six day period ending on the day of ovulation. Intercourse before this period will not leave viable sperm in the fallopian tubes for fertilization; later intercourse will not yield conception as the oocyte dies by 12 hours after ovulation if it is not fertilized. All of the fertility awareness methods rely on using observable signs to avoid intercourse during this six day period. Since the precise timing of ovulation is difficult to estimate by easily observable symptoms, all of the methods create a "buffer zone" around the estimated six day period to decrease the chances of pregnancy.

Efficacy

Fertility awareness methods can be a good choice for dedicated couples, since their use effectiveness is comparable to barrier methods. Perfect use failure rates for the first year are estimated at 9 percent for calendar method, 3 percent for cervical mucus method, 2 percent for basal body temperature and 2 to 3 percent for symptothermal method. Typical use for fertility awareness methods generally yields a 20 percent to 25 percent failure rate after the first year of use.

Guidance to Clients

All clients choosing a fertility awareness method should be given careful counseling as to how to use the method properly. The importance of correct and consistent use of the method must be stressed.

Clients choosing the calendar method should be instructed to keep a chart of the length of 6 to 12 cycles, recording the first day of menstrual bleeding as Day 1. Subtract 18 days from the length of the shortest cycle to find the first fertile day and subtract 11 days from the length of the longest menstrual cycle to find the last fertile day. For example, assume that after a ten month period the shortest cycle was 26 days and the longest cycle was 30 days. Beginning with first day of bleeding, the fertile period would be estimated as between Day 8 (26–18) and Day 19 (30–11). Intercourse should be avoided during the days 8 to 19 inclusive counting from the first day of menstrual bleeding.

Clients choosing the basal body temperature method should cease having intercourse on the day menstrual bleeding begins. Temperature should be recorded first thing upon awakening on each of the ten days following the beginning of menstruation. Note the highest temperature recorded during these ten days, excluding days of fever due to illness—this is called the "temperature line". Continue recording daily temperature upon awakening. When the daily temperature has exceeded the temperature line by at least $0.15°$ C for three days in succession, the fertile period has passed. Intercourse may occur from the evening of the third day until menstrual bleeding reappears.

Clients choosing the cervical mucus method must sample the mucus in the vaginal tract with their fingers to feel for moisture and consistency. Intercourse should be avoided during the menstrual period, since vaginal secretions will be hard to discern. A period of vaginal dryness, typically covering days 6 to 9 of the menstrual cycle, will then follow.

Intercourse may occur during this period of vaginal dryness. A period of abundant, slippery secretions will follow, usually from days 10 to 16. The woman must abstain from intercourse from the onset of the slippery secretions until four days after they end, which would be day 20 in a typical 28 day cycle. Intercourse may occur from day 21 until menstruation reappears.

Clients using the symptothermal method can use timing, temperature and vaginal secretions as "double-checks" to judge the fertile period. The coinciding of signs of the infertile period provides added assurance against the possibility of pregnancy.

Male Condoms[13,14,15]

Description

Condoms are sheaths made of latex, polyurethane or the intestinal caecum of lambs. The sheaths are placed over the erect penis and create a physical barrier to the passage of sperm. Only latex and polyurethane condoms create a barrier to the passage of many viruses, including HIV and hepatitis B. Lamb caecum condoms (also called "lambskin" or "natural membrane" condoms) are porous to viruses and therefore only suitable for use as contraceptives.

Some condom brands are treated with a spermicide, nonoxynol-9. There is little evidence that spermicidally treated condoms are more effective than untreated condoms in preventing pregnancy or infection. In addition, frequent use of treated condoms may irritate or ulcerate vaginal tissues, yielding them more susceptible to infection.

Efficacy

If condoms are used *perfectly*, they are highly effective as contraceptives, with a failure rate of only 3 percent. That is, if 100 couples used condoms consistently and correctly for one year, 3 of the women would become pregnant by the end of the year. However, the failure rate for typical use is about 14 percent, largely because of improper use of the condom. Condoms prevent many sexually transmitted diseases, but offer less protection against diseases, such as herpes or genital warts, that create lesions on the skin of the genital area that is not covered by the condom.

Common usage errors include failure to use a condom at every act of intercourse, placing the condom incorrectly on the penis, use of oil based lubricants that degrade latex, puncturing the condom with teeth or fingernails, failing to hold the condom in place during withdrawal after intercourse, and not wearing the condom throughout the act of intercourse.

Latex and polyurethane condoms rarely break if used properly, with most studies of condom use in vaginal intercourse showing breakage rates of less than 2 percent. Condoms are more likely to break if subjected to prolonged high temperatures, high humidity, sunlight or fluorescent light or coated with oil based lubricant. Slippage is somewhat more common— various studies of condom use during vaginal intercourse estimate that the condoms falls off the penis between 0.6 percent and 5.4 percent of the time, while partial slippage down the penile shaft occurs between 3.4 percent and 13.1 percent of the time.

Benefits and Risks

Condoms offer many advantages as a contraceptive device. They prevent many sexually transmitted diseases, as well as providing protection from unwanted pregnancy. They are very safe; except for those individuals with allergies to latex, there are no biological side effects. Use of the condom can be started at the discretion of the user, with no medical intervention needed. Condoms are usually easily accessible as they can be sold or distributed through a very wide array of outlets. Some people find that use of the condom increases sexual enjoyment because the condom prolongs intercourse due to decreased sensitivity, alleviates concerns about STD and pregnancy, and/or because placing the condom has been incorporated into foreplay.

Conversely, some people feel that the condom diminishes sexual enjoyment, because it interrupts the spontaneity of lovemaking, decreases male sensitivity, is messy and/or embarrassing to purchase, use or discuss. Many people associate condoms with STD, prostitution or infidelity. Reliance on the condom requires that a supply be available every time the partners wish to have sex. There is a preference for dry sex in some regions of the world and among some couples. Condoms are more likely to break during dry sex. A very small percentage of people are allergic to latex.

Guidance to Clients

Proper use of the condom is key to its effectiveness. Clients should be advised to:

- Use only latex or polyurethane condoms to avoid the risk of STD, including HIV.
- Keep a supply of condoms available and use a condom at EVERY act of intercourse.
- Put on the condom before the penis touches the vagina.
- Unroll the condom down to the base of the penis, while pinching the tip, leaving a small reservoir to contain the semen.
- Discard a condom if it is initially put on inside-out; reversing a condom that has touched the penis may expose the partner to sperm or infection.
- Avoid using oil-based lubricants with latex condoms (e.g., vegetable oils, mineral oil, petroleum jelly, suntan lotions, skin creams and lotions) and use only vaginal secretions or water-based lubricants (spermicides, glycerine, KY jelly, saliva, water).
- Keep the condom on throughout intercourse and hold the rim of the condom against the base of the penis during withdrawal.
- Dispose of the used condom properly and safely through burning, burial, placing in a pit latrine or in a secure trash receptacle.

Spermicides and Female Barrier Methods[16,17,18]

Description

Spermicides refer to a class of contraceptive gels, foams, creams, films, tablets and suppositories that are that are inserted vaginally and form a chemical barrier to the passage of sperm. Nonoxynol-9, octoxynol and benzalkonium chloride are among the most widely used active agents contained in spermicides. These agents typically act by breaking down the surface membrane of the sperm, thereby rendering it inactive.

Spermicides can be used alone, but are also commonly employed in conjunction with vaginal barrier methods. Vaginal barrier methods include:

- The *female condom*, marketed under the name the Reality Female Condom®, consists of a thin polyurethane sheath with a closed ring at one end and an open ring at the other. The female condom is inserted into the vagina with the closed end pressed against the cervix and the open end protruding from the vagina. The female condom is good for one-time use and can be inserted up to eight hours before intercourse. The female condom and the male condom are the only reliable barriers to the transmission of many sexually transmitted diseases, including HIV.
- The *diaphragm* is a dome-shaped, reusable latex device with a flexible ring at the base of the dome that rests against the cervix. The diaphragm provides a physical barrier to the passage of sperm that is enhanced by placing a spermicide inside the dome. The diaphragm provides contraceptive protection for up to six hours and must be left in place for six hours after intercourse. It should be removed within 24 hours of intercourse to avoid the risk of toxic shock syndrome.
- The *cervical cap* is made of rubber and rather resembles a thimble. Like the diaphragm, spermicide is placed inside the reusable cervical cap and the base of the cap is placed against the cervix, forming a physical and chemical barrier to the passage of sperm. The cervical cap provides contraceptive protection for forty-eight hours, but should not be kept in place for a longer period.
- The *sponge* is a pillow-shaped device impregnated with spermicide that rests against cervix. The sponge, which can only be used once, provides contraceptive protection for 24 hours and must be left in place for six hours after intercourse. The sponge should not be left in place for longer than 24 hours.

The male condom may be used in conjunction with the diaphragm, cervical cap or sponge to provide an extra measure contraceptive protection, as well as protection against sexually transmitted diseases. The male condom should not be used with the female condom, as the two devices adhere and both may become dislodged during intercourse.

Efficacy

Spermicides have a theoretical effectiveness of 94 percent; i.e., given correct and consistent use only 6 out of 100 women using spermicide for a year will become pregnant. In practice, spermicides are much less effective, with typical use effectiveness of 74 percent, largely due to the failure to use the spermicide correctly at every act of intercourse.

Vaginal barrier methods vary in efficacy, as shown in Table 6-2[19]. Because barrier methods require consistent and correct use at every act of intercourse, typical use rates are considerably higher than perfect use efficacy. For similar reasons, coital frequency affects efficacy, since a larger number of acts of intercourse increases the likelihood of user error. Parity also affects the efficacy of the cervical cap and sponge, both of which are less effective among women who have had children.

Benefits and Risks

Spermicides and barrier methods are, in general, quite safe and complications resulting from their use are relatively uncommon. Their principal benefit is placing control over use

TABLE 6-2. Typical Use Failure Rates of Vaginal Barrier Methods

Method	Typical use
Diaphragm	20
Female condom	21
Sponge (women having given birth)	40
Sponge (women with no births)	20
Cervical cap (women having given birth)	40
Cervical cap (women with no births)	20

of a method in the hands of the woman when the male partner is reluctant to use a condom. This is particularly advantageous to women who have only intermittent sexual relations. They also serve as a back-up method for women newly adopting hormonal contraceptives.

The female condom protects against bacterial STD and HIV. Spermicides may provide modest protection against some forms of bacterial STD, but not against HIV. The diaphragm is associated with a lower incidence of cervical cancer, since it may block the penetration of human papilloma virus.

The most common side effect of spermicides is irritation of the vaginal lining by the spermicidal agent (nonoxynol-9). This may actually increase the likelihood of HIV infection due to the increased vulnerability of the vaginal epithelium. Spermicide use alone or with barrier methods is associated with an increased risk of vaginal and urinary tract infections. In rare instances, vaginal barrier methods have been implicated as a contributing factor in toxic shock syndrome.

Spermicides and barrier methods may provoke an allergic reaction among women who have an allergy to latex, polyuretahane or spermicides.

Guidance to Clients

Women should wait 6 to 12 weeks after a birth or abortion before adopting a diaphragm or cervical cap to assure correct fitting of the devices. The diaphragm and cervical cap may be inappropriate for women with abnormalities of the vagina, cervix or uterus that would prevent fitting or retention of the devices. Women with a history of toxic shock syndrome should not use the diaphragm or cervical cap. Allergies to spermicides, latex or polyurethane would also preclude use of barrier methods and spermicides. Women with a medical condition that would make pregnancy particularly dangerous (e.g., heart disease, kidney disease, diabetes, hypertension) should be encouraged to consider more reliable methods.

Women should also carefully consider the probability of exposure to STD, including HIV. Of the woman controlled methods, only the female condom provides protection against STD/HIV. Women who believe they might be exposed to STD may wish to opt for the female condom if they cannot depend on use of the male condom.

Aside from the pospartum/post-abortion caution given above, women who can use spermicides and barrier methods may start using them at any time. Even if the woman is pregnant, there are no consequences for the fetus of using spermicides or barrier methods. Proper fitting of the diaphragm and cervical cap by the health provider is essential to their efficacy.

For all users of spermicides and barrier methods, the importance of correct and consistent use at every intercourse must be emphasized. Proper storage of spermicides must be emphasized as they degrade in hot weather, especially if exposed to moisture. If the spermicide is to be used alone, proper technique for use of the film, suppository, tablet, gel or foam product must be explained. Proper technique for inserting and removing a diaphragm or cervical cap should be explained and the client provided the opportunity to practice insertion and removal under the guidance of the health provider.

Clients should be alerted to the signs and symptoms of allergic reaction, vaginal irritation, urinary tract infection and toxic shock syndrome. Women experiencing such symptoms should seek prompt medical care. Women using the diaphragm or cervical cap should avoid use of oil based lubricants, which may degrade the latex. A substantial supply of spermicide should be provided upon adoption of the methods.

Combined Oral Contraceptives[20,21,22]

Description

Combined oral contraceptives (COCs) are pills containing a combination of estrogen and progestin. Many variants of the COC have been produced over the years and multiple brands are in the marketplace. The quantity of estrogen provided by a COC has declined over the years without loss of effectiveness. Today, a typical low-dose COC provides 30 or 35 micrograms (mcg) of ethinyl estradiol, an estrogen, plus a progestin. Ethinyl estradiol levels can vary from 20 mcg to 50 mcg. A few pills contain mestranol, which is converted to estrogen in the liver. Both the type and amount of progestin varies widely. COC are taken once daily for 21 days, followed by seven days of iron supplementation or respite, after which a new cycle of 21 COC pills is taken.

Mechanism of Action

COC induce three physiological effects that prevent pregnancy. First, they inhibit ovulation by inhibiting the release of FSH and LH. As was described earlier, FSH and LH must be released in sufficient quantity for the follicle to develop and for the ovum to be released from the follicle. The second effect of COC is to bring about changes in the properties of the endometrium, rendering it unsuitable to implantation in the event that the ovum is fertilized and reaches the uterine cavity. Third, and likely least important, is that sperm transport is inhibited through changes in the cervical mucous that mimic the luteal phase of the menstrual cycle.

COC do *not*, as is sometimes alleged, provoke abortions. Abortion is the removal of an implanted embryo or fetus from the uterus. Since the principal effect of COC is to inhibit ovulation, they prevent the development of a fertilized ovum. Secondarily, in the event of ovulation and fertilization, COC prevent implantation of the fertilized ovum, which usually occurs by the sixth day after fertilization.

Efficacy

COC are highly effective at preventing pregnancy when used properly. Perfect use of low-dose COC is 99.9 percent effective at preventing pregnancy (1 pregnancy per thousand women using the pill for a year), while typical use during the first year yields 95 percent effectiveness. However, discontinuation rates are relatively high, ranging from 25 percent to 50 percent after one year of use. Women choose to become pregnant, find the daily regimen of taking the pill inconvenient or expensive, have difficulty accessing COC on a regular basis, switch to another method, or experience side effects.

COC can also be used as a form of emergency contraception[23]. A woman who has sexual relations without benefit of contraception can take two high doses of COC. A first dose of 100–120 mcg of ethinyl estradiol within 72 hours after unprotected intercourse plus a second equal dose 12 hours later will inhibit ovulation. Administration of the emergency contraception regimen is unlikely to protect against pregnancy if ovulation has already occurred. Over all, use of COC for emergency contraception prevents 75 percent–80 percent of pregnancies that would otherwise have occurred.

Benefits and Risks

COC are a safe, effective form of contraception that have been widely studied over many years and in many contexts. COC are a sound option for most women, with the exception of those at high risk of cardiovascular disease, active liver disease or active breast cancer. In the general population, pregnancy carries a higher risk of mortality than use of COC.

COC have many beneficial health effects other than contraception. Women who use COC are less likely to develop ovarian or endometrial cancer, ovarian cysts, benign breast disease and symptomatic pelvic inflammatory disease (PID). Many women find that COC improve the menstrual cycle through decreased bleeding, reduced mid-cycle pain, lessened cramps and decreased premenstrual symptoms. The estrogen in COC tends to reduce low-density lipids and increase high-density lipids, and therefore may decrease the likelihood of developing atherosclerosis. Some women also experience benefits of decreased hirsutism and acne. COC may also provide protection against osteoporosis, endometriosis and rheumatoid arthritis.

The most important potential complication associated with COC use is exacerbating the likelihood that women with other risk factors will develop cardiovascular disease. Women who have significant risk factors for cardiovascular disease should not take COC. COC should therefore be avoided by women with heart or coronary artery disease, hypertension (blood pressure greater than 160/100), deep vein thrombosis, pulmonary embolism, severe headaches accompanied by focal neurological symptoms (vision problems, difficulty speaking or moving), or who are 35 and smoke more than twenty cigarettes per day.

COC may increase the likelihood of blood clots among women who are immobilized by injury or surgery. Therefore, women who experience prolonged immobilization, plan major surgery or undergo surgery on the legs should discuss COC use with their health provider.

COC may be a co-factor in the development of breast cancer among women under the age of 35, though this effect approaches zero by the time women reach age 55. Women who take COC are more likely to develop a benign liver tumor, though it must be emphasized that such tumors are rare. There is conflicting evidence as to whether COC increase the risk of liver and cervical cancer. Women with breast cancer or who have certain liver diseases (liver cancer, benign adenoma, viral hepatitis, severe cirrhosis) should not take COC.

COC increase the likelihood of chlamydial cervicitis in the event of exposure.

COC decrease milk supply during lactation and should not be used by women who are breastfeeding their children.

COC may hasten the development of gallbladder disease among women predisposed to such diseases.

Some women using COC will experience menstrual changes, nausea or vomiting, headaches, depression, decreased interest in sex, breast tenderness, increased facial pigmentation, acne, weight gain or hair loss. In many cases, these problems will resolve after a few cycles of pills have been completed.

There is no relationship between use of COC and malignant melanoma, kidney, colon or gallbladder cancer or pituitary tumors. COC do not have a significant impact on carbohydrate metabolism. COC do not cause birth defects, even if accidentally taken during the early stages of pregnancy.

There are a number of drugs that decrease the efficacy of COC, especially anticonvulsants, rifampin (used to treat tuberculosis and meningitis) and griseofulvin (used to treat fungal skin infections). Women taking these drugs should be advised to use a back-up method or switch to a different form of contraception

Guidance to Clients

Counseling with respect to COC use should focus on three basic issues: ensuring the client is an appropriate candidate for COC, ensuring correct use of COC and managing COC side effects.

Clients who meet one of the following conditions should not use COC:

- Age 35 or older and smokes cigarettes;
- Blood pressure in excess of 160/100;
- Breastfeeding or birth within the past 21 days;
- Cardiovascular disease;
- History of breast cancer;
- Liver disease;
- Severe headaches with focal neurological symptoms;
- Gallbladder disease;
- Diabetes accompanied by damage to vision, kidneys or nervous system;
- Pregnancy

A woman can start taking COC at any point during the menstrual cycle if she and the health provider are confident she is not pregnant. To protect against the possibility of pregnancy, it is best for the woman to begin taking COC on the first day of menstrual bleeding or during the first seven days after menstrual bleeding begins. COC may be started three to six weeks after childbirth if the woman is not breastfeeding, immediately after a miscarriage or abortion, or immediately upon stopping another contraceptive method. A back-up contraceptive method, such as condom or spermicide, should be used during the first seven days of COC use.

Clients should be given a generous supply of pills at the time of initial consultation – up to twelve cycles if local regulations allow. There is no reason to withhold pill cycles. Emphasis should be placed on good counseling and ensuring access to a qualified provider if management of side effects is needed.

COC are distributed in packs containing 21 or 28 pills. Both contain 21 COC pills, with the client expected to take one pill every day at the same time. The remaining seven pills in the 28 pill pack are an iron supplement, such as ferrous fumarate, or a placebo.

CONTRACEPTION

Many women find it easier to take a pill every day, rather than stopping for seven days and remembering to start a new cycle. COC compliance is often made easier by associating the pill with the woman's daily routine; e.g., taking a pill right after brushing her teeth in the morning or at bedtime.

Women using the 28-pill pack should finish the 21-day cycle of COC pills and then take one of the seven iron supplement pills or placebos each day. A new cycle of pills should then be started. Women using the 21-pill pack should take one COC pill each day for 21 days, stop taking pills for seven days and then start a new cycle.

A woman who forgets to take one COC pill should take the pill as soon as she remembers and then take the rest of the cycle normally. This may mean taking two pills on the same day or two at the same time.

A woman who forgets to take two or more COC pills must use a back-up contraceptive method for seven days. If the omission of two or more pills occurred during the first 14 days of the 21-day COC cycle, simply resume taking one pill per day. If the omission of the two or more pills occurs during the last seven days of the 21-day COC cycle, resume taking the pills once daily but do not allow a seven day respite after completing the cycle. Begin a new 21-day COC cycle immediately.

Omitting the iron supplement pills has no effect on the effectiveness of COC. A woman who forgets to take the iron supplement pills should simply throw the missed pills away.

It is very important that women receive accurate, comprehensible information about side effects of COC. Failure to advise women in advance of common side effects is a major reason for discontinuation. Common side effects include mild headaches, nausea, mood changes, breast tenderness, spotting between periods and irregular bleeding. These effects are not symptoms of a serious health problem. Women experiencing these side effects should be advised to take the COC pill at the same time each day and that the side effects usually disappear after a few months. If symptoms persist, then alternative COC formulations or another contraceptive method should be considered.

Potentially serious side effects of COC that may indicate severe disease can be summarized using the mnemonic ACHES:[24]

- Abdominal pain (severe);
- Chest pain (severe cough, shortness of breath, sharp pain on breathing in);
- Headaches (severe), dizziness, weakness, numbness, especially if one-sided;
- Eye problems (vision loss or blurring), speech problems;
- Severe pain in calf or thigh

Women experiencing one of the ACHES symptoms should consult a qualified clinician immediately, who may advise switching to another contraceptive method.

Progestin-Only Oral Contraceptives[25,26,27]

Description

Progestin-only pills (POP) are one of a class of contraceptives that rely on very low doses of synthetic progesterone to prevent pregnancy. A single POP would typically contain .03 mg of levonorgestrel or .35 mg. norethindrone. POP are taken every day, without respite.

The POP and other forms of progestin-only contraception are particularly well-suited for lactating women, since they have no effect on milk supply once lactation is established.

POP can also be used as a form of emergency contraception. The recommended dosage is .75 mg. of levonorgestrel within 72 hours of intercourse, followed by a second, equal dose 12 hours later.

Mechanism of Action

Like COC, POP prevent pregnancy by inhibiting ovulation, diminishing transport of the ovum through the fallopian tube, decreasing sperm transport and changing the character of the endometrium. In short, POP prevent the development of a fertilized ovum or its implantation. Progestin-only methods are not abortifacients

Efficacy

POP are slightly less effective than COC under conditions of perfect use: 99.5 percent versus 99.9 percent efficacy. Under conditions of typical use, first-year pregnancy rates range from about 1 percent to about 13 percent. The efficacy of POP are enhanced among lactating women due to the additional contraceptive effect of lactation.

Benefits and Risks

There are a number of benefits common to all progestin-only methods, including:

- Suitability for lactating women
- Absence of estrogen induced side effects associated with COC, including potential cardiovascular complications;
- Decreased risk, compared to non-contracepting women, of endometrial and ovarian cancer, benign breast disease and pelvic inflammatory disease;
- Decreased risk of ectopic pregnancy; and,
- Reduced menses and menstrual pain.

Some women will also experience decreased breast tenderness and premenstrual symptoms.

For women who are not breastfeeding, the most common side effects are irregularity in the menstrual cycle. Women may experience bleeding at various times during the cycle, amenorrhea or, less commonly, heavy bleeding at menstruation. These side effects are not serious from a medical point of view and do not indicate underlying disease. Nonetheless, they can prove very discomfiting to the client, especially where regularity of menses has psychological or cultural significance.

Another potentially important disadvantage of POP is that they demand rigorous adherence to a schedule—the pills must be taken at about the same time every day. Even a few hours delay can decrease efficacy, while COC are much more forgiving of client forgetfulness.

POP reduce the likelihood of ectopic pregnancies compared to non-contracepting women. However, a woman who does become pregnant while using POP is significantly more likely to experience an ectopic pregnancy. Hence, POP users must be counseled as to the warning signs of ectopic pregnancy.

In addition to menstrual cycle disturbances, some women will experience weight gain, breast tenderness or depression while taking POP. Women using POP are at increased risk of ovarian cysts, most of which will spontaneously regress.

As is the case with COC, certain medications decrease the efficacy of POP. Women taking anticonvulsants, rifampin or griseofulvin should not use POP.

Guidance to Clients

POP are a safe, effective form of contraception for women who can comply with necessary daily regiment and want an easily reversible method. POP are particularly indicated for women who are breastfeeding or who want to avoid a contraceptive containing estrogen.

Women meeting any of the following conditions should *not* take POP:

- History of breast cancer;
- Liver disease;
- Breastfeeding a child less than six weeks old;
- Pregnancy

Women who are taking anti-seizure medication, rifampin or griseofulvin can take POP, but should use also use condoms or spermicides as a back-up.

A woman can start taking POP at any point during the menstrual cycle if she and the health provider are confident she is not pregnant. To protect against the possibility of pregnancy, it is best for the woman to begin taking POP on the first day of menstrual bleeding or during the first five days after menstrual bleeding begins. POP may be started immediately after childbirth if the woman is not breastfeeding, immediately after a miscarriage or abortion, or immediately upon stopping another contraceptive method. A back-up contraceptive method, such as abstinence, condom or spermicide, should be used during the first cycle of POP use. Clients should be given a generous supply of pills at the time of initial consultation.

Women should be advised as to the importance of taking a pill every day at the same time. Unlike COC, there is no respite between POP cycles—a hormonal pill must be taken every day. A woman who forgets to take one POP pill should take the pill as soon as she remembers and then take the rest of the cycle normally. This may mean taking two pills on the same day or two at the same time. She should use a back-up method of contraception for at least 48 hours.

If a woman misses more than one pill she should take two pills every day until she "catches up" and can return to a one pill per day pattern. She should be certain to use abstinence, condoms or spermicides for at least 48 hours until the contraceptive effect of the POP is re-established. If she had unprotected intercourse and her period does not appear within 4–6 weeks she should seek a pregnancy test.

Women should be counseled in advance as to common side effects, especially menstrual cycle disturbances, and reassured that such disturbances are not harmful or symptomatic of serious illness.

Women should also be advised of symptoms that may signal a serious medical condition warranting a change in contraceptive method. These include:

- Severe lower abdominal pain, which may signal ovarian cysts or ectopic pregnancy;
- Severe, repeated headaches that begin or worsen after POP are started;
- Jaundice;
- Very heavy vaginal bleeding; i.e., twice as much or as long as a "normal" menstruation;
- Suspected pregnancy

Progestin Injection Contraceptives[28,29,30]

Description

There are three basic variants of the injectable contraceptive, which provide, respectively, 13 weeks, eight weeks and four weeks of contraceptive protection.

The DMPA injectable contraceptive, usually sold under the trade name Depo-Provera®, consists of a 150 mg. injection of depot-medroxyprogesterone acetate, a synthetic progesterone that provides reliable contraceptive protection for thirteen weeks, though its actual protective effect may extend up to 17 weeks.

The NET-EN injectable contraceptive, commonly marketed under the trade name Noristerat®, consists of a 200 mg. injection of norethindrone enanthate or norethisterone enanthate. NET-EN provides eight weeks of contraceptive protection, though the protective effect probably extends to ten weeks. The use, benefits and risks of NET-EN are very similar to DMPA, though it is somewhat less likely to induce amenorrhea.

A one-month form of injectable contraceptives, marketed under the trade names Cyclofem™ (formerly Cycloprovera) and Mesigyna®, is also available. The one-month variant is a combined contraceptive, containing both estrogen and progestin and is similar in its action to COC. Cyclofem combines DMPA with an estrogen, while Mesigyna combines NET-EN with an estrogen.

The following discussion is limited to the progestin-only contraceptives and does not consider the combined injectable contraceptive.

Mechanism of Action

Like POP, progestin injection contraceptives (PIC) act primarily by suppressing ovulation and inhibiting implantation through changes in the endometrium. PIC also inhibit sperm transport through changes in the cervical mucous and slowed transport in the fallopian tubes.

Efficacy

PIC are highly effective. Only about 0.3 percent of women using DMPA for a full year will experience a pregnancy. PIC take effect in less than twenty-four hours. A study of U.S. users of DMPA found a one-year continuation rate of just under 60 percent.

Benefits and Risks

Like POP, PIC do not have any estrogen side effects, such as the potential for exacerbating cardiovascular problems or suppressing milk production. They are more accessible and discreet than many other forms of contraception, since they require contact with a health provider only four times per year. In some cultures a woman may have to hide taking a

CONTRACEPTION

daily contraceptive pill, while an injection can be secured without the knowledge of other household members.

PIC decrease the risk of endometrial cancer, benign breast disease, sickle cell crises, ectopic pregnancy and pelvic inflammatory disease. PIC may also decrease anemia, menstrual bleeding and menstrual cramps.

The most common side effect of PIC is menstrual cycle disturbance. Over half of women using PIC will experience a period of amenorrhea and many will have spotting and bleeding between periods. In rare cases, women experience excessive vaginal bleeding. Weight gain is common and some women experience a period of mild headaches or breast tenderness. Upon cessation of DMPA, return to fertility takes an average of ten months and may be delayed by as much as twelve months.

Guidance to Clients

PIC should *not* be taken by women who are pregnant, breastfeeding an infant less than six weeks old, have cardiovascular disease, a history of breast cancer, diabetes with complications, or liver disease.

As is true for all hormonal methods, women who are pregnant or suspect they may be pregnant should not use PIC. To protect against the possibility of pregnancy, it is preferable to give the first injection of PIC during the first seven days of the menstrual cycle, within the first six weeks postpartum if the woman is not breastfeeding or within the first seven days after a miscarriage or abortion. An eligible woman may start PIC at any other time she is reasonably certain she is not pregnant.

Women should be advised of possible side effects and reassured that the most common side effects are transient and harmless.

Women should be advised to seek immediate medical attention if any of the following occur:

- Severe lower abdominal pain, which may signal ovarian cysts or ectopic pregnancy;
- Severe, repeated headaches that begin or worsen after PIC are started;
- Jaundice;
- Very heavy vaginal bleeding; i.e., twice as much or as long as a "normal" menstruation;
- Persistent pain, pus or bleeding at injection site;
- Suspected pregnancy

Contraceptive Implants[31,32,33,34]

Description

Contraceptive implants are another form of progestin-only contraceptive and come in two forms. Norplant® consists of six silicone tubes, each 34 mm. long and 2.4 mm in diameter, filled with levonorgestrel. Each Norplant® rod contains 36 mg. of levonorgestrel and is about the size of a matchstick. Jadelle® levonorgestrel rod implants consist of two silicone tubes containing 75 mg. each of levonorgestrel; each tube is 43 mm. long and 2.5 mm in diameter. In both cases, the tubes are surgically implanted into the underside of the upper arm. Norplant® preceded the Jadelle® Rods and there is substantially more field experience with Norplant® as of this writing. Progestin diffuses slowly through the walls of the silicone tubes.

The surgical procedure involves making a small incision (2 to 3 mm) in the upper arm under local anesthetic. The six Norplant® tubes are inserted in a fan like array under the skin through this single incision. A skilled provider can complete the insertion procedure in about ten minutes. Norplant® must also be removed surgically using local anesthesia. Because adhesions to the tubes form, the removal process is somewhat lengthier and more complex than insertion; removal can take as long as one hour, though techniques have been developed to greatly reduce removal time by experienced providers.

In the case of Jadelle® Rods, the two tubes are inserted in a similar manner, though the two tubes rest parallel upon insertion. Because two rather than six tubes are involved, insertion and removal of Jadelle® Rods is easier as compared to Norplant®.

Mechanism of Action

The mechanism of action of implants is similar to that of other progestin-only methods. Ovulation is suppressed in at least half the cycles. Progestin induced changes in the endometrium prevent implantation in the event the ovum is fertilized. Sperm transport through the cervix and the fallopian tubes is also inhibited.

Efficacy

Implants are extremely effective. Both the Norplant® and Jadelle® rods have a typical failure rate of 0.1 percent during the first year of use. Norplant® is effective for five years, with a five year cumulative pregnancy rate of 1.6 percent. The efficacy of Norplant® declines somewhat among women weighing more than 154 pounds, with a recorded cumulative five year pregnancy rate of 2.4 percent in this group. Jadelle® Rods are effective for at least three years; efficacy does not appear to be affected by the weight of the woman.

Continuation rates for implants are very high. Typically, one year continuation rates for Norplant® range from 76 percent to 90 percent, while half retain the implant for three years. Clinical trials found that 88 percent retained Jadelle® after one year and 61 percent after three years.

Benefits and Risks

Implants offer the same non-contraceptive benefits as PIC. Lactation is unaffected and there are no estrogen induced complications. Protection is provided against endometrial cancer, benign breast disease, ectopic pregnancy and some causes of PID. Implants may yield improvements in menstrual bleeding, menstrual cramps and anemia.

Implants tend to disrupt the menstrual cycle, which is the source of the most common client complaint about the method. Bleeding and spotting between periods and amenorrhea are a frequent side effect of implants. Some women will also experience headaches, enlargement of ovaries or ovarian cysts, dizziness, breast tenderness, nervousness, nausea, acne, weight gain or hirsutism. Though pregnancies are very rare while using implants, there is a high risk they will be ectopic (1 in 6).

Implants also have the disadvantage that the client is dependent upon access to a skilled provider to start or stop the method. This removes a measure of control for the woman that may be deleterious in some settings. Programs offering implants must be certain to guarantee that women can freely and meaningfully decide to accept, reject or cease any contraceptive method, including implants.

Like any surgical procedure, there is some discomfort associated with insertion of implants, as well as the danger of infection if proper procedure is not observed.

Guidance to Clients

While implants are safe and effective, many women experience side effects, especially menstrual cycle disturbances. It is therefore very important that women receive accurate, complete and comprehensible information before choosing implants or any other contraceptive method. Failure to prepare clients for possible side effects prior to insertion as part of an informed consent procedure is unethical, heightens client dissatisfaction, and increases the likelihood of discontinuation.

Women who are pregnant, breastfeeding a baby less than six weeks old, have active liver disease, a history of breast cancer or unexplained vaginal bleeding should *not* use Norplant® or Jadelle® Rods.

To protect against the possibility of pregnancy, it is best to insert implants during the first seven days after menstrual bleeding starts, within the first six weeks after childbirth if the woman is not breastfeeding, within the first six months if she is fully breastfeeding, within seven days of an abortion or miscarriage or immediately after stopping another contraceptive method. Eligible women may adopt implants at any time it is reasonably certain they are not pregnant.

Women taking anticonvulsants, rifampin or griseofulvin should use a back-up contraceptive method.

Women should be advised to keep the insertion site dry for four days and retain the adhesive bandage for five days and that a few days of soreness at the insertion site is normal. Prolonged soreness or other evidence of infection at the insertion site requires prompt medical attention.

A back-up method of contraception should be used for the first forty-eight hours after insertion.

A woman using an implant should seek immediate medical assistance if the insertion site appears infected, she believes she is pregnant, experiences severe lower abdominal pain, has very bad headaches, has very heavy menstrual bleeding or becomes jaundiced.

It is very important that women be provided with some means of remembering when the effective period for the implant has ended (three years after insertion for Jadelle® Rods and five years for Norplant®). This may involve giving her a plastic record she can keep or linking the end date with a memorable event, such as a child's birthday. Program managers must be certain that women will have ready access to providers who can remove the implant before beginning insertions.

Intrauterine Devices[35,36,37]

Description

Intrauterine devices (IUD) are small devices that are inserted in the uterus. A short string is appended to most IUD that protrudes from the cervical os into the vaginal canal.

There are three types of IUD:

- Unmedicated devices, which include the plastic Lippes Loop and Saf-T-Coil or a stainless steel ring. Unmedicated devices are no longer distributed outside of China and so are not discussed here.
- Copper-releasing devices, which have copper wire or a copper sleeve wrapped around a plastic core. Minute amounts of copper are continually released from the IUD. Among the most widely used copper releasing IUD are the Copper T 380A, Copper T 220C, Nova T, Multiload 375 and Multiload 250. Some variants of the IUD add silver to the copper, which appears to increase efficacy.
- Progestin-releasing devices, which include the Progestasert IUD and the LNg20 IUD. These consist of T-shaped devices that hold a reservoir of progestin in the vertical stem. A small amount of progestin is steadily released from the tube; 65 mcg/day of progestin is released from the Progestasert IUD and 20 mcg/day of levonorgestrel from the LNg IUD. Because these forms of the IUD are relatively expensive, they are rarely used in developing countries.

IUD are widely and successfully used as a contraceptive method; in 1995 over 106 million women were using an IUD.

Mechanism of Action

The primary mechanism of action for the copper-releasing IUD is prevention of fertilization. Copper IUD appear to inhibit sperm transport and damage sperm and ova in ways that prevent fertilization. Progestin-releasing IUD have a local, rather than systemic effect on progesterone levels. Changes in uterine levels of progesterone are believed to inhibit sperm transport through thickening of cervical mucous thereby preventing fertilization and/or to induce changes in the endometrial lining that prevent implantation. IUD are therefore not abortifacients.

Efficacy

Intrauterine devices are extremely effective contraceptives. The one year pregnancy rate for the Copper T 380A is only 0.7 percent and the cumulative seven year probability of pregnancy is only 1.7 percent. The LNg20 IUD has a one year pregnancy rate of just 0.1 percent and a cumulative seven year pregnancy rate of 1.1 percent. The Progestasert IUD has a one year pregnancy rate of 2.0 percent.

Continuation rates for the IUD are high compared to other reversible methods. For the Copper T 380A, the continuation rate is 77 percent after the first year of use, declining to a cumulative drop-out rate of 23 percent by the end of the third year.

The Copper T 380A remains effective for ten years, while the efficacy of the LNg20 IUD is effective for five years. The Progestasert IUD is only effective for one year and must be replaced every twelve months.

Benefits and Risks

Intrauterine devices are very effective and very safe for most women. Women who should not use hormonal contraceptives may benefit from the copper IUD. Estrogen, with its attendant potential side effects, is absent from both copper-releasing and progestin-releasing IUD. Once the IUD is inserted, little additional action by the client is needed to ensure safe, effective use. The LNg20 IUD is an effective treatment for excessively long menstrual bleeding (menorrhagia) and can prevent and treat Asherman's syndrome, a condition in which adhesions between the walls of the uterus develop.

The greatest health concern associated with the IUD is pelvic inflammatory disease (PID). Narrowly defined, PID is an infection of the fallopian tubes (salpingitis) usually caused by chlamydia or gonorrhea, though other infectious agents may be involved. The term PID is often used more broadly to encompass associated infections of the ovaries, uterus and peritoneal cavity. During the 1970s, there was significantly increased risk of IUD-associated PID, which was largely attributable to the now banned Dalkon Shield. The Dalkon Shield used a tailstring susceptible to capture and transport bacteria; no IUD now uses a tailstring with similar properties.

Currently, any increased risk of PID associated with IUD use is attributable to poor insertion technique, the presence of an STD at the time of insertion or exposure to sexually transmitted infections subsequent to insertion. Studies of women who have had an IUD inserted show that the increased risk of PID largely disappears after the first twenty days following insertion. Hence, careful practice of aseptic technique during IUD insertion and proper selection of suitable candidates for the IUD can largely eliminate the increased risk of PID. Women who are in a mutually monogamous relationship with an uninfected partner are ideal candidates for the IUD.

Women using only an IUD are at greater risk of being infected with an STD than women using a barrier or hormonal method. Women using the LNg20 IUD are at less risk of PID than women using a copper-releasing IUD, possibly due to the protective effect of the thickened cervical mucous engendered by progestins. Women who practice risky sexual behaviors or who have partners at risk of STD should use condoms consistently.

Pregnant women and women with any cancer of the reproductive tract, active genital tract infections, current or recent PID, a recent septic abortion, uterine abnormalities or fibroids that distort the uterus, unexplained vaginal bleeding or pelvic tuberculosis should not use an IUD. Since copper-releasing IUD increase menstrual bleeding, caution should be exercised in managing a client with anemia; if a copper-releasing IUD is selected anemia treatment is important. Progestin-releasing IUD actually decrease menstrual bleeding and may be indicated for women with anemia. A very small number of women suffer from Wilson's disease, which is an inability to properly metabolize copper; women afflicted with Wilson's disease should not use a copper-releasing IUD.

Between 2 percent and 10 percent of women will expel the IUD during the first year of use. This rate rises to 30 percent among women who have previously experienced an IUD expulsion.

Though IUD are very effective, a woman who becomes pregnant while carrying an IUD should have the IUD removed immediately. IUD significantly increase the risk of spontaneous abortion and PID during pregnancy. Pregnancies that occur to IUD users are also more likely to be ectopic.

Other than PID, expulsion or the rare case of pregnancy, women with an IUD may experience the following complications:

- Spotting, bleeding, anemia or hemorrhage;
- Cramping and pain, which usually disappear shortly after insertion, but may indicate more serious problems if prolonged or severe;
- Missing strings (which may indicate expulsion) or too long strings that irritate the partner;

- Perforation or embedding of the IUD in the uterine wall or through the cervix, which happens in about 0.1 percent of insertions;
- Genital actinomycosis, a bacterial infection which can, in an unusual cases, lead to PID.

The likelihood of serious complications from an IUD can be greatly reduced by ensuring that providers are properly trained, equipped and supervised. Women experiencing complications must have access to clinical assessment and attention. Hence, family planning managers must ensure that women have access to competent and adequately equipped providers for insertion, follow-up care and removal.

Guidance to Clients

Potential clients should be given accurate and comprehensible information about the IUD as one contraceptive option. Clients should be carefully screened to be certain there are no conditions that would preclude use of the IUD.

An IUD may be inserted at any point during the menstrual cycle provided the client and the provider are reasonably certain the woman is not pregnant. Insertion may take place within 48 hours after childbirth *if the provider has received special training in postpartum insertion.* Otherwise, copper-releasing IUD may be inserted four weeks after childbirth and progestin-releasing IUD six weeks after childbirth. Insertion may also occur immediately after an abortion or miscarriage provided there is no evidence of infection.

Women receiving an IUD should be advised of the type of IUD inserted, the duration of the IUD's efficacy and a written record on which this information is recorded. A woman receiving an IUD should be given the following information:

- She should return for a follow-up visit three to six weeks after insertion and at any time she has concerns about her IUD.
- She should check for the tailstring once a week during the first month, and after her menstrual period thereafter to be sure the IUD is still in place; medical attention should be sought if the string cannot be felt or is noticeably shorter.
- Some increase in menstrual flow, menstrual cramping, spotting between periods and mucous discharge are common during the first two to three months following IUD insertion.
- A missed period may indicate a pregnancy and requires immediate medical attention.
- Severe lower abdominal pain may indicate an ectopic pregnancy and requires immediate medical attention.
- Fever, chills, pelvic pain or tenderness, severe cramping or unusual vaginal bleeding may indicate PID.
- Possible exposure to a sexually transmitted disease increases the risk of PID.
- Health care providers should be informed that she has an IUD.

Female Sterilization[38,39,40]

Description

Female sterilization is a surgical procedure that prevents the joining of sperm and ovum in the fallopian tubes by cutting or blocking the tubes. There are two basic surgical procedures that are used to carry out female sterilization: minilaparotomy and laparascopy.

Minilaparotomy is carried out by making a small incision under local anesthesia just above the public hair line. The incision site will be higher if sterilization occurs in the post-abortion period and just below the navel if carried out in the 2 days following a birth. An instrument called an elevator is inserted vaginally into the cervix and used to move the uterus and fallopian tubes into position. The physician then grasps the fallopian tubes with a surgical hook or forceps and occludes the tubes.

Laparoscopy involves the insertion of a laparoscope into the abdomen through a small incision below the navel. The laparoscope is a stainless steel tube that has lenses permitting visualization of the internal organs and through which instruments are passed. Laparoscopy is done under general or local anesthesia.

To provide a clear line of sight and room to maneuver the instruments, the abdomen is inflated with a nitorus oxide, carbon dioxide or room air through a specially designed needle that is inserted into the abdominal cavity. Once the abdomen has been expanded, the physician inserts the laparoscope. Instruments are then passed through the laparoscope to grasp and occlude the fallopian tubes.

There are a number of different techniques for occluding the fallopian tubes. These include excising a portion of the tubes, placing a clip or ring on the tubes and electrocoagulation. Excision of a portion of the tubes is most commonly used with minilaparotomy, while a clip, ring or electrocoagulation is usually used with laparoscopy.

Whether to use minilaparotomy or laparoscopy depends upon the condition of the woman and the options available through the local health system. Laparoscopy is generally less painful and more convenient to the client and less apt to result in complications. Minilaparotomy is precluded when the fallopian tubes cannot be easily moved due to adhesions or visualized using the uterine elevator, such as when the woman is obese. However, minilaparotomy is technically simpler. Laparoscopy demands more in the way of specialized training, equipment and operating room facilities. Laparoscopy is also precluded in the immediate postpartum period.

Other sterilization techniques are available, such as the use of chemicals that block or scar the fallopian tubes and transcervical procedures. These are not yet demonstrated to be safe and effective. Hysterectomy should not be used as a contraceptive method, since it is less safe than minilaparotomy or laparoscopy.

Efficacy

Female sterilization is highly effective. While there are variations depending on the occlusion technique used, only about 0.5 percent of women undergoing a sterilization procedure will become pregnant by the end of the first year. A study that followed 10,685 women with tubal ligations for between 8 and 14 years showed that 143 women (1.3 percent) eventually became pregnant.[41]

Contraceptive failures associated with female sterilization are most commonly due to poor surgical technique (30 percent to 50 percent), pregnancy at the time of sterilization, failure of laparoscopy equipment, tears in the fallopian tubes when using electrocoagulation and spontaneous reconnecting of the cut ends of the tubes.

Benefits and Risks

Female sterilization is quite safe, with an estimated developing country mortality rate of 4.7 per 100,000 procedures. By way of comparison, there are 630 maternal deaths for every 100,000 births in the developing world. In addition to being highly effective, it requires no additional behaviors by the client or the partner. It is very cost effective, though the initial outlay can be high. There are no known long term negative health consequences.

Female sterilization should be considered permanent. Reversal is technically complex, uncertain, expensive and, for practical purposes, inaccessible in much of the world. The permanence of sterilization can be advantageous in that it frees the woman (and couple) from ever worrying about contraception. Conversely, hasty decisions or changing life circumstances may lead to client regret over a choice that cannot be reversed. Therefore, good counseling and informed consent are critical before performing sterilization.

Short-term complications are unusual but may arise as a result of the surgical procedure, including infection, damage to internal organs or reaction to the anesthesia. Proper surgical technique, including scrupulous asepsis, can help avoid most of these complications. Clients should be advised of the warning signs of surgical complications (see below) and health managers must be sure that health providers are trained and equipped to manage complications should they arise.

Pregnancies among women who have undergone a sterilization procedure carry a high risk of being ectopic pregnancies. Therefore, women who suspect pregnancy must seek immediate medical attention.

Guidance to Clients

Because of the permanence of sterilization, extra effort is needed to be certain potential clients understand the method and that informed consent is obtained. Clients should know the benefits, risks and alternatives. They should never be coerced or pushed into accepting sterilization. A complete explanation of the procedure must be provided and informed consent documented. Questions from the client should be encouraged and answered respectfully.

Most women can safely adopt sterilization. There is no medical condition that permanently precludes a woman from securing a tubal ligation. However, there are a number of health conditions that must be managed before sterilization is carried out or that may complicate the sterilization procedure. These include a number of cardiovascular conditions, obstetric and gynecological problems and chronic diseases, such as AIDS, liver disease and severe iron deficiency anemia. Potential sterilization clients must be properly screened to identify relevant health conditions that may require delay, referral or caution to be sure that such health problems are being properly managed.

Women should be given proper preoperative guidance, including the importance of washing the area between the navel and pubis, avoiding food and drink for eight hours before surgery, preparing for a period of pain and low workload, and the need for companionship and support for the trip home.

Postoperative instructions should focus on the need for rest, pain management and symptoms of infection. Women should return immediately if there is persistent or increasing pain, pus, fever or bleeding or fluid from the site of the incision. A missed period or severe lower abdominal pain may signal an ectopic pregnancy and requires immediate medical attention.

Vasectomy[42,43,44]

Description

Vasectomy is a surgical procedure in which the vas deferens is cut and occluded, thereby preventing transport of the sperm through the male reproductive tract. There are two basic variants of the vasectomy: conventional and no-scalpel.

The *conventional* procedure involves making one or two small incisions in the scrotum under local anesthesia using a scalpel. A small portion of the vas deferens is lifted through the incision and severed. The ends are then occluded using ligature or elecrocoagulation. The incision is closed using an absorbable suture.

The *no-scalpel* procedure was pioneered in China, where more than nine million men have undergone vasectomy. After application of local anesthesia, the vas deferens are grasped through the skin of the scrotum by a specially designed ring forceps. These hold the vasa in place, while a very small incision is made using sharp-tipped dissecting forceps. The vas deferens are then cut and occluded. Because the wound is so small, no sutures are used to close the wound.

Efficacy

The probability of a pregnancy during the first year after vasectomy is quite low, ranging from 0.1 percent to 0.15 percent. After a vasectomy, residual sperm can be found in the upper portion of the vas deferens and in the urethra. About 20 ejaculations are needed to clear the remaining sperm. The most common cause of vasectomy "failure" is unprotected intercourse prior to clearing the remaining sperm. Men should be counseled to use a condom or another family planning method until the remaining sperm have been cleared.

Vasectomy failure can also occur as a result of poor surgical technique, spontaneous recanalization of the vas deferens or the presence of an undetected additional vas deferens that appears in rare instances as a congenital anomaly.

Benefits and Risks

Vasectomy is a simple, safe and effective surgical procedure. The most serious risk of vasectomy is client regret over opting for a method that is, for practical purposes, irreversible in the developing world. Accordingly, the main consideration in providing a vasectomy is ensuring that the man clearly understands that vasectomy should be considered a permanent method of contraception and that this meets his needs.

In a small percentage of cases (< 3 percent), men may experience complications from the vasectomy. Possible complications include infection, hematoma from leakage of blood as a result of the procedure, granulomas (inflamed tissue mass) associated with sperm leakage from the cut end of the vas deferens and swelling of the epididymis. Some of these conditions, such as most hematoma and granuloma, will spontaneously resolve, while others will require medical intervention.

Vasectomy does not have any negative effect on sexual desire or performance or on secondary sex characteristics.

Guidance to Clients

Informed consent is critical. As is the case for female sterilization, there is very little possibility of a client in the developing country being able to effect a vasectomy reversal. Clients must understand the permanence of the method and their alternatives. Clients must be provided with comprehensible information about the risks and benefits and benefits of vasectomy.

Most men can safely opt for vasectomy. However, certain conditions must be treated before a vasectomy is provided or require special management. Men with an active STD; infections of the penis, testicles or scrotum; acute systemic infection, significant gastroenteritis, filariasis or elephantiasis need treatment before a vasectomy is carried out. Men with a inguinal hernia (hernia of the groin), undescended testicles on both sides, AIDS or coagulation disorders need special handling and so should be treated only by physicians with appropriate capacity.

Clients should be provided with preoperative and postoperative instructions. Men should clip their scrotal hair, wash the genital area thoroughly and wear clean, loose-fitting clothing on the day of the procedure. They should not take any medication during the 24 hours prior to undergoing vasectomy without consulting the health provider.

Men should be advised that a period of discomfort lasting 2 to 3 days will follow the procedure, often accompanied by swelling, bruising, bleeding and pain. At least two days of rest are needed following the procedure and heavy lifting or strenuous exercise should be avoided for a week. The incision should be kept clean and dry for at least two days. Cold compresses, support for the scrotum (such as snug underwear) and over the counter pain killers (aspirin, ibuprofen, acetaminophen) will help lessen discomfort and speed recuperation.

Men should be advised that twenty ejaculations are needed to clear any remaining sperm from the reproductive tract. An alternate form of birth control or masturbation must be used until this has been accomplished. Ideally, a semen sample can be provided for examination under a microscope to detect if sperm are still present.

It is very important that clients return immediately if there is any sign of infection, such as high fever during the four weeks following the procedure, bleeding or pus from the wound, or pain that does not subside or worsens after the first 2–3 days.

7

Maternal Health Care

This chapter follows the woman through the phases of pregnancy: the prenatal, intrapartum and post-partum periods. The physiological changes, objectives of care, essential interventions and complications associated with each period are discussed. Methods of abortion are also discussed, as well as post-abortion contraception. The chapter concludes with a review of essential newborn care during the post-partum period.

PRENATAL PERIOD

Maternal Adaptation and Fetal Growth[1]

The uterus undergoes spectacular growth during pregnancy, increasing in weight 20-fold from two ounces to two pounds and increasing from 10 milliliters to between 2 and 10 liters. Growth of the uterine muscle is concentrated in the upper part or fundus of the uterus, which prepares for the downward pressure on the fetus during labor. The uterus rises in the pelvis and rotates to the right after the twelfth week of pregnancy, while maintaining a longitudinal lie relative to the pelvic axis. The wall of the abdomen supports the uterus. Hormonal changes induce a relaxation of the joints, which helps the body manage the shifting center of gravity as the uterus grows. The uterus will tip towards the spine if the woman lies on her back, which compresses the vena cava and aorta. This decreases blood flow to the brain and uterus, inducing supine hypotensive syndrome.

Blood flow increases to the cervix and vagina. The cervix extrudes a thick mucus that fills the cervical canal and serves as a barrier to infection (often called the mucus plug). The vaginal canal becomes increasingly acidic, which also has an antimicrobial function.

In response to the secretion of progesterone, prolactin and adrenal steroids, the breasts change in size, sensitivity and structure in preparation for lactation. Colostrum production begins in the second half of pregnancy.

There are major changes in the cardiovascular system that have vital consequences for maternal health. The heart increases in size, rate and output; cardiac output will increase 40 percent to 60 percent over the non-pregnant state. Blood volume increases, including a

50 percent increase in plasma and 15–20 percent increase in red cell volume. Production of red cells accelerates. Systolic and diastolic pressure decrease slightly during the first half of pregnancy and then rise to pre-pregnancy levels. Peripheral circulatory resistance decreases. Blood flow to the uterus increases markedly. Anemia, hypertension and hypotension serve to decrease blood flow to the uterus.

Respiration is deeper during pregnancy as women take in more oxygen to accommodate the needs of the fetus. The lower ribs flare to accommodate the diaphragm, which rises as the uterus grows.

Kidney function changes to filter the increase in maternal blood volume and fetal waste. The bladder is pushed upwards and forwards. Decreased blood flow and swelling of the bladder render it more susceptible to injury and infection. Fluid retention increases, with characteristic swelling of the ankles and fingers. This normal pregnancy induced edema must be distinguished from swelling of the face and arms that signals pre-eclampsia.

Major changes in hormone production accompany pregnancy. There is a very large increase in the secretion of estrogen and progesterone, which accomplishes a wide range of essential functions, including uterine growth and maintenance, preparing the breasts for lactation, relaxation of smooth muscle and stimulation of the respiratory system. The placenta secretes the protein hormones HCG, which is critical to estrogen production and sex differentiation in the fetus, and HPL, which helps regulate the availability of nutrients for the fetus. Prostaglandins stimulate the cardiovascular changes needed to sustain pregnancy. Thyroid hormone levels also change in response to the increased presence of estrogen.

Fetal development can be divided into three stages: the pre-embryonic period, the embryonic period and the fetal period.

- *The pre-embryonic period* lasts from conception through the third week of pregnancy. During this period the fertilized ovum (zygote) passes through the fallopian tube and begins to divide and differentiate. Implantation of the multi-cell conceptus, now termed a blastocyst, into the uterine wall occurs by day 6. By the end of the second week the placenta has begun to form. The placenta will transfer oxygen, nutrition and maternal anitbodies to the fetus, while removing waste products. The placenta also serves as a protective barrier against harmful substances and secretes hormones, including estrogen, progesterone, HCG and HPL. Primitive organ formation has also begun.
- *The embryonic period*, from weeks 4 to 8, is a period of extermely rapid development, as well as high sensitivity to trauma and teratogenic agents. The major organs and organ systems are formed, a primitive circulatory system has emerged and the fetal heartbeat begins. The limb buds appear and bones and muscle have begun to form.
- *The fetal period* lasts from weeks 9 to 40 and is principally devoted to the growth and development of the organs and organ systems. The face emerges by the end of the third month. The brain and spinal cord are connected by the end of the twelfth week. Genital differentiation and spleen function occur by the end of week 12. By the end of week 16 the embryo is recognizable as human and the kidneys have begun to function. The mother begins to feel fetal movements between weeks 16 and 20.

Objectives of Prenatal Care

Identifying the optimal frequency and content of prenatal care is a difficult matter in a circumstance where prenatal contact is often limited and the resources of both the woman and the health provider are seriously constrained. Hence, the challenge is to craft the package of interventions that will have the greatest impact on maternal health given local realities. To this end, we must be clear as to the objectives of prenatal care, which are threefold:

1. To monitor the progress of the pregnancy, with emphasis on detecting and managing life threatening obstetrical emergencies and threats to the health of the fetus.
2. To help women and households prepare for, detect and manage complications of pregnancy, with special emphasis on life threatening obstetrical emergencies.
3. To optimize nutritional status during pregnancy.

Emphasis should be given to measures that address obstetrical complications and emergencies. This implies de-emphasizing the "risk factor" approach that has played such a large role in conventional prenatal care[2,3,4,5,6,7]. Risk factors indicate that an individual pregnant woman is at higher relative risk of having complications. They include poor obstetric history, short stature, very young maternal age, nulliparity or grand multiparity, extreme deprivation, unwanted pregnancy, size-date discrepancy and multiple gestation. While they are of use to the individual clinician, they are of very little public health utility. About fifteen percent of all women will experience an obstetric emergency. The risk factors are very poor predictors of which women will find themselves among the fifteen percent. Many women with risk factors will have a perfectly normal pregnancy and delivery, while women without obvious risk factors are still in jeopardy of experiencing an obstetrical emergency.

Women with a range of pre-existing medical conditions are also at greater individual risk. These conditions include malnutrition, anemia, hypertension, sexually transmitted infections, malaria, intestinal parasites, sickle cell disease, diabetes, heart disease or epilepsy. Treating women with these conditions decreases the likelihood of their suffering a related obstetrical emergency. What must be remembered, however, is that women without such conditions are also susceptible to obstetrical emergencies.

The key challenge to the risk factor approach is the inability to provide the requisite follow-up care to at-risk women and the potential neglect of obstetrical emergencies among women without risk factors. Risk factors are useful in contexts where most or all women receive regular prenatal care and deliver in hospitals. They provide signals for appropriate care, heightened awareness and precautionary steps, which can help and certainly do no harm in an uneventful pregnancy and delivery. Women without risk factors in developed countries are also carefully monitored to capture unanticipated obstetrical emergencies.

In developing countries, prenatal care and the health infrastructure are limited, and births occur at home. Under these conditions, the argument for the risk factor approach becomes extremely tenuous. Many more women than could be handled by the infrastructure fall into the "at risk" category. Women without risk factors may have the implied, but false, assurance of a pregnancy without the likelihood of an emergency. Every woman can experience an obstetrical emergency, whether or not they exhibit one of the risk factors. As a consequence, the strategy of "every woman should watch for danger signs" has replaced the "identify women with risk factors" strategy as more appropriate to developing country contexts.

The principal danger signs in pregnancy and their significance are presented in Table 7-1[8].

Of the conditions listed in Table 7-1, hemorrhage, eclampsia and infection account for the vast majority of deaths.

TABLE 7-1. Danger Signs during the Prenatal Period

Danger signs	Possible significance
Severe vomiting, inability to retain food or liquid	Hyperemesis gravidarum
Bleeding during early pregnancy	May indicate ectopic pregnancy, spontaneous abortion, hydatidiform mole or cervical pathology
Lower abdominal pain during early pregnancy, abdominal tenderness, with shoulder pain	Ectopic pregnancy
Bleeding during late pregnancy	Placenta previa, placenta abruptio, vasa previa
Swelling of hands and face, severe headache, tinnitus, visual disturbances, vomiting, clonus, hyper-reflexia, epigastric or right upper quadrant pain, convulsions	Pre-eclampsia/eclampsia
High fever, chills, pain, nausea, vomiting	Infection
Increased thirst, increased urination, weight loss	Diabetes
Pallor, easily fatigued and breathlessness on mild exertion	Anemia

Monitoring Progress during Pregnancy

The World Health Organization has recommended a minimum of four prenatal visits of at least 20 minutes each, to take place in accordance with the following schedule[9]:

- Visit #1—by the end of the fourth month
- Visit #2—in the sixth or seventh month
- Visit #3—in the eighth month
- Visit #4—at 36 weeks gestation

As will be remembered from the earlier discussion of patterns of prenatal care, only a small fraction of women actually receive four visits. In many, if not most settings of high maternal mortality, access to laboratory and diagnostic equipment is absent or extremely limited. Simply increasing contact between trained health providers and pregnant women would be a major change in health behaviors. It is therefore vital that the most effective possible use is made of limited prenatal care and that efforts focus on practical steps that can be implemented with a minimum of resources. Priorities for the prenatal visits are:

- Helping each household develop an individualized birth plan, which is discussed in greater detail below.
- Early detection and management of hemorrhage.
- Early detection and management of pre-eclampsia.
- Early detection and management of infection, especially urinary tract infections, malaria, sexually transmitted infections and hookworm.
- Tetanus toxoid immunization.
- Micronutrient supplementation and nutrition counseling.
- Monitoring fetal growth and position.

Complications of the Prenatal Period[10]

Women are subject to a range of diseases and disorders during pregnancy. Some pose immediate, grave risks to maternal survival and demand rapid action. This section briefly reviews the major abnormalities and complications of pregnancy, giving special attention to prenatal emergencies that require prompt medical intervention.

Hyperemesis Gravidarum

Some women will begin to vomit uncontrollably and will be unable to retain food or liquids. This condition, known as hyperemesis gravidarum, must be distinguished from nausea or "morning sickness" commonly associated with pregnancy. Hyperemesis gravidarum can lead to dehydration, weight loss, ketosis and rapid deterioration of the woman's condition. The most likely cause of severe vomiting in pregnancy is urinary tract infection, but it may also be indicative of pregnancy-induced hypertension or polyhydramnios, a condition of excessive amniotic fluid. A variety of other conditions may also lead to vomiting. Vomiting in late pregnancy is almost always indicative of a pathological condition that requires medical intervention.

Hyperemesis gravidarum requires, at minimum, intravenous infusion of fluids (dextrose and Hartmann's solution) and anti-emetic therapy to control the vomiting. The underlying cause of the vomiting must be determined and treated.

Hemorrhage

Bleeding at any time during pregnancy is cause for concern and requires medical monitoring and intervention. Vaginal bleeding may occur in as much as 50 percent of all pregnancies and light bleeding in early pregnancy may be without significance. Bleeding during early pregnancy (first or second trimester) may be due to any of the following conditions:

- *Ectopic pregnancy*: the fertilized egg will sometimes fail to be transported into the uterus and begin to grow inside the fallopian tube. Untreated, the tube will rupture, leading to hemorrhage, infection and death. The woman will complain of severe lower abdominal pain and vaginal bleeding or a dark brown discharge. The woman may be dizzy, experience shoulder pain and the lower abdomen will be tender if palpated. Ectopic pregnancy requires immediate treatment. Surgery and blood transfusion will be needed to remove the ectopic pregnancy, repair damage to the fallopian tube and restore lost blood.
- *Spontaneous abortion*: anywhere from 10 to 30 percent of all pregnancies will end in spontaneous abortion[11]. Most spontaneous abortions are complete and occur without complication. Inevitable abortions manifest as bleeding, pain and uterine contractions over a prolonged period without expulsion of the fetus. Incomplete abortions are those in which the fetal tissue is only partially expelled, while missed abortions refer to those in which the fetus dies *in utero* but the placenta and fetus are not expelled. These forms of spontaneous abortion can lead to hemorrhage, infection and coagulopathy. Therefore, medical management of the abortion is required. Control of the bleeding, treatment for infection and removal of any retained products of conception are the priorities for medical intervention.
- *Hydatidiform mole*: in some instances, the embryo will die early in pregnancy, but the placenta will undergo uncontrolled growth. The placenta becomes, in effect, a form of tumor that is highly susceptible to blood loss. Symptoms include vaginal bleeding, vomiting and pregnancy induced hypertension (PIH) before the 24th week. Removal of the hyaditiform mole is essential to the woman's survival. Women experiencing a hydatidiform mole should be followed up for a two year period during which pregnancy should be avoided, as there is increased risk of choriocarcinoma.
- *Cervical pathology*: early bleeding may be indicative of a problem with the cervix, such as polyps, or erosion (cervical ectopy). Neither condition requires intervention. Rarely, cervical cancer may be present during pregnancy and lead to bleeding.

Bleeding after the 24th week of pregnancy is likely to differ in cause from that associated with early pregnancy. Causes of bleeding in the last 14–20 weeks include:

- *Placenta previa*: the placenta normally grows in the upper or fundal portion of the uterus. In less than one percent of pregnancies, the placenta will attach to the lower part of the uterus and partially or totally cover the cervical os. As a result, the growing fetus exerts increasing pressure on the placenta, which will begin to bleed. Painless vaginal bleeding after the 24th week of pregnancy is highly indicative of placenta previa. Vaginal or rectal exams, as well as labor and vaginal delivery can provoke severe hemorrhage and death. Bed rest and close monitoring of the woman are required, with the objective of prolonging the pregnancy as long as possible to increase the chances of neonatal survival. Cesarean section is the only option for delivery in cases of placenta previa and must be carried out immediately at any stage of pregnancy, without regard to prospects for fetal survival, if bleeding becomes heavy. Placental adherence to the uterine wall is sometimes a complication of Cesarean section in cases of placenta previa.
- *Placenta abruptio*: in about 2 percent of pregnancies, the placenta will spontaneously separate from the uterine wall, causing bleeding at the point of separation. Abdominal pain and uterine tenderness usually accompany placenta abruptio. As blood accumulates in the space between the placenta and the uterine wall, further dislodging of the placenta may occur. Placenta abruptio can be insidious because blood loss may be may be concealed between the placenta and the uterine wall. There are different grades of severity of placenta abruptio, which reflect the degree of blood loss. Severe blood loss requires transfusion, treatment for shock and immediate Cesarean delivery.
- *Vasa previa*: is an uncommon condition in which the blood vessels of the umbilical cord cover the cervical os and are therefore susceptible to rupture. Cesarean delivery is indicated in the event of hemorrhage from the umbilical vessels.

Eclampsia

Pregnancy-induced hypertension (PIH) is a systemic disease involving spasming and constriction of the peripheral blood vessels. It therefore affects virtually every major organ system in the body. Impacts on the central nervous system can include damage to the endothelial cells of the brain, swelling and blood clots (thrombosis). The heart is subjected to unusual strain as it tries to push blood through constricted vessels, while simultaneously receiving less blood to pump. The platelet count in the blood decreases (thrombocytopenia), which may lead to disseminated bleeding. Pulmonary edema is common. Kidney damage results from the constriction of the blood vessels; protein will accumulate in the urine as renal function is disrupted and urine output will decline. Lesions on the liver may develop.

PIH may be divided in two stages: pre-eclampsia and eclampsia, with the dividing line being the appearance of convulsions and coma. Convulsions are most likely to occur in the first 24 hours postpartum, but can occur before, during or after labor.

The signs and symptoms of pre-eclampsia are broad, reflecting the involvement of multiple organs. Visible manifestations include swelling of the hands and face, visual disturbances, severe headaches, ringing in the ears (tinnitus), and altered mentation (especially lethargy and somnolence). Hypertension (BP>140/90 or increases of 30 mm in systolic or 15 mm in diastolic pressure) and proteinuria (reading of 1+ or greater on urine dipstick) are also likely to be present. It must be emphasized, however, that severe PIH can be asymptomatic unless eclampsia is near. Twenty percent of women experiencing eclampsia will have no warning sign or symptom, with normal prior blood pressure and proteinuria findings.

Signs and symptoms of imminent eclampsia include severe headache, visual disturbances, vomiting, spontaneous contraction and relaxation of a muscle group (clonus), unusual brisk reflex responses (hyper-reflexia) and epigastric or right upper quadrant pain.

The only cure for pregnancy-induced hypertension is delivery of the baby. Hypotensive drugs, such as methyl dopa, can be used to control the effects of known PIH, but the object must be safe delivery of the baby at the earliest opportunity.

Imminent or actual eclampsia is life-threatening and requires immediate action. The objective of emergency treatment of eclampsia is to maintain an airway and prevent or stop the convulsions. The woman must be prevented from choking on her tongue, which may be accomplished by placing a padded bite stick in the mouth or through use of a plastic oral airway. Anti-convulsives (magnesium sulfate or diazepam) are used control seizures. An anti-hypertensive, such as hydralazine, is also needed. Controlled administration of fluids is essential. At the village level, oral rehydration therapy can be used to combat dehydration.

Infections in Pregnancy

- *Urinary tract infections*: Urinary tract infections are relatively common in pregnancy—approximately six percent of women will have an asymptomatic bacterial infection, which is detectable only through urinalysis. Untreated urinary tract infection can have pernicious consequences, of which the most serious is acute pyelonephritis, an acute infection of the kidney characterized by high fever, chills, pain, nausea and vomiting. Pyelonephritis can lead to maternal sepsis, premature labor and intrauterine growth retardation. Treatment with antibiotics (ampicillin or amoxicillin, cephalosporin, nitrofurantoin or trimethoprin) is essential.
- *Sexually transmitted diseases*: Sexually transmitted disease (STD) can lead to a variety of serious consequences for both mother and child. STD that have a particularly grave impact on maternal and neonatal health in the developing world include:
  — *Gonorrhea*: untreated gonorrhea can lead to pelvic inflammatory disease, pre-term labor, chorioamnionits and postpartum endometritis. Infection of the neonate can lead to blindness as the infection tends to localize in the eyes (gonococcal opthalmia neonatorum).
  — *Syphilis*: untreated syphilis leads to the systemic form of the disease that has widespread organ effects, including impact on the cardiovascular and central nervous system, eventually leading to death. Syphilis in the mother can lead to spontaneous abortion, intrauterine demise, intrauterine growth retardation, preterm labor, and infection of the neonate. All pregnant women should be tested for syphilis using the Rapid Plasma Reagin (RPR) test and treated appropriately upon positive finding.
  — *Chlamydia*: causes infection of the eyes in newborns (opthalmia neonatorum) and has been linked to ectopic pregnancy, postpartum infection and post-abortion infection; there is conflicting evidence as to its impact on premature rupture of membranes, preterm birth and low birth weight.
  — *Human immunodeficiency virus*: the progression of HIV/AIDS may be accelerated by pregnancy. There is a 15 to 30 percent chance of transmission to the baby during pregnancy and another 10 to 20 percent chance of infection through breast feeding in the absence of treatment[12].

Other STD, such as trichomoniasis, bacterial vaginosis, herpes genitalis and genital warts have also been linked to adverse pregnancy outcomes. However, prevention and treatment of the above four are priorities for the developing world in light of their prevalence, severity of consequence and feasibility of mounting cost-effective interventions. Chapter 8 discusses pregnancy and STD in greater detail.

- *Malaria*: Women in their first or, to a lesser degree, second pregnancy who live in malaria endemic areas tend to lose the immunity gained during childhood because the parasite crosses the placental barrier. Malaria increases the probability of maternal anemia, abortion, stillbirth, premature birth and low birth weight. Research in east Africa has demonstrated the efficacy and cost-effectiveness of using sulfadoxine-pyrimethamine (SP, Fansidar) to treat malaria during pregnancy[13]. The SP trials showed the efficacy of providing one dose in each of the second and third trimesters. The anti-malarial of choice will vary depending on the malaria resistance in specific geographic areas. However, there is now a consensus that anti-malarials should be provided during pregnancy with special emphasis on targeting first and second pregnancies.

- *Helminthic infection*: In many parts of the world hookworms are endemic. Hookworms exacerbate the problems associated with iron deficiency anemia. While the only effective long-term solution to helminths is sanitation and a clean water supply, antihelminthic drugs can help protect women from increased risk of anemia. Antihelminthic drugs should not be provided during the first trimester of pregnancy. In areas where the prevalence is 20 percent to 50 percent a single dose should be provided during the second trimester; in areas where prevalence exceeds 50 percent a second dose should be given during the third trimester. One of the following drugs can be used[14]:
  - Albendazole: 400 mg single dose
  - Mebendazole : 500 mg single dose or 100 mg twice daily for three days
  - Levamisole: 2.5 mg/kg single dose, best if a second dose is given after 7 days
  - Pyrantel: 10 mg/kg single dose, best if dose is repeated on next two consecutive days

- *Tetanus*: All pregnant women should receive tetanus toxoid immunization. A schedule of five immunizations is needed to provide lifetime protection against tetanus, but two injections during pregnancy received four weeks apart will confer protection against maternal and neonatal tetanus.

- *Other infections*: There are a number of other infectious agents that can adversely affect pregnancy. Table 7-2 briefly summarizes these infections and the steps that can be taken to prevent or treat them.

TABLE 7-2. Systemic and Teratogenic Infections in Pregnancy

Maternal infection	Consequence	Intervention
Hepatitis B	Liver dysfunction in mother and neonate	Vaccination of mother and neonate to prevent perinatal transmission
Tuberculosis	Eventually fatal to mother; airborne infection of the neonate	Treatment of mother
Rubella	Abortion, fetal defects	Vaccination of mother
Varicella zoster (Chicken pox)	Birth defects, neonatal mortality	Maternal vaccination prior to pregnancy
Streptococcus B	Neonatal sepsis and meningitis	Antibiotic treatment of mother

Diabetes

Approximately 2 to 3 percent of all women will develop gestational diabetes mellitus during pregnancy. Diabetes is an inability produce or use insulin, which is essential to the transport of glucose across cell membranes. Blood sugar levels arise and fats and proteins are catabolized to meet the energy needs that would otherwise be derived from glucose. As fats are metabolized, ketones are released into the body, which can lead to diabetic ketoacidosis, a potentially fatal condition. Diabetes is linked to a variety of other complications of pregnancy, including hypertension, greater susceptibility to urinary tract infections, birth defects and abnormally large babies (fetal macrosomia). This latter condition increases the probability of obstructed labor. Neonatal morbidity and mortality are also more common among children of diabetic women. The signs of diabetes are increased appetite, increased thirst, increased urine output and loss of weight and muscle. Management of diabetes requires control of diet, physical activity and insulin levels.

Helping Households Plan for Obstetrical Emergencies

The first and foremost responsibility of the health provider is to help the woman and other important members of the household plan for, recognize and manage complications of pregnancy. Empowering women to take active control of their pregnancy and its outcomes is fundamental to reducing maternal mortality. It is obstetrical emergencies that kill women. Since every pregnant woman is at risk of an obstetrical emergency, all women need a strategy for managing emergencies.

As a first step, every pregnant woman must know the danger signs of pregnancy. Because hemorrhage, infection and eclampsia account for the vast majority of prenatal deaths, the danger signs of the prenatal period can be boiled down to a very simple message, "If you have vaginal bleeding, fever, lower abdominal pain, blurred vision, severe headaches or swollen face and hands or feel very weak or tired during pregnancy – SEEK HELP IMMEDIATELY!"

The key to preventing and managing complications is for the woman and her family to develop an **individualized birth plan**. The birth plan should cover the following elements:

- Adjusting the diet and workload of the woman to increase weight gain and energy resources.
- Teaching the woman and all key family members (husbands, in-laws) the danger signs of hemorrhage, PIH, obstructed labor and infection.
- Strongly encouraging the woman and her family to seek the services of a trained, skilled birth attendant.
- Insisting on aseptic practices. All births must adhere to the six cleans: attendant with clean hands, clean surface for the birth, clean string to tie the cord, clean blade to cut the cord, clean cloth for the mother and clean cloth for the baby.
- Identifying the facility that will be used in case of an emergency.
- Developing a plan for transport to the facility.
- Securing the cash needed to pay for services, drugs and commodities in the event of an emergency.
- Encouraging immediate and exclusive breastfeeding.
- Educating the woman and her partner on the importance of birth spacing and family planning options.

Some of the above can be undertaken at the household level. However, as discussed earlier, many require collective action at the community level, including emergency transport and emergency funds. Community mobilization is a necessary adjunct to developing household birth plans. Similarly, birth planning assumes the availability of competent providers and equipped facilities, which is the goal of institutional capacity building.

Nutrition and Pregnancy

As should be evident from the very brief description of maternal adaptation and fetal growth, a healthy pregnancy demands changes in the woman's nutritional status. The requirements for protein and energy rise in order to accommodate the growth of the placenta and fetus. A complex interplay of micronutrients, which is not well understood, affects maternal and fetal health.

Caloric requirements vary by age, pre-pregnancy weight, workload, metabolic rate, general health status and other factors. By way of example, a 25-year-old woman weighing 50 kilograms with the heavy physical workload typical in most developing countries would need 2080 kilocalories per day in the absence of pregnancy.[15] Pregnancy requires 55,000 kilocalories of energy above and beyond the basic needs of the non-pregnant woman, with the additional energy requirement largely concentrated in the last two trimesters. This means pregnant women should be consuming about 300 kilocalories per day in addition to their baseline energy requirement. In our example, this would raise the energy requirement in the last six months of pregnancy to 2380 kilocalories per day.

One index of weight is the Body Mass Index (BMI), which is obtained by dividing the weight in kilograms by the height in meters. Table 7-3 shows the recommended weight gain for different BMI categories[16].

Though precise figures are hard to obtain, it is likely that very high proportions of women in the developing world enter pregnancy consuming too few calories to meet their energy requirements prior to pregnancy. Approximately 450 million adult women are stunted due to long term malnutrition.[17] Pregnancy places an additional toll on under-nourished women. As a consequence, it is commonplace for women to gain less than the minimum of five to nine kilograms recommended by the World Health Organization[18]. Gains of as much as 18 kilograms are unrealistic in many settings. Hence, additional effort is needed to improve the pre-conception growth of girls and women to ensure higher weights before pregnancy.

Poverty partially explains the very large number of women who are under-nourished during pregnancy. However, other factors play an important role as well. In some cultures dietary habits preclude the consumption of meat and/or raise a variety of taboos to the consumption of specific foods during pregnancy. Women often have heavy workloads, which

TABLE 7-3. Recommended Pregnancy Weight Gain by Body Mass Index

Body mass index	Recommended weight gain in kilograms
Low (BMI < 19.8)	12.5–18
Normal (BMI 19.8 to 26.0)	11.5–16
High (BMI > 26.0)	7.0–11.5

further drains energy resources. In some instances, women fear having a large baby that may result in obstructed labor and so deliberately under-consume. Because of their low status in the household, women are often the last to gain access to the family meal, eating after the males have taken their fill.

Pre-pregnancy height and weight, in combination with inadequate caloric intake during pregnancy, explain more than 50 percent of the observed incidence of low birth weight in the developing world.[19] Nearly 1 out of 5 babies in the developing world are born weighing less than 2500 grams, which dramatically increases the likelihood of infant mortality. In sub-Saharan Africa, 16 percent of newborns are low birth weight, while 34 percent of newborns in South Asia are low birth weight.[20] The high proportion of low birth weight newborns is indicative of the stresses placed on the energy stores of under-nourished women.

Protein requirements also increase during pregnancy. Protein is needed for fetal development, blood volume expansion and growth of the uterus and breasts. To return to our example, the 25-year-old, 50 kilogram woman would need 40 grams of protein per day to meet her nutritional needs prior to pregnancy. This figure would jump to 60 grams per day of protein during pregnancy.[21] Developing country diets are frequently deficient in protein, particularly where poverty or dietary custom preclude meat consumption.

Micronutrients also play an essential role in pregnancy, though there is a surprising paucity of research on the effects of micronutrient malnutrition on maternal health. Most of the research on micronutrients during pregnancy has focused on outcomes for the fetus and infant rather than the mother.[22]

- *Iron deficiency anemia* is a serious and globally endemic problem. Pregnancy places heavy demands on iron consumption. A full term pregnancy of a single fetus requires 1000 mg of iron. The fetus will absorb maternal iron stores, even if the mother is highly iron deficient, thereby exacerbating any pre-existing anemia. Anemia afflicts over 50 percent of pregnant women.[23] The prevalence of anemia is especially high in South Asia (64–75 percent), followed by Southeast Asia (56–63 percent), Africa (52 percent) and the Caribbean (52 percent – 90 percent). The causes of anemia are complex, beginning with insufficient consumption of iron, complicated by the deficiencies in other micronutrients—especially folate, Vitamin B_{12} and Vitamin C - that are needed for efficient use of iron. Malaria, helminth infection and sickle cell disease further contribute to the prevalence of anemia. Anemia contributes to as much as 20 percent of maternal deaths by increasing the likelihood of infection and making it more likely that hemorrhage will lead to shock and death. Anemia also contributes to stillbirths, pre-term births and low birth weight. Iron stores in women tend to be low as a result of menstruation, so iron supplementation is needed both before and during pregnancy. The WHO recommends a daily dose of 60 mg of ferrous iron for 100 days, usually in the form of ferrous fumarate, ferrous sulfate or ferrous gluconate, plus 400 mcg of folic acid. A weekly dose of iron and folic acid is more common than daily dosage, given difficulties in compliance with daily dosage. If the one hundred day duration of treatment is not feasible, then the dose can be increased to 120 mg per day.[24] Iron supplementation during pregnancy will not cure pre-existing anemia; however, it does help prevent further deterioration of iron stores. Women with anemia need higher doses of iron and folic acid. Those with moderate anemia should increase the supplement to 120 mg of iron plus 500 mcg of folic acid. Women with severe anemia will need 180 mg of iron and 750 mcg per day of folic acid for four weeks, followed by 120 mg/day of iron and 500 mcg/day of folic acid. Women should be encouraged to eat foods rich in Vitamin C, such as citrus fruits, which aid in the uptake of iron and avoid tea and coffee, which inhibit the biological use of iron.

- *Vitamin A deficiency*, which is quite common among women in developing countries, can compromise fetal and placental growth, lead to night blindness in the woman and undermine the immune response. A well-designed study among rural under-nourished women in Nepal demonstrated that supplementation with low doses of Vitamin A or beta-carotene can have a significant impact on maternal mortality[25]. The randomized control trial in Nepal found that mortality was reduced by 40 percent among women receiving Vitamin A and 49 percent among beta-carotene recipients relative to women receiving a placebo. Low to moderate doses are safe, but high doses of Vitamin A can have a teratogenic effect, so proper management of supplementation is important. All pregnant women living in areas of endemic Vitamin A deficiency should receive 10,000 IU daily or 25,000 IU weekly of supplementary Vitamin A.[26] Breastfeeding women should receive a single high dose supplement of 200,000 IU of supplementary Vitamin A within the first eight weeks post-delivery.
- *Iodine deficiency* can lead to fetal wastage, mental retardation and cretinism in the child.[27] Consumption of iodized oil supplements or iodized salt is needed to redress iodine deficiency.[28] Major progress has been made in iodizing salt throughout much of the world and this has been shown to be an effective strategy for reducing the prevalence of iodine deficiency. Women should be encouraged to consume iodized salt prior to and during pregnancy.
- *Folic acid deficiency* has been associated with spontaneous abortion, bleeding, placenta abruptio, pre-eclampsia, poor fetal growth and fetal neural tube defects. Supplementation of the maternal diet with folate during pregnancy has been shown to reduce neural tube defects, but there is more uncertainty as to the impact of supplementation on other pregnancy outcomes.[29]
- *Zinc deficiency* has been linked to longer labor, spontaneous abortion and congenital malformations, especially of the central nervous system.[30,31] Animal protein, milk, wheat germ and legumes are good natural sources of zinc. Experimental studies with zinc supplementation have shown a decrease in pregnancy complications.
- *Calcium* is needed for fetal bone development.[32] The fetus will react to maternal calcium deficiency by de-calcifying the woman's skeleton. Calcium also seems to play a role in pregnancy-induced hypertension, principally by altering the contractile properties of smooth muscles, such as those that line blood vessels and the uterus. Trials of calcium supplementation suggest that it can reduce blood pressure and the incidence of pre-eclampsia among women with significant calcium deficiency.[33]
- *Magnesium deficiency* has been implicated in PIH.[34] Administration of magnesium sulphate is an established part of treating PIH, as well as an agent to reduce uterine activity in the event of premature rupture of membranes. Pregnant women should be consuming 320 mg per day of magnesium in their diet or through supplementation.[35] Trials of magnesium supplementation have indicated that it may reduce PIH, pre-term deliveries, premature rupture of membranes and intra-uterine growth retardation among magnesium deficient women.[36]
- *Other vitamins and minerals*:[37] Vitamin C deficiency may lead to premature rupture of membranes and premature delivery. Vitamin D stabilizes calcium levels and is therefore essential to fetal bone growth. Deficiencies in the B-complex vitamins (thiamine, B_6, B_{12}) can adversely affect intrauterine growth, fetal development, iron stores and full term delivery. Copper deficiency may be implicated in pre-term delivery and selenium deficiency may yield low birth weight.

Table 7-4 provides the recommended dietary allowances for micronutrients[38].

The policy question remains as to the ideal micronutrient supplementation schedule. Contact with pregnant women in developing countries is often very limited and resource constraints almost always render impractical a full schedule of supplementation. Micronutrient deficiencies are often context specific, so different levels or types of supplementation may be needed for different populations. Most programs have focused on supplementation

TABLE 7-4. Micronutrient Recommended Daily Allowance for Pregnant Women

Micronutrient	Recommended dietary allowance for pregnant women
Vitamin A	800 mcg retinol equivalents
Vitamin D	10 mcg
Vitamin E	10 mcg tocopherol equivalents
Vitamin K	65 mcg
Vitamin C	70 mg
Thiamine	1.5 mg
Riboflavin	1.6 mg
Niacin	17 mg
Folacin	400 mcg
Vitamin B_{12}	2.2 mcg
Vitamin B_6	2.2 mcg
Calcium	1200 mg
Phosphorous	1200 mg
Magnesium	320 mg
Iron	30 mg
Zinc	15 mg
Iodine	175 mg

of iron, folic acid and Vitamin A due to their prevalence and severe consequence. There is very little research on the impact of multivitamin-mineral supplements.

INTRAPARTUM PERIOD[39]

Physiology of Normal Labor

Labor is usually divided into three stages[40], beginning with the onset of labor and culminating in the birth of the infant. The first stage of labor begins with the appearance of contractions and ends when the cervix is completely dilated at approximately ten centimeters. The first stage is conventionally subdivided into the latent, active and transition phases. During the latent phase contractions are 10 to 20 minutes apart, last 15 to 30 seconds and are relatively mild in intensity. The latent phase ends when the cervix has dilated to three to four centimeters. During the active phase the cervix dilates to seven centimeters and the pace and intensity of contractions accelerates. The interval between contractions will diminish to three to five minutes. Contractions will increase in duration (45 to 60 seconds) and intensity. The transition phase completes dilation to ten centimeters. Uterine contractions now come every two to three minutes, last sixty to ninety seconds and are increasingly intense.

The second stage of labor begins when the cervix is completely dilated and ends when the neonate is born. Contractions may decrease in intensity and duration during the beginning of the second stage and then accelerate. Contractions will then become as frequent as every one to two minutes and become very intense. The membranes may rupture at any previous point in time, but must rupture for the birth to occur. If necessary, the birth attendant will rupture the membranes when the cervix is completely dilated.

The third stage of labor lasts from the birth until the delivery of the placenta. Contractions resume within a few minutes of the birth, initiating the *separation phase*. During the separation phase the uterus collapses, moving into the space occupied by the fetus. This forces the placenta to separate from the wall of the uterus. As placental separation occurs, contractions in the middle layer of uterine muscle serve to seal the severed blood vessels. Placental separation is usually accompanied by a gush of blood from the vagina, a change in the size and shape of the uterus and lengthening of the umbilical cord. Uterine contractions and the accumulation of blood between the uterine wall and the placenta force the placenta loose. After an interval lasting up to 30 minutes after birth, *expulsion* of the placenta occurs.

Care during Labor and Delivery

The objectives of care during labor and delivery are twofold:

1. To ensure a safe, supportive, clean delivery for mother and child with the minimum level of intervention needed to achieve this end.
2. To rapidly identify and manage emerging complications in accordance with a pre-established birth plan.

In accordance with these objectives, the optimal practices for a *normal* birth may be subdivided into the following categories: psychosocial support for the woman during labor and delivery, essential interventions, and qualifications of the birth attendant.

Psychosocial Support

During labor and delivery a woman is under great physical and psychological stress. Heart rate, blood pressure and respiration will increase. In the absence of anesthesia, which applies to most births, pain intensifies throughout the process. Concern or fear as to her safety and that of the baby are likely to be present. She may feel her privacy or modesty are invaded. She may be subjected to over-stimulus as the attention of attendants and family members are added to the inherent stresses or, conversely, feel lonely or isolated where local culture mandates minimal contact with the birthing woman.

So as to provide a more supportive environment for birth, every woman experiencing a normal birth has the right to the following:

- To make an informed choice as to the location of the birth.
- To have her privacy and modesty respected.
- To receive empathetic support from caregivers.
- To receive accurate, comprehensible information that helps her manage labor and delivery and/or responds to her queries.
- To have present the partner or companions that she finds helpful and supportive.
- To be free to move about during labor and delivery and to assume the position she finds most comfortable, while avoiding a supine position that may contribute to hypotension.

Essential Interventions

Birth is a natural process that should not be subjected to unnecessary interventions. However, WHO has identified a minimal set of interventions that have clear, demonstrable benefits and should be actively encouraged[41]. These include:

- Continuing assessment of maternal well-being to rapidly identify and manage the onset of a complication in keeping with the pre-established birth plan.
- Monitoring the progress of labor and delivery using the WHO partograph, which serves as a simple tool for recording duration and key events during labor. Events that exceed the parameters indicated on the partograph, such as fetal heart rate or duration of labor, mandate additional intervention and help delineate complicated from normal births.
- Offering oral fluids during labor and delivery. Restriction of oral intake has been the norm in many settings as a precaution in the event that anesthesia may be needed. Stomach contents might then be aspirated. This must be balanced against the danger of dehydration and ketosis in settings where women are unlikely to have access to intravenous infusion of fluids. WHO has therefore recommended that women in labor be permitted oral fluids in the absence of clear indication that anesthesia will be necessary.
- Use of non-invasive, non-pharmocological methods of pain relief. Touch, massage, patterned breathing and culturally appropriate, harmless, psychosomatic methods should be encouraged to alleviate maternal discomfort.
- Use of aseptic techniques, with specific focus on the "six cleans" (clean hands, clean surface for the birth, clean string to tie the cord, clean blade to cut the cord, clean cloth for the mother and clean cloth for the baby). If available, clean gloves should be used during vaginal examinations and delivery of the baby, as well as in handling the placenta to prevent infection of the attendant. Invasive techniques, such as episiotomy, should be kept to a minimum to minimize the chances for infection.
- Monitoring the well-being of the fetus regularly during labor. One visible sign of fetal well-being is the color and viscosity of the amniotic fluid. The amniotic fluids should be clear. Green or brown fluids indicate that the fetal intestinal contents (meconium) have been voided, which is a sign of distress. Aspiration of meconium during the birthing process can lead to asphyixa of the newborn, so immediate suctioning of the fetal airway is essential. Red amniotic fluids signal the presence of blood. If a stethoscope is available, the fetal heart rate can be monitored. Sustained heart rates of over 160 beats per minute or under 120 beats per minute are indicative of fetal distress. Fetal distress is a signal for urgent delivery of the baby.
- Use of prophylactic oxytocin in the third stage of labor with women at risk of postpartum hemorrhage or who may be endangered by even small blood loss. While this procedure would not be applied to healthy women experiencing normal blood loss, WHO recommends this step in light of the high prevalence of anemia in the developing world. Note that the use of oxytocin rather than ergometrine is recommended.
- Preventing hypothermia in the newborn. The baby should be gently wiped but not washed with water (which can rapidly decrease body temperature), wrapped in a clean cloth and placed in contact with the mother's body within one hour post-partum to initiate breastfeeding.
- Routine examination of the placenta and membranes. Any indication that a piece of the placenta is missing is a danger sign, since it has been retained in the uterus. The likely consequence is infection and provision must be made immediately to explore the uterine cavity and retrieve the missing pieces.

Use of a Trained Birth Attendant

The importance of a trained birth attendant to reducing maternal mortality and serious morbidity cannot be over-estimated. The trained and properly equipped midwife is the lynchpin to a system for preventing maternal mortality. As has been stressed throughout, obstetrical emergencies can arise quickly and require skilled intervention.

Approximately 60 million births per year—over half the total—occur without the assistance of a trained attendant. In these cases women give birth alone or with the assistance of a family member or traditional birth attendant. Training and equipping traditional birth attendants can contribute to maternal health by reducing harmful practices, promoting asepsis, encouraging prompt recognition of obstetrical emergencies and increasing recourse to obstetric first aid in the event of an emergency. However, traditional birth attendants cannot be expected to manage emergencies alone. Drugs, transfusions and surgery are necessary to handle obstetric emergencies. Traditional birth attendants must be linked to a facility that can provide the requisite care if lives are to be saved.

A trained birth attendant is, at minimum, able to provide the following services:

- Maintain an aseptic environment for the birth; i.e., practice the "six cleans"
- Provide empathetic psychological and social support to the woman, her partner and family during labor, birth and the postpartum care period;
- Perform minor interventions, such as amniotomy or episiotomy if needed;
- Monitor and assess both the woman and the infant during labor, delivery and the post-partum period to detect complications;
- Administer life-saving interventions if needed in the event of an emergency pending access to a higher level of care; i.e., uterine massage and administration of oxytocics to control bleeding, administration of magnesium sulfate or diazepam to control seizures, administration of an initial course of antibiotics to control infection.
- Facilitate referral and transport of the woman in event of an emergency in keeping with the pre-established birth plan.
- Avoid/discourage harmful practices, such as enemas, pubic shaving, rectal exams, inappropriate use of oxytocics and ergometrine, pressure on the uterus during the second stage of labor, massage of the perineum, routine uterine lavage and routine post-partum uterine exploration.
- Provide essential newborn care; i.e., prevention of asphyxia, hypothermia and sepsis.

Complications of the Intrapartum Period[42]

Women are subject to a variety of complications during labor and delivery. Many of the potential complications of the prenatal period – eclampsia, hemorrhage, infection, exacerbation of pre-existing conditions – are more likely to appear during labor and delivery. Labor and delivery also bring a new set of potential problems that bear careful attention, notably infection associated with rupture of the membranes, obstructed labor and threats to the well-being of the fetus. Eclampsia was discussed earlier and a detailed discussion of hemorrhage is included in the section on the postpartum period.

Women, families and birth attendants must be aware of the danger signs during labor and delivery, which are presented in Table 7-5. **The appearance of a danger sign is the signal for immediate action in accordance with the birth plan developed during the prenatal period.**

Infection in the intrapartum period

- *Premature Rupture of Membranes*: Rupture of the membranes one or more hours before the onset of contractions is termed premature rupture of membranes (PROM), which occurs in 10 to 12 percent of pregnancies. PROM increases the risk of infection and cord prolapse. Vaginal examination of women experiencing PROM should therefore be avoided to reduce the likelihood of infection. They should be monitored carefully for signs of infection, which should be treated aggressively with antibiotics. WHO recommends prophylactic

TABLE 7-5. Danger Signs During the Intrapartum Period

Danger sign	Significance
Heavy bleeding (more than 500 ml.)	Hemorrhage
Severe headache, tinnitus, visual disturbances, vomiting, clonus, hyper-reflexia, epigastric or right upper quadrant pain, convulsions	Eclampsia
Labor longer than 12 hours, malpresentation of the fetus	Dystocia (Obstructed or prolonged labor)
High fever, chills, pain, nausea, vomiting, foul smelling vaginal discharge	Infection
Placenta retained for more than 30 minutes	Very high risk of hemorrhage

administration of antibiotics if the membranes have been ruptured for more than 12 hours without delivery. Most women will go into spontaneous labor within 48 hours of the rupture of membranes.

- *Chorioamnionitis*: Chorioamnionitis is an infection of the chorion, amnion, amniotic fluid and fetus. Chorioamnionitis is transmitted in three ways: ascending infections across ruptured or inflamed membranes, transplacental infection as a result of maternal blood borne infection, and descending infections from the abdominal cavity and fallopian tubes. Bacteria, protozoa and parasites have all been identified as causative agents in chorioamnionitis. As many as 20 percent of women with PROM will be subjected to chorioamnionitis, which reinforces the importance of watching for infection in a woman who has experienced premature rupture of membranes. In other instances, inflammation of the membranes during labor, even in the absence of rupture, may render them more susceptible to permeation by infectious agents. Malnutrition in pregnant women also increases the likelihood of the disease. Women experiencing chorioamnionitis will become very ill if untreated. Symptoms will include general malaise, fever, chills, elevated heart rate and respiration and uterine tenderness. Dehydration is common. The infection affects the uterus, resulting in weak (hypotonic) contractions. As a consequence, vaginal delivery is impeded and augmentation with oxytocics or Cesarean section may be necessary. The infection may spread to other parts of the body. Both the woman and the fetus are at risk in the event of chorioamnionitis. Prompt treatment of the mother with antibiotics and rehydration are needed. The neonate should be closely monitored for sepsis and prophylactic treatment of the newborn with antibiotics is warranted.

Dystocia: Obstructed or Prolonged Labor

Obstructed labor is defined as labor that is prevented from progressing due to a mechanical obstruction, such as malpresentation or disproportion between fetal size and the pelvic opening. Prolonged labor consists of active labor with regular uterine contractions and progressive cervical dilation for more than twelve hours. Dystocia can lead to maternal exhaustion, dehydration, ketosis or uterine rupture. The key element in protecting maternal health is prompt recognition by the birth attendant that a difficult labor is manifesting. The woman must be transported to a facility that can provide assisted delivery. Dystocia may arise from a number of causes:

- *Fetal dystocia*: Dystocia may be due to fetal characteristics that prevent normal passage through the pelvis. The fetus may be unusually large. The head may be too large for the pelvic opening, a condition known as cephalopelvic disproportion. While the head normally presents the widest diameter, there are anomalies in which the shoulders or chest may be wider and inhibit passage. In rare cases, hydrocephalus (large head due to the accumulation of cerebrospinal fluid) or anencephaly (failure of the cerebrum and cranium to develop) may cause prolonged labor. Fetal dystocia may also result from malpresentation. In 95 percent of births, the head enters the pelvis first, which is known as a vertex or cephalic presentation. In a normal birth the skull is positioned such that the small possible diameter is presented to the pelvic inlet, which also requires that the fetal face be positioned towards the rear of the maternal pelvis (occiptoanterior position). A vertex lie may be accompanied by presentation of the brow or face, thereby increasing the diameter that must pass through the pelvis. The head may be rotated such that the back of the skull, rather than the face, is closest to the rear of the maternal pelvis (occiptoposterior position). The birth may be complicated by a breech presentation, such that the buttocks, legs or feet enter the pelvis first. In rare instances, the fetal shoulder may enter the pelvis first, with the fetus lying perpendicular to the mother's spine. In some instances of fetal dystocia, a vaginal delivery may be possible. However, a Cesarean section will usually be necessary. This is a decision that needs to be made in a hospital by a qualified physician. Waiting too long or attempting to deliver a malpresented fetus can result in the death of the mother and the child.

- *Uterine dystocia*: A successful birth depends on strong, regular contractions that are focalized in the fundus. Approximately 5 percent of labors will suffer from some form of uterine dystocia. Variations of this problem include:
  — *Constriction rings*, which are rigid bands of muscle, in the middle to lower part of the uterus. These constriction rings work against the muscles in the fundus, which are attempting to push the fetus towards the pelvis. The woman is usually in excruciating pain while little progress towards descent of the fetus occurs. Pathologic constriction rings are a precursor to uterine rupture. A tocolytic agent, such as terbutaline, is needed to reduce uterine activity and a Cesarean section is required.
  — *Hypotonic labor* in which contractions are too weak to effect birth or which do not occur in the requisite pattern. Instead of sweeping down with appropriate pressure from the fundus, contractions may occur sporadically or weakly at different points along the uterine wall. Hypotonic labor is almost invariably prolonged. In the absence of some form of pelvic or fetal dystocia, hypotonic labor may be treated with oxytocin. However, Cesarean section may be needed if there are complicating factors.
  — *Hypertonic labor*, which is characterized by an unusually tense uterus that does not relax between contractions and a lack of fundal dominance. The woman experiences frequent, painful contractions with little progress and quickly becomes dehydrated and exhausted. Rehydration, amniotomy and oxytocin may redress the situation or a Cesarean section may be needed.
  — *Structural abnormalities of the uterus* that impede the progress of labor. Some women will suffer from variations of the uterine shape that constrict the space available to the fetus and/or provoke dysfunction during labor. Cesarean delivery is usually required in these instances.
- *Pelvic dystocia*: The pelvis may be too narrow or distorted along any of its dimensions. As a result, normal descent of the fetus will be impeded. Cesarean delivery is required in these instances.
- *Cervical failure*: Failure of the cervix to dilate adequately can also obstruct delivery. The norm for cervical dilation is 1 cm/hour for primiparous women and 2 cm/hour for multiparous women. Dilation to 10 centimeters should occur within 10 hours for primiparous and 6 hours for multiparous women. Prolonged labor is usually caused by a dysfunction of the myometrium, the innermost layer of uterine muscle. This can be complicated by obstructions that prevent the fetus from exerting sufficient pressure on the cervix. Barring obstructions or uterine dystocia, cervical dilation and delivery can sometimes be hastened through oxytocics, nipple

stimulation and amniotomy. However, Cesarean section may be required. Failure of cervical dilation is occasionally combined with precipitous labor, in which full fetal descent occurs in less than three hours. Such cases can lead to uterine rupture and laceration of the genital tract.

The duration of labor can vary widely. The average duration of the latent phase is just under nine hours for primiparous women and just over five hours for multiparas. The upper limit for the latent phase in a normal birth is 20 hours for a primipara and 14 hours for a mulipara. The active phase in a normal birth averages just under six hours for primiparas and 2.5 hours for multiparas, with normal upper limits of 12 and 6 hours, respectively. Second stage labor in a normal birth averages a little less than one hour for primiparas and 18 minutes for multiparas, with normal upper limits of 2.5 hours and 50 minutes, respectively.

Assessing the significance and cause of a longer than usual labor is likely to prove difficult in a home setting. Transport time must also be factored into the decision to move the woman to a medical facility; many hours may elapse between the decision to transport and the moment care is initiated. Latent phase labor lasting longer than eight hours should alert the family and the provider that prolonged or obstructed labor may be occurring. **WHO recommends that any woman who has been in labor for longer than 12 hours be transported to a hospital that can provide the full range of services, including Cesarean section**[43]. A woman who has been in labor for longer than 12 hours may have a normal vaginal delivery. However, prudence dictates transport after 12 hours since dystocia accounts for eight percent of maternal deaths. A trained attendant can use the partograph to help chart the course of labor.

Retained or Incomplete Placenta

The placenta should normally be expelled within 30 minutes of delivery, accompanied by a gush of blood, lengthening of the umbilical cord and contraction of the uterus. Expulsion can be aided by having the woman squat and push, nipple stimulation (by initiating breastfeeding or rolling the nipples) and ensuring that the bladder is voided. Administration of 10 mg. of oxytocin will help expel the placenta, as well as help prevent postpartum hemorrhage.

The placenta and the membranes must be carefully checked to ensure that no pieces are missing. Retained or incomplete placenta is a recipe for hemorrhage and infection. In some cases, the retained placenta will have separated and very gentle traction on the umbilical cord will suffice to remove the placenta. However, in approximately one of every 7000 deliveries, the placenta will be embedded in the myometrium (inner wall of the uterus) and surgical removal will be needed. Pulling on the umbilical cord in these instances can cause massive hemorrhage. This form of placental adherence carries a high risk of maternal mortality due to hemorrhage and infection and requires immediate transport to a hospital.

Shock

Shock is a serious illness that results from any condition causing an inadequate flow of blood through the body. It may result from rapid blood loss, sepsis, heart failure, disorders of the nervous system or allergic reactions. If shock is not reversed there is progressive loss of oxygenation, leading eventually to failure of vital organs. Signs of shock include rapid heart rate, rapid respiration, cool, clammy skin, confusion and fainting. Because women giving birth in the developing world are prey to anemia, hemorrhage and infection, they are particularly vulnerable to shock. Intervening early to prevent the emergence of shock is the best way to save lives. Treatment for shock requires replacing the lost fluids, increasing the flow of oxygen and correction of the underlying condition. In a village setting, oral or rectal rehydration, clearing the airway of an unconscious woman and immediate transport to a medical facility are required.

Disseminated Intravascular Coagulation

Disseminated intravascular coagulation (DIC) is a disorder of the blood clotting function brought on by a severe physiological insult. Rather than focusing the clotting on the site of the injury, diffuse clotting occurs throughout the body. As a result, the clotting factors are expended and hemorrhage at the site of the injury occurs. Symptoms include diffuse bruising and bleeding from the gums and other unusual sites. DIC can result from eclampsia, placental or uterine bleeding or intra-uterine fetal demise. Blood transfusion and replacement of the blood clotting factor (fibrinogen) are needed to preserve the woman's life.

Uterine Rupture

Uterine rupture is a tearing of the uterine wall and may be complete or incomplete, ranging from a small tear that is asymptomatic to a major tear through all layers of the uterus leading to rapid exsanguination. Uterine rupture results from failure to properly manage dystocia, improper obstetrical technique or a weakness in the uterine wall, usually from previous trauma, such as Cesarean section. Signs and symptoms will vary according to the degree of rupture. Serious ruptures manifest as cessation of contractions, severe pain, bleeding and shock. Treatment requires replacements of lost blood and fluids and immediate surgery to repair or remove the uterus.

Intrapartum Complications of the Fetus

There are a variety of fetal anomalies that can result in an emergency during delivery. These include:

- *Multiple gestation* : Multiple gestation carries heightened risk at the time of labor and delivery. PIH, placenta previa, placenta abruptio, hemorrhage, infection, PROM, umbilical cord problems, polyhydramnios, oligohydramnios and intrauterine growth retardation are more likely in cases of multiple gestation. Infants from multiple gestation are more likely to be low birth weight, which significantly increases the likelihood of infant mortality. Surgical delivery is often required in multiple gestations. Hypotonic contractions are common due to the distension of the uterus. There is a greater likelihood that one or more of the fetuses may be malpresented as compared to a singleton birth. Both circumstances will often necessitate Cesarean section. Early detection and hospital delivery is the best strategy in cases of multiple gestation.
- *Umbilical cord abnormalities*: Complications involving the umbilical cord can pose a serious threat to the mother and the fetus. *Umbilical cord prolapse* is a condition in which the cord is interposed between the presenting part of the fetus and the cervix. As a consequence, the cord

is compressed during fetal descent, depriving the fetus of oxygen. The fetus is then apt to void meconium, which may be aspirated during birth. The birth attendant must try to relieve pressure on the cord, while hastening the delivery of the fetus. A quick Cesarean section is often the only way to prevent the demise or severe injury of the fetus. *Unusual cord length* can also precipitate a crisis. Normal cord length at term is between 32 cm and 100 cm. A too short umbilical cord can result in placenta abruptio as the fetus descends, with consequent hemorrhage. A cord that is too long may become knotted or wrapped around the baby's neck during fetal descent. Hypoxia will then result. Cord length cannot be changed. In the event that the cord is too long the birth attendant must be prepared to remove the cord from the child's neck. A short cord requires the ability to manage hemorrhage.

- *Post-term gestation*: Post-term gestation is defined as gestation beyond 42 weeks. Placental aging, characterized by decreasing flow of blood and oxygen, begins gradually at 38 weeks gestation. Post-term gestation runs the risk of fetal hypoxia, starvation and meconium aspiration when birth occurs. Tracking the duration of pregnancy is important to managing post-term gestation. Induced delivery once the 42nd week is reached is the most common strategy for managing post-term gestation.

POSTPARTUM PERIOD[44]

The postpartum period is a period of enormous and rapid change that provides a crucial opportunity for safeguarding the health of the mother and the neonate. As described earlier, the great majority of maternal deaths occur during the postpartum period. Moreover, a high and increasing proportion of all deaths under age five occur during the neonatal period. Proper care and education of the household during the postpartum period could have a significant impact on maternal and neonatal mortality.

Unfortunately, the postpartum period has been virtually neglected in both maternal and child survival programs until very recently. Maternal health programs have focused largely on prenatal care and training birth attendants on the specious assumption that this would prevent obstetrical emergencies. Child survival interventions largely take effect after the neonatal period. A new norm that mandates regular care in the immediate and early postpartum period is needed to achieve gains in maternal and neonatal survival.

Changes in the Postpartum Period

The postpartum period may be divided into three stages: immediate post-partim (the first 24 hours), early postpartum (24 hours to the end of the first week) and late postpartum (2 weeks to 6 weeks).

Women undergo significant physiological and psychological changes during the postpartum period as they recuperate from pregnancy and childbirth, while caring for a new child.

- *Changes in vial signs*: temperature may be elevated during the first 24 hours but should return to normal thereafter. Fever after the first 24 hours signals infection. Women may experience chills immediately after delivery, which are without significance in the absence of fever. Pulse during the first 24 hours is usually in the range of 50–90 beats per minute and respiration at 16–24 breaths per minute. Rapid respiration (more than 24 bpm) indicates one of several complications, including infection or blood loss. Blood pressure should remain stable. A decrease in blood pressure (down 15 to 20 mm Hg) may indicate blood loss or shock, while an increase of 30 mm systolic or 15 mm diastolic suggests the onset of eclampsia.

- *Pain and discomfort*: pain from perineal lacerations, episiotomy, hemorrhoids and breast engorgement is common. These should decline during the late postpartum period.
- *Cardiovascular changes*: cardiac output increases during the first 48 hours as blood is withdrawn from the uteroplacental bed, but then decreases over the next four weeks to prepregnancy levels. A relatively slow heartbeat (50 to 70 bpm) during the early postpartum period compensates for increased cardiac output. Tachycardia (pulse in excess of 90–100 bpm) is a warning sign and may be due to infection or hemorrhage.
- *Uterine involution*: rapid involution of the uterus should occur. The uterus should contract to the size of a large grapefruit within 1–2 hours of birth and have a firm tone. The fundus should be 1 cm above the umbilicus after 12 hours, 3 cm below the umbilicus after 3 days and 9 cm below the umbilicus by the ninth day. By 5 to 6 weeks the uterus should have returned to its pre-pregnancy size. A soft uterus that fails to involute quickly is highly prone to hemorrhage. Gentle uterine massage can be applied to help restore uterine tone.
- *Discharge of lochia*: the remaining uterine contents are emptied during the first ten days postpartum via a vaginal discharge called lochia. The lochia will be red during the first 3 days, pink to brown during days 4–9 and yellow to white thereafter. Unusually heavy, bloody lochia (soaking more than one thick pad or cloth every fifteen minutes) is a warning sign of hemorrhage and foul smelling lochia at any point indicates infection.
- *Breast engorgement*: the breasts will secrete colostrum during the first 2–3 days postpartum after which milk production should be firmly established. Women may experience breast tenderness or pain and are susceptible to cracking or infection of the skin around the nipples.
- *Psychological and behavioral adaptations*: the latter stages of pregnancy, labor and delivery are likely to have depleted maternal energy reserves, which are typically stressed by the poor nutritional state and heavy work load of women in developing countries. A period of rest and sleep is needed in order to optimize maternal recuperation and adaptation to caring for a newborn. Bonding between the mother and newborn, with appropriate caring behaviors is essential if the newborn is to thrive. For a combination of reasons, affective disorders, ranging from "baby blues" to clinical depression are common during the postpartum period. In most cases these are transient but they may lead to serious mental illness. Depression among women in developing countries is a serious and largely ignored phenomenon.

Care in the Postpartum Period

The objectives of care during the postpartum period are as follows:

1. Early detection and prompt management of postpartum complications giving special attention to the immediate and early postpartum periods, since the great majority of deaths occur during the first week.
2. Counseling of the mother in self-care.
3. Newborn care, with special attention to preventing neonatal mortality.
4. Counseling in family planning for the mother and her partner.

The American College of Nurse-Midwives has recommended the following schedule of postpartum visits[45]:

- First visit—six hours after birth
- Second visit—3 days after birth
- Third visit—14 days after birth
- Fourth visit—40 days after birth

MATERNAL HEALTH CARE

This level of postpartum assessment and care would constitute a radical change in most parts of the world. Care has focused largely on the intrapartum and prenatal periods. However, the pattern of maternal mortality dictates a significant alteration in caregiving if maternal mortality is to be reduced.

At minimum, a visit during the first 24 hours to assess for hemorrhage and eclampsia and during the third to fifth day to check for infection is needed. The visit must be by an attendant who has been trained to detect an obstetrical emergency and who can undertake life saving interventions pending transfer to a medical facility. Complications of the postpartum period are discussed below.

Postpartum care should cover the following points:

- Assessing the uterus to ensure that normal involution is occurring
- Monitoring postpartum bleeding to ensure it is within normal limits
- Assessing the lochia to monitor for hemorrhage and infection
- Monitoring for signs of infection
- Monitoring for signs of pre-eclampsia/eclampsia
- Encouraging voiding of the bladder and monitoring for bladder or urinary tract infection
- Assessing the condition of the lower extremities to monitor for signs of thromboembolism (warmth and pain in the calf, feeling of heaviness in the leg)
- Encouraging proper nutrition during the postpartum period. Lactation and maternal recuperation place additional demands on both energy and micronutrient stores. Iron and folic acid supplementation should continue, as should supplementation with zinc and calcium. A single oral dose of 200,000 IU of Vitamin A should be provided during the first month postpartum[46]. Consumption of iodized salt should be encouraged.
- Counseling on care of the perineum, with emphasis on proper hygiene (gentle rinsing with warm, clean, soapy water) to help prevent infection.
- Counseling on the woman's need for rest during the first six weeks postpartum.
- Counseling on the importance of immediate and exclusive breastfeeding and breast care
- Counseling on family planning, emphasizing the importance of birth spacing to protect infant health. Contraceptive options should be discussed and postpartum family planning initiated as soon as feasible.
- Newborn care, which is discussed in detail later in this chapter.

Complications in the Postpartum Period[47]

All women, households and birth attendants should be trained to watch for danger signs during the postpartum period. Hemorrhage, eclampsia and infection are the major threats to maternal health during this period. The importance of proper management of the postpartum period cannot be over-emphasized, since it is the time when the great majority of maternal deaths occur. Table 7-6 provides a quick guide to danger signs during the postpartum period.

Eclampsia

Eclampsia has been discussed earlier. It is more likely to emerge during the first 24 hours postpartum than during the prenatal period. Prompt emergency treatment of eclampsia coupled with rapid transport to a medical facility is essential.

TABLE 7-6. Danger Signs during the Postpartum Period

Danger sign	Significance
Heavy bleeding (more than 500 ml.)	Hemorrhage
Severe headache, tinnitus, visual disturbances, vomiting, clonus, hyper-reflexia, epigastric or right upper quadrant pain, convulsions	Eclampsia
High fever, chills, pain, nausea, vomiting, foul smelling vaginal discharge	Infection

Postpartum Hemorrhage

Postpartum hemorrhage is defined as losing more than 500 ml of blood subsequent to birth. Visual assessment of blood loss is notoriously unreliable and different crude measures have been suggested for field application. For example, 500 ml has been compared to two cupfuls. Alternatively, soaking through more than 1 or 2 thick cloths per hour has been proposed as a barometer of blood loss.[48] Experienced birth attendants may have an intuitive sense of whether blood loss is normal or excessive. Bright red bleeding should stop within about an hour, though discharge of bloody lochia will continue for several days. Women experiencing hemorrhage are likely to show signs of shock—rapid breathing, rapid heart rate, cool, clammy skin, thirst, feeling faint or dizzy, decreased urine output. Postpartum hemorrhage can lead to death within a matter of a few hours so urgent action is needed once hemorrhage is suspected.

Postpartum hemorrhage is classified as *early* if it occurs during the first 24 hours and is usually due to uterine atony, lacerations, hematomas or uterine prolapse. *Late* postpartum hemorrhage occurs after the first 24 hours and is typically caused by infection, failure of the uterus to involute completely and retained placental fragments. The treatment of postpartum hemorrhage depends on the cause of bleeding, though uterine atony is the most common culprit. Blood transfusion and intravenous replacement of fluids may be needed irrespective of the cause of hemorrhage.

- *Uterine atony*, in which the uterus has failed to properly contract and the vessels that fed the placenta remain open, accounts for the great majority of cases of postpartum hemorrhage. The uterus remains soft and "boggy" to the touch. Measures to treat hemorrhage due to uterine atony include:
    — Nursing by the neonate or nipple stimulation to induce uterine contraction.
    — Uterine massage, in which the fundus is massaged with one hand, while the lower portion of the uterus is supported with the other hand. Massage should end once bleeding has stopped and be resumed if necessary.
    — Bimanual compression, in which one hand is inserted vaginally and pressed, in the form of a fist, against the bottom of the uterus while the other hand squeezes the fundus towards the pubis so as to compress the uterus. Bimanual compression is used if external massage fails.
    — Administration of oxyotcin or ergometrine to induce uterine contraction.
    — Blood transfusion and fluid replacement.
- *Trauma and lacerations* are common as a consequence of birth. Minor lacerations are usually self-healing and not dangerous if they remain uninfected. However, deep tears can extend from the vagina into the muscles of the perineum, the anal sphincter and the rectum. These can create permanent disabilities at best and life threatening hemorrhages at worst. Continued

bleeding in the presence of a contracted uterus usually signals hemorrhage due to laceration. Treatment requires compression of the wound with gauze packs or other clean compress and suturing of the wound with absorbable sutures (chromic catgut). A catheter is usually inserted to aid in voiding the bladder.

- *Hematomas* occur as a result of difficult or prolonged second stage labor or invasive procedures that damage the tissue surrounding the vaginal wall. These forms of hemorrhage can be particularly insidious since bleeding may be concealed. The woman will usually complain of extreme pain and pressure and exhibit signs of shock. Draining of the hematoma and closing the bleeding vessels are needed to arrest hemorrhage.
- *Uterine inversion* is the total or partial collapse of the uterus towards or into the vaginal canal. The inner wall of the uterus will move towards the cervix and may actually protrude through the vagina. The uterus is atonic and highly susceptible to massive blood loss and infection. The uterus must be immediately returned to its natural position and shape by manual pressure – the uterus is literally pushed back into place. A tocolytic agent may be needed to relax the uterus so it can be placed in its normal position and then oxytocin or ergmetrine used to contract the uterus. Antiobiotic therapy is initiated to prevent infection. Hysterectomy may be needed if drug therapy fails to restore uterine tone.

Bleeding that *begins* after the first 24 hours is a sign of hemorrhage most likely due to retained placental fragments. Continued soaking of pads with blood or a continuous small flow of blood are danger signs. The uterus will not have contracted properly and corollary infection may have set in. Nipple stimulation, external uterine massage, ergometrine and antibiotics are needed to redress postpartum hemorrhage. If placental fragments are still not expelled then curettage of the uterus will be needed.

Postpartum Infection

The most important tool in managing postpartum infection is *prevention*. Asepsis during labor and delivery and cleanliness in the postpartum period can eliminate many sources of infection. Cleansing after voiding or defecating, changing of perineal pads, gentle cleaning of perineum and frequent voiding of the bladder can also contribute to reducing infection.

Postpartum infection is suspected whenever fever appears during any two of the first ten days postpartum. Fever with chills, pain and tenderness in the abdomen and/or foul smelling vaginal discharge should lead to a presumptive diagnosis of postpartum infection. Postpartum infection can take many forms:

- Infections of the perineum and vagina emanating from lacerations suffered during birth or from an episiotomy;
- Infections of the reproductive tract resulting from bacterial invasion of the uterus during labor, delivery or the postpartum period; these infections can spread from the reproductive organs to the abdominal lining and cavity;
- Urinary tract infection, which is facilitated by difficulty or reluctance to urinate in the immediate postpartum period;
- Infection of a Cesarean section incision.

All of these forms of infection can be deadly or have very serious consequences if not treated promptly and effectively. Postpartum infections are usually polymicrobial. In addition, laboratory identification of the infectious agent will usually be impossible in most developing country settings. Accordingly, combination therapy drawing on broad spectrum antimcrobial drugs from different families is usually prescribed; e.g., a combination of antibacterial and anti-protozoa drugs.

INDUCED ABORTION[49]

Abortion remains intensively controversial and is severely restricted in many countries. Unsafe abortion remains a major contributor to maternal mortality and morbidity. The Programme of Action adopted at the 1994 United Nations International Conference on Population and Development calls on all countries to ensure that abortion is safe where it is legal. Hence, health providers in countries where abortion is legal should help ensure that it is safe and accessible.

Where abortion is legally permissible, the decision must be made by the woman and must be informed and voluntary. Good, nonjudgmental counseling must be made available to the woman so she can make a free and informed choice. Counseling should be age and culturally appropriate, as well as taking into account the woman's emotional state. She should be presented with factual information, her options should be explained, and she must be allowed to explore her feelings about carrying out the abortion. Under no circumstances should a woman feel pressured or coerced in making a choice about abortion.

First Trimester Methods

The surgical technique of choice for first trimester abortion in most developing country settings is manual vacuum aspiration. A narrow cannula is inserted into the uterus through the cervix and negative pressure is created, evacuating the contents of the uterus. A vacuum is created in the barrel of the syringe, to which the cannula is attached, by drawing back on the plunger. The contents of the uterus are aspirated into the transparent barrel of the syringe, permitting easy identification of pregnancy tissue. Vacuum aspiration using an electric vacuum pump is also used, though it makes pregnancy tissue more difficult to verify as the uterine contents are passed through a filter into a receptacle. A local anesthetic (lidocaine) is injected into the cervix to prevent pain and analgesics should be provided for post-abortion pain management. Failure to provide proper pain management, including anesthetics and supportive counseling, can make abortion a terrible ordeal for women.

Dilation and curettage (D&C) is still widely used as an abortion procedure in the developing world, though it has largely been abandoned in the United States and other developed countries. The D&C technique involves dilating the cervix and inserting a metal rod with a curette (loop) on the end into the uterus. The lining of the uterus is scraped with the curette to remove fetal and placental tissue. D&C should be performed under anesthesia, which, in practice, is often unavailable. Vacuum aspiration has many advantages over D&C and manual vacuum aspiration provides a practical, safer, easier, less costly alternative.

The use of abortifacient drugs during the first trimester has gained increasing currency. There are two drug regimens for first trimester abortion. One involves a combination of mifepristone and misoprostol and the other combines methotrexate and misoprostol.

Mifepristone acts as an antagonist to progesterone, which is needed to sustain the pregnancy. Misoprostol serves to enhance the efficacy of mifepristone. The mifepristone-misoprostol regimen requires three visits to the providers. Six hundred milligrams of mifepristone is provided during the first visit, followed by 400 micrograms of misoprostol two days later, after which the woman is kept under observation for four hours. A follow-up visit two weeks later is used to ensure the abortion was complete.

The mifepristone-misoprostol regimen is 95 percent effective during the first seven weeks after the last menstrual period (LMP) and 80 percent effective in the ninth week LMP. Efficacy beyond nine weeks has not been established. The mifepristone-misoprostol regimen is therefore best suited to early abortion.

Most women using the mifepristone-misoprostol regimen experience cramping and bleeding. The observed blood loss can provoke concern among women, but it is usually without clinical significance (i.e., less than 100 ml). One percent of women will need follow-up curettage and 0.1 percent will need transfusion. Analgesics (acetaminophen, acetaminophen with codeine) are important to managing pain from cramping.

An alternative drug regimen consists of a combination of methotrexate and misoprostol. Methotrexate acts by inhibiting the ability of fetal cells to divide, thereby provoking an abortion. The methotrexate-misoprostol regimen is less widely used because methotrexate is more expensive, the protocol is less clearly established and there are concerns about the toxicity of methotrexate. The regimen requires the intra-muscular injection of methotrexate (50 mg per square meter of body surface) followed 3 to 7 days later by vaginal insertion of 800 micrograms of misoprostol. The methotrexate-misoprostol regimen is 95 percent effective during early pregnancy. Cramping and bleeding are common, with use of acetaminophen with codeine for pain management. A follow-up visit is needed, though recommendations as to the timing of the visit vary from 3 to 7 days.

Second Trimester Methods

The surgical method of choice for abortion from 13 to 20 weeks is dilation and evacuation. Subsequent to administration of local anesthesia, the cervix is dilated using laminaria (a dried seaweed that slowly expands) or synthetic dilators. Once the cervix has been dilated, vacuum aspiration is used to empty the uterus. Oxytocin or vasopresin are sometimes used to contract the uterus, reducing the amount of bleeding.

There are drug regimens available for second trimester abortions. However, they have generally fallen into disfavor relative to dilation and evacuation, which is safer, faster and less expensive. Hypertonic agents (saline solution or hypertonic urea) are feticides that are injected into the amniotic fluid. Alternatively, prostaglandins (dinoprostone and misoprostol) are inserted as vaginal suppositories to provoke an abortion through induction of labor.

Managing Complications of Unsafe Abortion

Complications of unsafe abortion should be handled as an obstetric emergency. Most post-abortion complications are due to incomplete abortions. These complications manifest as hemorrhage, infection and trauma and should be handled in accordance with the general procedures described earlier. Of particular importance as a public health strategy is making manual vacuum aspiration widely available. Evacuation of uterine contents is essential to managing incomplete abortions. MVA presents a practical method for managing incomplete abortions that can be applied widely in the developing world.

D&C is still widely used to manage incomplete abortions. Providers of post-abortion care in the developing world should be encouraged to switch from D&C to manual vacuum aspiration (MVA) with local anesthesia. MVA is a simple, low-cost practical alternative that can expand access to safe, efective post-abortion care. MVA combined with local anesthesia obviates the need for general anesthesia, requires no electricity and little equipment, has a significantly lower rate of complications and is less costly.

Post-abortion Contraception[50]

Women undergoing an induced abortion will usually want to avoid a quick return to pregnancy. It is very important that women be aware of their susceptibility to pregnancy almost immediately after an abortion and that the health care system is oriented to post abortion family planning services.

Return to fertility can occur as quickly as ten days after an abortion. Seventy-five percent of women will ovulate within six weeks of an abortion. This stands in marked contrast to the normal 4–6 months that elapses after a birth before ovulation re-commences. Women receiving an abortion or treated for post-abortion complications must receive counseling at the time of treatment. Counseling should inform the woman of the probability of conception in the immediate aftermath of abortion, ascertain the woman's fertility desires and inform the woman of her contraceptive options.

Most health systems do a poor job of providing contraceptive services post-abortion or to women treated for abortion complications. Family planning services are rarely linked to the abortion care providers. Providers often focus on the immediate problem of resolving the abortion or complication without follow-up counseling on family planning. Women are also often subjected to insensitive or harsh conduct from the providers, rather than supportive counseling on fertility management.

Abortion care providers should systematically refer women undergoing an abortion or treatment for complication of an unsafe abortion to a family planning counselor. Quality of care standards should be observed in delivering post-abortion contraceptive services (see Chapter 5). Women experiencing an uncomplicated abortion and wishing to avoid pregnancy should start use of contraception immediately if they are having sex. Women who have had an uncomplicated abortion can use any method of contraception that is not otherwise contraindicated. An important caveat to this general statement is that women opting for natural family planning methods should practice abstinence until a normal menstrual pattern returns.

Complications from unsafe abortion constrain contraceptive options. Infections must be resolved before IUD insertion or sterilization can proceed. Trauma to the genital tract requires delaying sterilization until the trauma has healed and IUD insertion must be delayed in cases of uterine perforation. Barrier methods and spermicides may be inappropriate for women with vaginal or cervical lacerations. Women who have experienced serious blood loss or have severe anemia will be poor candidates for sterilization or copper-bearing IUD, both of which will entail additional blood loss. Short-term methods should be provided to victims of hemorrhage until their condition permits use of sterilization or IUD. Second trimester abortions preclude the use of diaphragms or cervical caps until the uterus involutes to normal position at 6 weeks post-abortion. Displacement of the fallopian tubes until the uterus returns to pre-pregnancy position may also complicate sterilization. IUD expulsion rates are higher if insertion occurs before six weeks post-partum.

Because post-abortion contraception poses special problems, relevant training is needed for family planning and abortion care providers. The training should emphasize both supportive counseling for the woman and the technical constraints to contraceptive choice emanating from abortion complications.

NEWBORN CARE

Of the approximately 11 million deaths of children under five that occur each year, about 3.3 million are to children 30 days or less.[51] Neonatal mortality is a huge contributor to the over-all rate of child mortality and its importance is growing. Thanks to the success of other child survival interventions, such as immunization and oral rehydration therapy, child deaths are increasingly concentrated in the neonatal period. Like maternal mortality, many neonatal deaths occur during the first seven days post-partum. Hence, an increased focus on post-partum care for the mother also creates a splendid opportunity for saving the lives of children.

The barriers to saving newborn lives are much the same as the barriers to reducing maternal mortality. Newborns get very sick very fast. Illness in the newborn must often be recognized and treated within hours. The sequence of delays that blocks maternal care also tends to result in neonatal mortality. Similar efforts to induce rapid recognition, transport and treatment are needed to reduce newborn mortality.

Fortunately, there are a number of technically simple and low cost interventions that could have a major impact on neonatal mortality. Approximately 85 percent of neonatal mortality is attributable to infections (septicemia, pneumonia and tetanus), birth asphyxia and birth trauma.[52] This permits the delineation of effective interventions:

1. *Prevent tetanus*: Tetanus, which kills 500,000 neonates per year, can be prevented through tetanus toxoid injection of the mother.[53] Using a clean razor to cut the umbilical cord, keeping the umbilical stump clean and avoiding traditional practices of placing a poultice on the stump can also prevent tetanus. Tetanus can be treated with penicillin, tetanus antitoxin and anticonvulsives, but prompt recognition and care are needed for care to be effective.[54]
2. *Avoid prolonged labor*: Obstructed labor is damaging to the child as well as the mother. Prompt recognition, referral and treatment in cases of obstructed labor can minimize birth trauma and consequently reduce neonatal mortality.
3. *Keep the baby clean, dry and warm*: Neonates are highly susceptible to hypothermia. In many cultures it is the practice to wash the baby immediately (usually in cold water). Simply wiping the baby clean suffices, without use of cold water. Practicing the six cleans at birth can help reduce the probability of infection. Wrapping the child in a clean cloth and placing the child in the "kangaroo position" next to the mother's skin will help keep the baby warm.
4. *Immediate treatment of birth asphyxia*: Newborns who fail to cry or breathe immediately after birth are likely to have the respiratory passages clogged with meconium. A simple, very inexpensive suction bulb can be used to clear the breathing passage. This often suffices, but mouth-to-mouth breathing may also be needed. The child should be watched for signs of infection.

5. *Practice immediate and exclusive breastfeeding*: Breast milk consists of colostrum during the first few days after birth. Restricting the baby's intake to colostrum is very helpful in preventing infection and ensures proper nutrition.
6. *Prophylactic treatment to prevent opthalmia neonatorum*: Ocular infection with gonorrhea can be prevented. Alternative regimens for ocular prophylaxis are single applications of 1 percent silver nitrate eye drops, 1 percent tetracycline eye ointment or 0.5 percent erythromycin eye ointment.[55] Conjunctivitis in newborns should be assumed to be due to gonorrhea and/or chlamydia and be treated immediately.
7. *Monitor for rapid respiration and immediate treatment for presumptive pneumonia*: A respiration rate of more than 60 breaths per minute or severe chest indrawing indicates pneumonia.[56] Community health workers and mothers can be trained to watch for rapid respiration. Children with presumed pneumonia should receive a dose of co-trimoxazole immediately from the community health worker[57] or intramuscular injection of gentamicin and benzylpenicillin from the clinical provider[58] and be referred to the hospital. The key to saving lives is prompt recognition and treatment.
8. *Monitoring for other infections*: Septicemia and meningitis are the other major killers of newborns. Symptoms of meningitis include fever, stiff neck and back, bulging fontanel, vomiting, convulsions and a weak, odd cry.[59] Meningitis must be treated immediately with ampicillin or gentamicin. Signs of septicemia include failure to suckle, lethargy, pallor, vomiting, fever, swollen belly, jaundice and convulsions.[60] Ampicillin and gentamicin are also used to treat septicemia.
9. *Immunization of newborns*: Newborns should receive polio, BCG and hepatitis B vaccination during the first week of life.

In sum, a handful of feasible interventions could have a major impact on saving newborn lives. Instituting a new norm of immediate post-partum care would thus have a major impact on both maternal and newborn survival.

8

HIV/AIDS and Sexually Transmitted Diseases

This chapter focuses on the application of health technologies to preventing and treating sexually transmitted diseases, with an emphasis on HIV/AIDS. The greatest public health impact will come from preventing new cases of sexually transmitted disease. The behavior change and community empowerment strategies discussed in earlier chapters are therefore central to any effort to reduce the burden of disease from STD. However, we must also avoid a false dichotomy between prevention and treatment. Treating and counseling those already infected is essential to slowing the spread of disease, as well as providing relief to the affected client.

There are five basic steps that health managers can take to reduce the burden imposed by sexually transmitted diseases:

1. Increase the percentage of infected individuals who seek and receive appropriate treatment.
2. Increase the use of syndromic management of STD, an approach adapted to resource poor settings.
3. Provide appropriate, low-cost care for people living with AIDS that will reduce the spread of opportunistic infections, alleviate suffering and prolong life. Access to anti-retroviral therapy (ART) is likely to increase in the developing world, so a primer on ART is also provided.
4. Prevent and manage maternal to child transmission of STD, including HIV.
5. Prevent STD transmission through blood transfusion.

The chapter concludes with a look at options for detecting and managing cervical cancer, which is attributable to sexual transmission of human papillomavirus (HPV).

A QUICK GUIDE TO SEXUALLY TRANSMITTED DISEASES

There are a wide array of sexually transmitted diseases (STD), varying in etiology, consequence and treatment. Table 8-1 provides a an overview of STD.[1]

TABLE 8-1. A Quick Guide to Sexually Transmitted Diseases

Disease	Infectious agent	Signs & symptoms
AIDS	Human immunodeficiency virus (HIV)	Multiple signs of immune deficiency including tuberculosis, wasting, diarrheal disease, PCP
	Diseases Characterized by Genital Ulcers	
Syphilis	Treponema pallidum	1. Primary syphilis—genital chancre that is often hidden in women; lymphadenopathy 2. Secondary syphilis—rash, cutaneous lesions, wide array of organ involvement 3. Tertiary syphilis—lesions of cardiovascular, central nervous and other organs 4. Congenital syphilis—nasal discharge, skin rashes, damage to eyes, teeth, hearing
Chancroid	Haemophilus ducreyi	Painful, irregular ulcer that extrudes a yellow-gray exudate and bleeds easily. Often accompanied by painful enlargement of regional lymph nodes
Genital herpes	Genital herpes simplex virus	Pustular or ulcerative lesions that persist for 4 to 15 days accompanied by itching and pain before scabbing or healing
Granuloma inguinale (Donovanosis)	Calymmatobacterium granulomatis	Highly vascular, painless, progressive lesions that bleed easily on contact, without regional lymphadenopathy
Lymphogranuloma venereum	Chlamydia trachomatis, immunotypes L-1, L-2 and L-3	Small painless lesion on penis or vulva that is frequently unnoticed. Manifests as inguinal buboes on men and pelvic node inflammation in women.
	Diseases Characterized by Urethritis and Cervicitis	
Chlamydia	Chlamydia trachomatis	Men: scanty to moderate mucopurulent discharge from penis, urethral itching, burning on urination Women: Largely asymptomatic, but may include mucopurulent discharge from cervix and easily induced bleeding from endocervix.
Gonorrhea	Neisseria gonorrhea	Men: abundant, purulent discharge from penis; burning on urination Women: Largely asymptomatic, but may include mucopurulent discharge from cervix, burning on urination, changes in vaginal secretion/discharge, painful intercourse, redness of the vulva

Bacterial vaginosis	High concentrations of anaerobic bacteria	White, noninflammatory discharge and a fishy odor.
Trichomoniasis	Trichomonas vaginalis	Men are largely asymptomatic, while women usually have a malodorous yellow-green discharge
Vulvovaginal candidiasis	Candida albicans	Vaginal discharge and itching
Ectoparasitic infections		
Pediculosis pubis	Pubic lice (Phthirus pubis)	Visible lice, itching
Scabies	Sarcoptes scabiei	Itching
Other Sexually Transmitted Diseases		
Genital warts	Human papilloma virus	Visible genital warts
Cervical cancer	Human papilloma virus	Usually detected via gynecological examination
Hepatitis A and B	Hepatitis A and B viruses	Jaundice, liver disease
Pelvic inflammatory disease	Neisseria gonorrhea, chlamydia trachomatis are most common causes, but vaginal flora can also cause PID	Lower abdominal tenderness, adnexal tenderness, cervical motion tenderness, fever
Epididymitis	Neisseria gonorrhea, chlamydia trachomatis are most common causes	Testicular pain, swelling of the epididymis

CASE DETECTION AND MANAGEMENT

Detecting and managing cases of STD serves to alleviate the suffering of the person afflicted and reduce transmission to other people. Delays in detection and treatment greatly increase the likelihood that the infected individual will suffer serious consequences from the disease. Most STD are progressive; the longer the disease goes untreated, the worse the outcome for the infected individual and the more difficult the treatment. Delays in treatment after infection also increase the probability of transmission to sexual partners. Recall the discussion of the epidemiology of STD transmission in Chapter 2. The likelihood of transmission is partly a function of the number of times an infected person has sex with an uninfected partner. Delaying treatment will typically mean a higher number of exposures. The problem is exacerbated among untreated people with multiple partners.

Early detection is particularly important to preventing the spread of HIV. Viral load is highest during the period shortly after infection, which increases the likelihood of transmission, and then wanes until the disease takes hold some years later.

Prompt case detection and management are therefore central to preventing STD and minimizing their impact on the infected. However, asking the question, "Who has an STD and which STD has been contracted?" reveals a host of difficulties facing health providers and health managers. Figure 8-1 illustrates the difficulties in case detection and management[2].

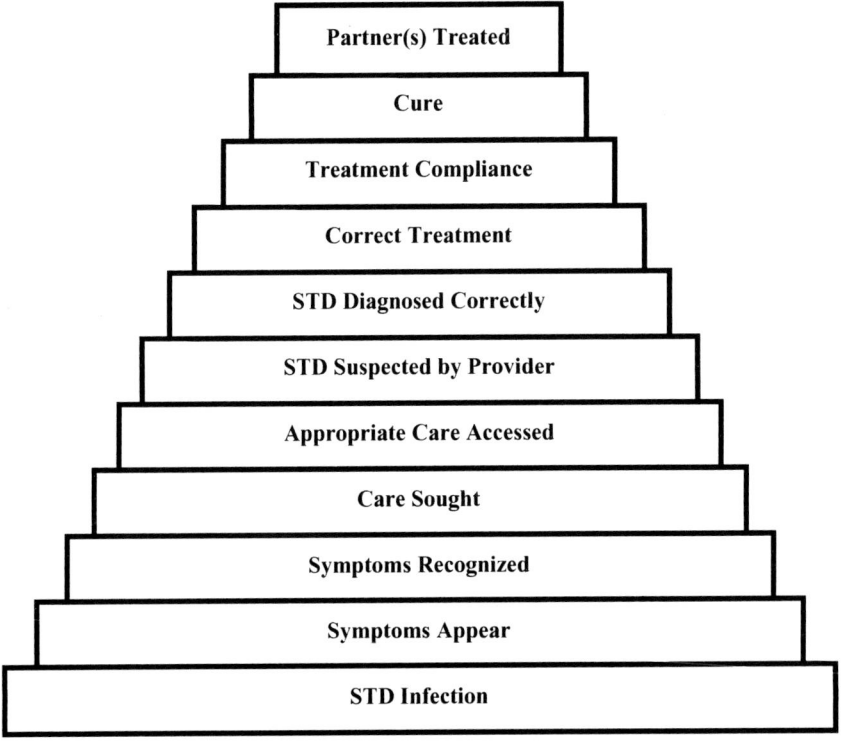

FIGURE 8-1. Potential losses to STD detection and treatment.

Moving from top to bottom, each succeeding rung in the inverted period represents a proportion of the total number of STD cases lost to detection or treatment. STD are often asymptomatic or present symptoms easily confused with other diseases or disorders. Hence, only a fraction of those infected may suspect they have an STD. Physical, economic, psychological and social barriers mean that only a portion of those who fear they are infected will seek and access appropriate care. Health care providers encountering patients for other reasons, such as prenatal care or family planning, may also fail to look for or detect an STD. Diagnosis is often difficult because providers are poorly trained and laboratory support is usually not available. Of those properly diagnosed, an even lesser fraction of those infected will complete successful treatment and fewer still will refer their sexual contacts for treatment. The stigma and shame often associated with STD make it particularly difficult for infected individuals, who often have difficulty accessing health care for any reason, to seek and comply with treatment.

Detecting People with an STD

Health managers have a number of strategies at their disposal for increasing the likelihood that those infected will seek and receive treatment:

- *Ease access to trained health providers and drugs*: Health seeking behavior and case detection is in part a function of ease of access to competent providers. Training primary health care health providers at the lowest levels of the health system to recognize the signs and symptoms of STD is an important aide to case detection. Chapter 5 suggested that managers develop a Provider/Services Matrix that specifies the services to be offered at every level in the health system. Table 5.1 suggested, for example, that community level services include promoting behavior change, condom distribution, referral for care and testing, access to antibiotics, prophylactic treatment against gonococcal opthalmia neonatorum and social support to people living with AIDS. Making basic services easily accessible increases the likelihood of an infected individual seeking care. Drugs for STD treatment must be readily available, so systems for drug supply down to the village level must be strengthened. The choice of STD drugs in any given setting depends on the prevalence of various syndromes, efficacy, cost, toxicity, antimicrobial resistance, mode of administration (oral is preferred), and teratogenic effects.[3]
- *Encourage care seeking through behavior change and community empowerment*: Behavior change and community mobilization programs should systematically incorporate efforts to encourage use of STD care services. The act of seeking care implies that an individual has a modicum of knowledge about STD, believes he or she is at personal risk of contracting an STD, has overcome the fear or embarrassment associated with seeking care, and that the perceived benefits of seeking care exceed the perceived costs. Ease of access and high quality care serve to reduce the costs of health seeking behavior. Communication programs can serve to increase the sense of personal vulnerability and awareness of the signs and symptoms of STD, including HIV/AIDS. Community mobilization can help create a more supportive environment for care seeking. A shared sense of vulnerability to STD as a result of a participatory process can help spur action. Commitment of community resources to increase access to care sends an important signal and reduces the cost to individuals. Support or opprobrium from the individual's community, social network and leaders is likely to play a role in the decision to seek care.
- *Voluntary counseling and testing*: Voluntary counseling and testing (VCT) has become a key element of the HIV/AIDS control strategy of both UNAIDS and the U.S. Centers for Disease Control and Prevention.[4,5] The essence of this approach is to combine increased knowledge of

HIV status with effective counseling for the purpose of inducing behavior change. Counseling is specifically directed at helping the individual or couple adopt risk reducing behaviors, including the development of the requisite knowledge and skills. Knowledge of HIV status combined with counseling can help people plan for the future, prevent maternal-to-child transmission, seek appropriate medical care, identify support groups, and adopt family planning, as well as change behavior that reduces risk to oneself and partners.

Well designed VCT programs have been shown to be effective as a risk reduction strategy. A controlled trial of the efficacy of VCT compared to dissemination of health information in Kenya, Tanzania and Trinidad found that VCT yielded significant declines in unprotected intercourse among both men (35 percent versus 13 percent) and women (39 percent versus 17 percent).[6] VCT has also been shown to be a cost-effective public health intervention compared to both standards suggested by the World Bank and other, widely used primary health care interventions.[7]

Effective VCT programs have a number of essential characteristics and failing to adhere to these parameters helps explain why the record of counseling is more mixed than the exemplary trial cited.[8] A review of 35 studies of HIV counseling found that while many programs provided some evidence of behavioral impact, others did not.[9] Implementation of VCT should be preceded by securing community and political support. Reducing stigma is critical to encouraging clients to seek VCT. VCT programs must be voluntary; coercion or pressure to enter programs is both unethical and counter-productive. Counseling practice must be of high quality and based on sound principles, such as those described in Chapter 3, that will help the clients adopt new behaviors. Confidentiality must be assured for the client, partners and families. There should be continuity of counseling so that clients see the same counselor before and after testing. For both HIV positive and negative clients, VCT must be linked to a context appropriate package of services that includes continued counseling, medical care, support groups and social and services. The public health impact of VCT is also likely to be greatest when it is targeted to clients at high risk.

- *Target active case finding to high risk groups and other populations of public health significance*: Some countries have adopted an assertive approach of STD screening among known core transmitter groups. In Thailand, for example, brothel owners are required to make regular STD screening available to their employees[10]. Many context-appropriate tactics have been used to make screening and treatment services easily available to sex workers. Men living away from home, such as miners[11] or truck drivers[12], have also been the beneficiaries of targeted programs aimed at increasing health services utilization. Adolescents[13], drug users[14] and men having sex with men[15] have also been targeted for active case finding, usually through the use of peer educators. While pregnant women *per se* are not generally considered core transmitters, a large proportion will have contact with the medical system. Capturing pregnant women with an STD is important both for the woman's sake and to prevent potential damage to the child. At minimum, prenatal screening for syphilis should be part of all maternal health programs.

- *Increase use of risk assessment protocols*: As a general matter, the protocols and procedures for patient intake are often weak in developing countries. Improving the quality of the initial patient interview is needed for many reasons, one of which would be to ask about STD risk behaviors. Using two to five minutes, a provider might ask questions along the following lines, "Are you married or have you had a sexual partner during the past year? If so, with how many people? Have you ever had a sexually transmitted disease? Do you use condoms during sex? If so, with which of your partners? Have you ever given yourself an injection or received an injection from someone other than a health provider? Do you have reason to believe that your spouse or sexual partner may have other partners? Have you or your partner experienced sores on your genitals or discharge?"[16] The specific questions would have to be adapted to the context. A program in Tanzania, for example, tested the utility of a simple five question protocol to screen at-risk antenatal patients.[17]

- *Trace and treat partners of individuals with an STD*[18,19]: Contact tracing, otherwise known as partner notification, is one of the cornerstones of STD case management. Once a patient has been diagnosed with an STD, the health provider has a responsibility to reach as many of the patient's sexual partners as possible. Many STD are asymptomatic, especially in women. People who are asymptomatic are less likely to seek care than those with symptoms, unless they believe they are at risk. Many infected people do not seek care even in the presence of symptoms; they may not understand their significance or be too embarrassed to approach a health provider. Tracing sexual contact is therefore a key mechanism for finding and treating infected individuals, which serves to reduce the rate of transmission. Educating the STD client as to the importance of partner notification is a critical component of case detection and management. The STD client should be advised that the disease is transmitted sexually, that partner(s) may be infected even if asymptomatic, that there are potentially serious consequences for the health of the partner, and that the client may become re-infected if the partner is not treated.

  Contact tracing to reach partners who practice high-risk behaviors is particularly important; cases of STD often cluster around a node of relatively few people engaged in high-risk behaviors. Unfortunately, tracing partners who engage in the highest risk behavior is also often much more difficult than finding a spouse or steady partner.

  Because resources are usually very limited, health managers may choose to target contact tracing to high priority STD in the population served. This will vary in response to local epidemiology. In general, however, priorities for contact tracing include HIV, syphilis, gonorrhea and chlamydia or syndromes indicative of these agents, such as pelvic inflammatory disease or opthalmia neonatorum.

  The two basic strategies for contact tracing are patient referral and provider referral. Under the former approach the patient notifies each sexual contact that they may have contracted an STD and encourages them to seek care. The index patient is sometimes provided with a pre-printed card. The card has two sections, each with the same unique identification number. The provider keeps one section, which identifies the index patient and the diagnosis. The other section has a message stating that he or she may be infected and how to get medical help. By discreetly delivering the card, the index patient can avoid a direct confrontation with a potentially infected partner. A much less frequently used approach is provider referral, which requires obtaining partner contact information (names, addresses) from the index patient. The provider uses this information to make contact with the partner. It must be remembered that only a fraction of partners will be infected so the initial contact messages, whether provided by the index patient or the provider, must be worded carefully.

  Partner notification must take place within a framework of ethics and sensitivity to the local context. The confidentiality of the index patient and all contacts must always be maintained. Patients must never be coerced into revealing the names of contacts. Providers must also be aware of the possibility of violence or other abusive behavior. Women are often justly afraid that telling their husbands or partners may result in their being abused.

- *Mass treatment in high prevalence communities or groups*: One alternative to seeking out and treating individual clients is mass treatment of communities or groups where STD prevalence is high. In some instances, there is clear epidemiological evidence that an STD has reached very high prevalence levels among a specific group or in a specific community. In these instances, some public health authorities have elected mass treatment of the entire group or community. This clearly has the short-term effect of extending the reach of the STD control program. Mass treatment has been shown to achieve reductions of STD prevalence among targeted groups in Uganda, Greenland, Philippines, California, Indonesia and South Africa[20]. However, it is unlikely to be a useful control measure unless accompanied by other efforts to prevent reintroduction of the infection. Since such mass treatment programs tend to target core transmitters, repetition of past behaviors quickly leads to renewed high levels of prevalence. Mass treatment also tends to be relatively expensive and demands substantial logistical support. Hence, mass treatment is not a widely used strategy unless there is clear evidence that it will be accompanied by behavior change and/or regular screening and treatment of the at-risk population.

Managing Patients in Resource Poor Settings

Once a patient presents with a suspected STD, the health provider has three options: (1) secure a laboratory diagnosis and prescribe treatment; (2) attempt a diagnosis of a specific STD on the basis of clinical findings without laboratory confirmation; or, (3) treat a syndrome indicative of one or more STD without narrowing the diagnosis to a specific disease.

Access to laboratory diagnosis is very limited in most developing country settings. To be useful in a typical primary health care setting, a diagnostic test would have to be inexpensive, technically simple to carry out, rapid enough to obviate the need for a return visit by the patient, use an easily collectable sample, have a long shelf life, be stable under high temperatures and accurate.[21] Very few tests come close to meeting these criteria. Tests that are appropriate to a typical primary health care setting are the rapid plasma reagin (RPR) test for syphilis and microscopic examination of specimens for gonorrhea, trichomoniasis, candidiasis and bacterial vaginosis[22]. Access to these diagnostic tests should be expanded, with special attention given to screening pregnant women as part of prenatal care. However, most health providers will have to forego reliance on laboratory tests as an aid in patient management. Table 8-2 shows the WHO recommendation as to the level of laboratory diagnostic capacity that should be available at each level of the health system[23].

Simple, inexpensive and technically simple tests are becoming increasingly available, particularly for HIV. Increasing provider access to diagnostic tests at all levels is an important long-term goal for all health managers. However, progress will be incremental at best and most providers will have to rely on diagnostic procedures that do not rely on laboratory tests.

Diagnosis of a specific disease on the basis of clinical examination can be subject to a high degree of inaccuracy, depending on the disease and the skill of the clinician. Some diseases,

TABLE 8-2. WHO Recommended Level of Laboratory Diagnostic Capacity

Disease	Peripheral level	Intermediate level	Hospital/STD Center
Gonorrhea	✓	✓	✓
Chlamydia		✓	✓
Syphilis	✓	✓	✓
Chancroid			✓
Genital herpes			✓
Granuloma inguinale			✓
Trichomoniasis	✓	✓	✓
Canididiasis	✓	✓	✓
Bacterial vaginosis	✓	✓	✓
HIV		✓	✓
Human papillomavirus		✓	✓

such as candidiasis or genital herpes, present signs and symptoms that are distinguishing. However, others present signs and symptoms, such as genital ulcers, cervicitis, urethritis, vaginal discharge or epididymitis, which may be caused by two or more infectious agents. These agents can also be present simultaneously in a patient, each generating the same clinical signs. It is therefore difficult for a health provider to develop a treatment plan that presumes identification of a single causative agent.

Because of difficulties in diagnosing an infectious agent under field conditions, the most appropriate approach to STD management in many settings is *syndromic management*. Syndromic management means applying a broad treatment that will handle all or most of the causes of a clinically observable set of signs and symptoms, rather than trying to narrow down the cause to a specific agent. Syndromic management is discussed in detail below.

Patient management always requires client counseling to encourage compliance with the treatment regimen and safer sex. Treating an STD may require more than a single dose administered under the supervision of a health provider. Unfortunately, patient compliance with the required treatment is often poor. Many patients do not secure the necessary medication or finish taking their medicine. As a result, a cure is not affected, transmission continues and antimicrobial resistance increases when a prescribed drug regimen is only partially completed. Alternatively, clients take their medication, but do not practice safer sex, leading to transmission of the disease and/or they return to risky behaviors that lead to re-infection. Hence, counseling has the dual objectives of compliance with the treatment regimen and safer sex to avoid transmission and re-infection.

In carrying out client counseling it is important to apply the behavior change principles discussed in Chapter 3. Lecturing a client is not counseling nor is it a strategy for achieving behavior change. The elements of effective counseling must be respected – recapitulation of the situation by the client, offering technically sound information and advice, negotiating a plan and eliciting a commitment. These steps require that the client have a good understanding of what is needed to protect herself or himself against risk, that she or he has the confidence to undertake the necessary steps, and that the costs do not outweigh the benefits. If buying medication will mean a woman's depriving her family of food or risking a beating from her husband, then no amount of "education" will help. Rather the counselor and the client must engage in a genuine, non-judgmental dialogue that helps the client negotiate the barriers to risk reduction.

Syndromic Management

Syndromic management relies on using observable signs and symptoms to prescribe treatment for a patient. For each syndrome, context appropriate algorithms are developed by health authorities to guide patient management. The diagnostic component of the algorithm is designed in response to an understanding of the prevalence and manifestation of relevant STDs. The algorithm also provides guidance in prescribing drugs suitable to the local setting in terms of antimicrobial resistance, efficacy, availability and cost. Table 8-3 show the syndromes that present and common causative agents in the developing world.[24,25,26]

WHO has developed flowcharts that guide patient management for each of the syndromes. These flowcharts or algorithms may need to be adapted in specific contexts. Figure 8-2 gives an example of a flowchart for managing a patient presenting with a urethral discharge[27].

TABLE 8-3. STD Syndromes and Common Causative Agents (developing world)

Syndrome	Causative agents
Urethral discharge	Gonorrhea, chlamydia. Ureaplasma urealyticum is found mostly in the developed world.
Swollen scrotum	Gonorrhea, chlamydia. Can also be caused by tuberculosis, non-infectious trauma, especially in younger boys, or a tumor
Genital ulcers	Chancroid, syphilis, herpes are most common. More rarely—lymphogranuloma venereum (Africa) and donovanosis (Papua New Guinea)
Inguinal lymphadenopathy (enlarged lymph glands in groin area)	Chancroid, lymphogranuloma venereum (LGV)
Vaginal discharge	Trichomoniasis, gonorrhea and chlamydia can all lead to discharge. Candidiasis and bacterial vaginosis also present with discharge, though they are often not sexually transmitted.
Lower abdominal pain in women	Gonorrhea, chlamydia; may also indicate ectopic pregnancy
Neonatal conjunctivitis	Gonorrhea, chlamydia

As the above flowchart demonstrates, diagnosis and treatment of the symptomatic patient using the syndromic management algorithm is only one part of case management. Effective management of STD clients requires, in addition to diagnosis and treatment, assiduous attention to the "4 Cs" of STD client management, which are Compliance, Contact tracing, Counseling and Condom distribution and promotion[28]. Diagnosis and prescription alone are not enough to achieve either clinical or public health impact. Clients must receive appropriate counseling. They must be helped to adhere to the drug regimen needed for a cure to be effectuated. Sexual partners must be traced and treated. Use of condoms should be encouraged and condoms made easily available. Syndromic management provides a logical structure for covering the multiple aspects of client management.

An understanding of the local context is important in developing and applying algorithms. Factors that may influence the design and application of flow charts include:

- The prevalence and incidence of sexually transmitted disease in the local context will influence the application of the algorithms. Local etiologies of syndromes may vary and the flowchart will have to be adapted accordingly.
- The pattern of antimicrobial resistance can influence the content of the flowchart. Drug resistance will obviously influence the protocol for patient management.
- The availability of drugs.
- The diagnostic capacity at different levels at different levels in the health system, especially the availability of laboratory tests.
- The skill level of staff.
- The acceptability of the questions and examinations required by the algorithm to clients.

Small scale pilot tests and/or periodic adaptation of the algorithms is therefore essential to effective syndromic management. This caveat, however, should not be seen as a barrier to action. Extant flowcharts for urethral discharge and genital ulcers have been shown to have wide applicability, obviating the need for context specific assessments of their validity[29]. WHO and the U.S. Centers for Disease Control and Prevention (CDC) provide regular updates on treatment guidelines. National authorities, WHO, and CDC can be consulted

HIV/AIDS AND SEXUALLY TRANSMITTED DISEASES

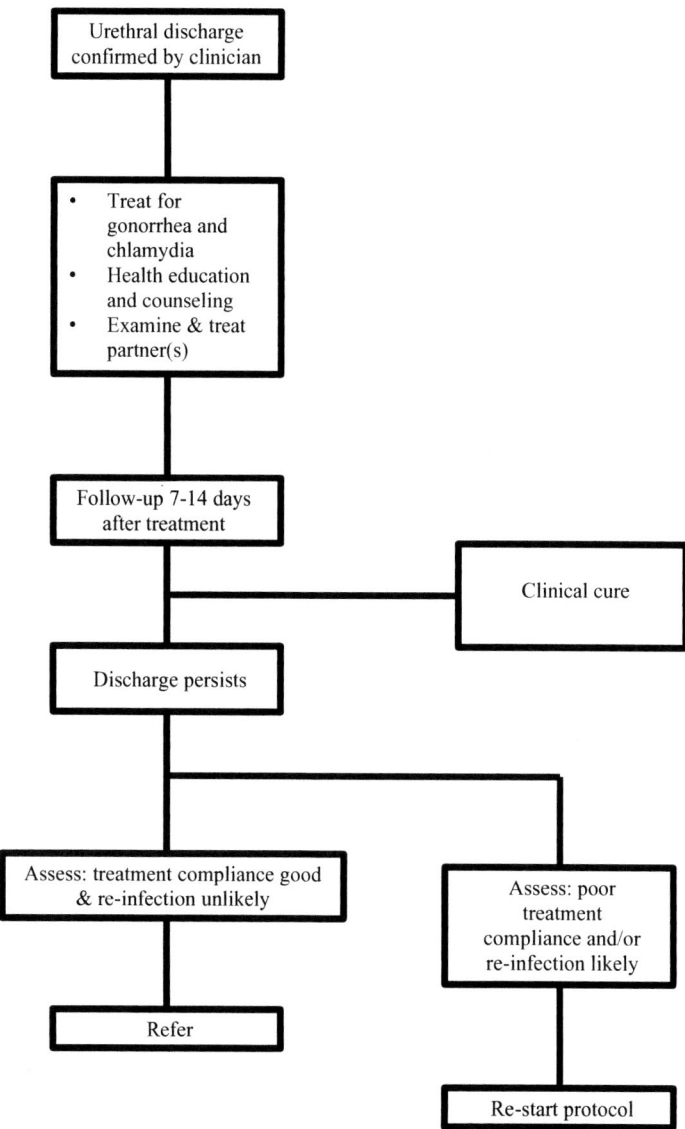

FIGURE 8-2. Flowchart for managing urethral discharge in absence of laboratory support.

as to the applicability of flowcharts to specific contexts. Table 8-4 gives the current WHO recommendation for treating STD syndromes.[30]

In resource poor settings, syndromic management has proven to be a useful tool in treating men with discharge or painful urination, treatable genital ulcers in both men and women, epididymitis and pelvic inflammatory disease.[31,32] The obvious weakness to syndromic management is that it only applies to people with observable symptoms. Women infected with gonorrhea and chlamydia are typically asymptomatic. Conversely, vaginal discharge may occur in the absence of an STD. Treating women on the basis of vaginal

TABLE 8-4. WHO Recommendation for STD Syndrome Treatment

Syndrome	Treatment
Urethral discharge	Treat for gonorrhea and chlamydia *Gonorrhea*: • Ciprofloxacin 500 mg tab as single oral dose *or* • Ceftriaxone 250 mg IM as single dose *or* • Cefixime 400 mg tab as single oral dose *or* • Spectinomycin 2 g IM as single dose Where resistant gonoccoci strains are present, alternative regimens are: • Kanamycin, 2g IM as single dose *or* • Co-trimoxazole, 480 mg tabs (80 mg trimethoprim + 400 mg sulfamethoxazole), 10 tablets orally for 3 days *Chlamydia*: • Doxycycline 100 mg tab orally twice daily for 7 days *or* • Tetracycline 500 mg tab orally 4 times daily for 7 days *or* • If tetracyclines are contraindicated then erythomycin 500 mg tab orally 4 times daily for 7 days
Swollen scrotum	Eliminate non-infectious origin, then treat for gonorrhea and chlamydia
Genital ulcers	If herpes is excluded, treat for syphilis and chancroid *Syphilis*: • Benzathine penicillin G 2.4 million units IM in a single session *or* • Aqueous procaine penicillin G 1.2 million units IM daily for 10 consecutive days *Chancroid*: • Erythromycin 500 mg tab orally 3 times daily for 7 days *or* • Ciprofloxacin 500 mg tab as single oral dose *or* • Ceftriaxone 250 mg IM as a single dose *or* • Spectinomycin 2 g IM as a single dose *or* • Co-trimoxazole 480 mg tab—2 tabs, twice daily for 7 days
Inguinal lymphadenopathy	If genital ulcer is present, treat for syphilis and chancroid. Otherwise, treat for LGV: doxycycline 100 mg orally twice daily for 14 days *or* tetracycline hydrochloride 500 mg orally 4 times daily for 14 days
Vaginal discharge	Treat for gonorrhea/chlamydia if examination reveals mucopurulent cervicitis or if patient history indicates high risk or if local prevalence of gonorrhea and/or chlamydia exceeds 10–20% AND Treat for candidiasis, trichomoniasis and bacterial vaginosis. For *candidiasis*: • Nystatin 100,000 units intravaginally daily for 14 days *or* • Miconazole or clotrimazole 200 mg intravginally daily for 3 days *or* • Clotrimazole 500 mg intravaginally as a single dose For *trichomoniasis and bacterial vaginosis*: • Metronidazole 2 g orally in a single dose *or* 400–500 mg orally twice daily for 7 days
Lower abdominal pain in women	Eliminate alternative causes (e.g., ectopic pregnancy), then treat for gonorrhea and chlamydia

discharge will mean that many women not infected with an STD are treated and that the stresses of partner notification may be induced needlessly.

The limitations of syndromic management underscore the importance of capitalizing on other opportunities for screening, such as prenatal care and of notifying the partners of the symptomatic patient. Nonetheless, syndromic management is an important tool in combating STD, providing a practical means of meeting the health needs of a significant fraction of STD clients in resource poor settings.

STD Treatment and HIV Control

There is very strong evidence that the presence of other sexually transmitted diseases significantly enhances the likelihood of HIV transmission. Genital ulcerative disease (herpes and syphilis) has been causally related to acquiring HIV.[33,34] Chlamydia has also been identified as a co-factor in becoming infected with HIV[35], as have gonorrhea and trichomoniasis.[36] The presence of these diseases makes the infected individual more vulnerable to acquiring HIV by creating lesions and inflammation that facilitate entry of the virus.

STD also make it more likely that an infected individual will transmit HIV. HIV-positive men with urethritis have been found to have a higher concentration of HIV in their semen than HIV positive men without urethritis.[37] Women with gonorrhea, chlamydia or cervical or vaginal ulcer have also been shown to shed a higher concentration of HIV.[38]

As a result, STD control has been proposed as an important strategy for reducing the spread of HIV. Two interesting studies have tested the utility of this approach. Between 1991 and 1994, a randomized trial of the impact of syndromic management of STD on HIV incidence was conducted in Mwanza, Tanzania.[39] The communities targeted for the intervention benefited from the establishment of an STD referral clinic, staff training, regular supply of drugs, regular supervisory visits to the health facilities and an STD education campaign. Key to the approach was the continued and systematic availability of syndromic management of STD, as well as continuous campaigns to encourage people to seek treatment. The control communities continued to receive the unimproved services available at the start of trial. The Mwanza trial yielded a significant decline in syphilis prevalence and symptomatic urethritis in the intervention group. There were no significant reductions in gonorrhea, chlamydia, asymptomatic urethritis nor in the prevalence of STD among pregnant women attending prenatal clinics. Very importantly, the Mwanza experiment reduced HIV incidence in the intervention group by 38 percent.

A counterpoint, with useful lessons for policy and practice, can be found in a test of a mass treatment approach in Rakai, Uganda.[40] In this experiment, the intervention group received mass treatment every ten months with broad spectrum antibiotics, while the control group received vitamins and anti-helminthics. This experiment yielded reductions in syphilis, trichomoniasis and bacterial vaginosis in the intervention group, as compared to the control group. There were no reductions in gonorrhea, chlamydia, or urethritis. There were significant reductions in the prevalence of trichomoniasis, gonorrhea, chlamydia and bacterial vaginosis in the cohort of pregnant women. Unfortunately, there was no significant decline in the incidence of HIV in the intervention group.

What explains the difference in outcomes? The lead researchers of the two trials have suggested some useful hypotheses and lessons learned:[41]

- The prevalence of HIV was much higher at baseline in Rakai (16 percent) as compared to Mwanza (4 percent). This suggests that the relative importance of STD treatment in preventing new infections may be less in high HIV prevalence settings.
- Rakai appears to have had a significantly higher prevalence of untreatable genital herpes. As discussed above, ulcerative disease is a co-factor in HIV transmission. The antibiotics used in Rakai would have had no impact on the prevalence or incidence of herpes.

- Because of its design, the Mwanza trial targeted symptomatic disease. It may be that symptomatic disease has a greater impact on HIV transmission, compared to asymptomatic infection.
- Both targeted populations were susceptible to re-infection with STD. However, the availability of continuous treatment in Mwanza made it more likely that the newly infected would receive prompt treatment, as compared to the Rakai population, which received treatment only once every ten months.
- Treatable and symptomatic STD may simply have been more prevalent and therefore played a greater role in HIV transmission in Mwanza, as compared to Rakai.

STD control is a useful and important component of a strategy for reducing HIV transmission. The Mwanza and Rakai trials tested two different approaches to achieving STD control in populations that appear to have had significantly different characteristics. The STD control strategy must be carefully tailored to the population being served. Mass treatment of groups with high prevalence of treatable STD and relatively moderate HIV prevalence may be a useful control strategy when combined with efforts to prevent re-infection. Syndromic management can be helpful as an HIV control strategy in situations where more sophisticated approaches to case management are unavailable, though the impact will probably vary depending on the stage of the HIV epidemic and the specific pattern of other STD. It must also be remembered that in any given population there are usually sub-groups, such as adolescents, for whom an appropriately designed STD control intervention can help reduce the incidence of HIV.

CARE FOR PEOPLE LIVING WITH HIV/AIDS[42]

The goals of caring for people living with HIV/AIDS (PLWHA) are to prolong life, reduce suffering, prevent transmission of HIV and opportunistic infections (especially tuberculosis) and lessen the impact of the disease on the welfare of the household by using limited resources efficiently. Feasible, cost-effective strategies are available to pursue these goals. These strategies focus on strengthening social support to PLWHA, providing palliative care and treating opportunistic infections. Antiretrovirals, which have been prohibitively expensive, may become more readily available in the developing countries.

From a broad public health perspective, expenditures to care for PLWHA must be compared to those spent on other serious health problems. During the 1990s, annual per capita expenditures for health averaged $33 in sub-Saharan Africa and $17 in South Asia[43]. Both household and public sector expenditures must be judged relative to the constraints on health financing in resource poor settings.

Alleviating Stigma and Strengthening Social Support

The first step in responding to PLWHA is alleviating the social stigma associated with the disease. HIV and others STD carry a measure of blame and shame unlike that associated with any other disease. PLWHA are often viewed as being "at fault" and somehow deserving of illness. The degree of social stigma associated with sexually transmitted diseases is quite different in degree and kind from many other diseases that have a behavioral etiology. PLWHA are often ostracized, expelled from their homes, lose jobs and/or are subjected to

violence, especially if they are women. Testing, counseling and care become very difficult in a hostile environment.

Support groups and non-governmental organizations can play a particularly important role in alleviating social stigma. These groups serve the dual role of encouraging problem solving by their members and legitimizing public discussion of HIV/AIDS. By bringing together people with a common concern, support groups can serve as a forum for a variety of critical functions:[44]

- Encouraging adherence to drug regimens;
- Sharing practical, experience based strategies for managing the disease and its consequences;
- Addressing ethical dilemmas about disease transmission;
- Promoting behavior change;
- Receiving accurate technical information about disease management; and,
- Receiving emotional support and emotional release.

Non-governmental organizations can encompass support groups, but often include additional functions. These include advocacy with community and political leaders, community education about PLWHA, securing resources for services to PLWHA and direct service delivery to PLWHA. Non-governmental organizations that serve PLWHA as advocates or service providers may or may not be primarily devoted to AIDS issues. Some organizations, such as TASO in Uganda and KASAKA in the Philippines, were born as community based responses to the local AIDS crisis. Organizations with a different, broader mission have also incorporated AIDS advocacy, education and service. Women's groups, health organizations, religious groups and development organizations have all played a significant role in broadening the dialogue about HIV/AIDS. Effective NGOs tend to have very strong roots in the communities they serve, understanding the norms, power structure and communication channels[45]. Through dialogue with community leaders and members, they help alleviate the stigma associated with HIV/AIDS.

Social support to PLWHA also extends to ensuring access to basic needs. As the condition of a person with AIDS worsens, he or she is increasingly hard pressed to acquire food, water, personal hygiene and basic nursing. Shelter and clothing may also become problematic. The extended family usually has primary responsibility in securing these essentials, but this safety net does not always function in very poor communities or in households burdened by AIDS. Community based organizations and non-governmental organizations are increasingly called upon to help with these functions.

CARE-Thailand, for example, supports the Living with AIDS Project, which is implemented in cooperation with the Faculty of Nursing, Chiang Mai University, the Ministry of Public Health and the Ministry of Education. The project aims to create an accepting and caring environment for people with HIV/AIDS and their families living in poor rural villages in northern Thailand. The project trains village volunteers who organize activities to reduce the stigma towards people with HIV/AIDS. The direct support includes medical costs, food for infants, education for children, and occupational support.

Palliative Care and Opportunistic Infections

PLWHA suffer from a variety of opportunistic infections that are amenable to low cost, low technology treatments. Among the more common syndromes are diarrhea, skin

TABLE 8-5. Essential Drugs for Palliative Care and Managing Opportunistic Infections in People Living with AIDS

Drug	Function
Isoniazid, rifampin, pyrazinamide, ethambutol, streptomycin	Tuberculosis control
Cotrimoxazole	Systemic antibacterial; e.g., treatment of pneumococcal infection, chronic diarrhea
Ketoconazole	Fungal and yeast infections
Metronidazole	Protozoal diseases such as giardiasis, amoebaisis and trichomoniasis
Broad spectrum antibiotic	Bacterial infections
Nystatin	Oral antifungal; e.g., treatment of candidiasis
Gentian violet	Fungal infections, especially thrush
Hydrocortisone cream	Skin rashes
Calamine lotion	Skin rashes
Multivitamin	Nutritional supplementation
Aspirin	Pain and fever
Paracetamol	Pain and fever
Codeine	Pain control
Morphine	Pain control
Chlorpromazine	Tranquilizer, antipsychotic
Diazepam	Sedation

rashes, respiratory infections, nausea, tuberculosis, pneumocystosis and fungal infections. The World Bank estimates that these problems could be managed at a cost of $20–$30 per year and add one to four years of life[46]. This is a level that would be affordable in many settings through a combination of household and public sector expenditure. There is a particularly compelling case to be made for investment in tuberculosis control, which is highly cost-effective. Tuberculosis incidence has been growing rapidly as a result of the HIV pandemic; annual incidence in the year 2000 is estimated at 11 million, with 14 percent due to HIV infection[47]. Proper nutrition can also play an important role in prolonging life and improving the quality of life.

As AIDS progresses other opportunistic infections emerge that are more difficult and/or expensive to treat and that will usually be beyond the means of poor families and developing country health systems. In the final stages of AIDS, patients often suffer from dementia and extreme pain. Inadequate use is made of inexpensive sedatives and analgesics, such as diazepam, codeine and morphine, to alleviate pain and suffering. Concerns over drug abuse have limited access to these drugs. However, this must be weighed against the suffering of terminal AIDS patients.

Table 8-5 provides a list of essential drugs for palliative care and opportunistic infection and their functions[48].

Antiretroviral Treatment

The advent of highly active antiretroviral therapy (HAART), which consists of a combination of three antiretroviral drugs, has yielded a stunning decline in AIDS-related mortality in the more developed countries. In the United States, for example, the number of AIDS deaths and cases has declined dramatically, with the number of deaths due to HIV declining from about 46,000 in 1995 to about 14,000 per year by the end of decade, about the same level as in 1987.[49,50] Age-adjusted death rates due to HIV/AIDS declined from almost 18/100,000 to about 5/100,000. The number of new AIDS cases also declined precipitously. Life expectancy after diagnosis of HIV has increased significantly. The number of new cases and deaths now appears to have reached a plateau. These changes are largely attributable to the widespread use of HAART and not because of behavior change. Halting the progression of the disease in those infected also yields important gains in prevention.

HAART has been prohibitively expensive for developing countries until very recently, with the cost of triple combination therapy exceeding US $10,000 per year per patient.[51] Prices have since plummeted with generic alternatives of selected combinations now available for $300–$400 per year.[52] This still remains very high relative to total per capita health expenditures in low income countries. Public spending in sub-Saharan Africa is only about $8.00, so the purchase of HAART drugs alone would be a manifold increase in costs.[53] Annual expenditures per PLWHA average $1250 in eight Latin American countries. The cost of drugs is only one part of actually delivering therapy. The U.S. Medicaid system, for example, spends over $35,000 per PLWHA. Nonetheless, rapid declines in drug prices are placing HAART within the reach of middle income countries and hold out the prospect for increasing access even in low income nations.

HAART Fundamentals[54]

The antiretrovirals used in HAART all function by blocking the action of enzymes essential to the replication of HIV (reverse transcriptase and protease). The fifteen available antiretroviral drugs fall into three categories: protease inhibitors (PI), nucleoside analogue reverse transcriptase inhibitors (NRTI) and nonnucleoside analogue reverse transcriptase inhibitors (NNRTI). Table 8-6 summarizes the available drugs by class.

As an initial course of treatment, the drugs are used in triple-combination therapy under one of three possible regimens:

1. A protease inhibitor in combination with two NRTI;
2. Two NNRTI plus an NRTI; or
3. Three NRTI

Use of any one drug alone or any combination of two drugs is ineffective and ultimately dangerous.

TABLE 8-6. Antiretroviral Drugs Used in Treating HIV (generic names)

PI	NRTI	NNRTI
• Indinavir	• Zidovudine (ZVD, AZT)	• Nevirapine
• Ritonavir	• Didanosine (ddI)	• Delavirdine
• Nelfinavir	• Zalcitabine (ddC)	• Efavirenze
• Saquinavir	• Tenofovir*	
• Amprenavir	• Stavudine (d4T)	
• Lopinavir + Ritonavir	• Lamivudine (3TC)	
	• Abacavir (ABC)	

* As of this writing insufficient data exist to recommend or discourage use of this drug as part of HAART.

Each of the three combinations serves to "spare" a class of drugs for later use. HIV tends to mutate rapidly and the emergence of drug resistance is not uncommon. Each of the three regimens holds a class of drugs in reserve that can be used to combat the virus in the event of drug resistance. In addition, the drugs have pronounced side effects that patients may not be able to tolerate, so reserving an alternative class of drugs increases the options available to the physician.

HAART does not "cure" HIV infection or AIDS. There is no cure for this HIV/AIDS. When effective, HAART suppresses the replication of HIV to undetectable levels and thereby halts the progression of the disease. The goal of HAART is therefore to suppress the presence of HIV in blood plasma to undetectable levels.

In addition to cost, HAART poses a number of technical and logistical problems that will have to be addressed in resource poor settings:

- *Lifetime use*: HIV infects and destroys CD4+ lymphocytes, which are essential to triggering the body's response to infectious disease. HIV can remain latent in CD4+ cells indefinitely and treatment must therefore be continued for life. Discontinuation of HAART has been documented to lead to recrudescence of HIV.
- *Diagnosis and monitoring*: In more developed countries, the decision to initiate therapy rests upon an assessment of the level of HIV in the blood (viral load) and the concentration of CD4+ cells. In the United States the current standard is to initiate therapy in asymptomatic individuals with a CD4+ count of < 350 cells/mm^3 or a viral load of > 55,000 copies/ml.[55] People undergoing HAART should be regularly tested for both viral load and CD4+ count to ensure that the therapy is remaining effective. Declines in CD4+ or increases in viral load are key markers for the decision to change the therapeutic regimen. Testing for CD4+ and viral load requires the availability of appropriate laboratory tests. Many, if not most, resource poor settings will lack the requisite capacity. There has been an interesting small-scale pilot in Haiti to test a syndromic approach to initiating HAART.[56] This pilot uses such signs and symptoms as recurrent HIV associated opportunistic infections, wasting, HIV related neurological complications and blood disorders as clinical markers for initiating therapy. The validity and replicability of this approach remains to be seen.
- *Adherence*: Adherence to the HAART regimen is essential both to achieving efficacy and to avoiding the emergence and spread of drug resistant variants. The HAART regimen is complex. Multiple pills must be taken at least twice a day and there are food requirements associated with the pills. Encouraging adherence is a major challenge in any setting and works best when accompanied by good counseling, a multi-dimensional health team, community support and supportive family and friends. The Haiti pilot described above used a form of directly observed therapy by community workers to encourage adherence.
- *Toxicity*: The drugs used in HAART can have a wide range of serious side effects that discourage adherence, damage health and reduce quality of life. Complications include lactic acidosis, liver disorders, diabetes, fat mal-distribution, elevation of cholesterol and triglycerides, bone disorders and skin rashes. Counseling and management of these side effects are an essential part of therapy, with adjustment of the HAART regimen as needed.
- *Need for trained and experienced health providers*: Choosing, adapting and supporting the HAART regimen to the needs of individual patients requires a skilled and experienced health team, working closely with the client over a sustained period. Introducing HAART will mean considerable skill building, often in those countries that have the weakest public health infrastructure.

HAART has been demonstrated to be a life saving response to HIV/AIDS in the more developed countries. Financial, technical and logistical barriers will have to be overcome to make it widely available in the worst afflicted developing countries.

MATERNAL TO CHILD TRANSMISSION OF HIV AND STD

As was described in Chapter 7, STD infection during pregnancy can have grave consequences for the health of the child. Of particular concern are HIV, syphilis, gonorrhea and chlamydia. These diseases are widely prevalent and can have a particularly devastating impact on child health, in addition to the consequences for the women affected. This section focuses on prevention and management of maternal to child transmission (MTCT) of STD.

HIV

Studies of maternal to child transmission among children born to untreated HIV positive mothers have found that from 14 percent to 25 percent of children are born infected and an additional 15 percent to 20 percent are infected through breastfeeding[57]. The likelihood of transmission depends on a number of factors, including the stage of the infection, the viral strain, the duration of breastfeeding, preterm birth, the integrity of the infant's gastrointestinal tract and the mother's vitamin A status. Over five hundred thousand infants are infected each year.[58]

Zidovudine (ZDV) has been found to reduce maternal to child transmission of HIV. A study carried out in the United States and France found that maternal to child transmission was reduced from 25.5 percent in the placebo group to 8.3 percent in the ZDV treated group[59]. A study in Thailand showed that transmission was reduced in half (18 percent versus 9 percent) through ZDV administration[60]. Other studies of ZDV efficacy in Cote d'Ivoire, Burkina Faso and Thailand have shown reductions of 37–38 percent in breastfeeding populations and 50 percent in non-breastfeeding populations[61,62,63].

In the United States, a three part regimen of ZDV that begins at 14 weeks gestation and continues through the first six weeks of the life of the newborn is used.[64] This includes oral administration of ZDV during pregnancy, intravenous administration intrapartum and oral administration to the newborn. This regimen yields a 66 percent reduction in maternal to child transmission of HIV. Combining antiretroviral therapy with Cesarean section and reducing the duration of ruptured membranes can reduce the total risk of perinatal transmission to less than two percent.[65]

However, in developing countries a large proportion of women are not seen by a clinician until the third trimester of pregnancy. In addition, the three part ZDV regimen is costly and complex. Accordingly, a short course of ZDV has also been tested. A trial in Thailand found that beginning administration of ZDV at 36 weeks pregnancy (300 mg. twice daily) and during labor (300 mg. orally every 3 hours) reduced transmission by 50 percent compared to a placebo.[66]

A trial of the drug nevirapine in Uganda was found to reduce maternal to child transmission at 14–16 weeks postpartum by approximately 50 percent as compared to intrapartum and postpartum administration of ZDV[67]. Nevirapine is also simpler to administer than

ZDV and much less expensive. Only a single dose is required consisting of a 200 mg tablet for the mother administered at the onset of labor and a 2 mg/kg suspension dose for the baby within 72 hours of birth. (The short course of ZDV used in the Uganda study consisted of giving the mother two 300 mg. tablets at the onset of labor, followed by one 300 mg tablet every 3 hours during labor and 4 mg/kg of ZDV syrup twice a day for 7 days to the neonate.) Nevirapine was well tolerated in the study population and did not appear to elicit adverse effects. The requisite dose costs U.S. $4.00, to which must be added the cost of counseling and testing, estimated at $5.00 per patient in Uganda[68]. This holds promise of a feasible strategy at an affordable cost for high HIV prevalence countries.

Expanding the use of nevirpaine will require significant investment and major changes in the pattern of maternal health care. As we saw in Chapter 7, maternal health care is often inadequate. Large proportions of women do not receive prenatal care and many, if not most, deliver their babies with the help of a traditional birth attendant. Many women are reluctant to ascertain their HIV status and resist testing. Training, supervision and supply of maternal health providers would be needed to support delivery of nevirapine.

There is also the fundamental ethical dilemma of supporting an intervention that saves the child, while leaving the mother untreated. The net effect of a successful effort to prevent maternal to child transmission of HIV may be to increase the number of AIDS orphans, who then have heightened susceptibility to mortality from other causes. While this should not be a barrier to making available a cost-effective treatment for saving lives, it does highlight the wrenching social problems generated by AIDS.

One major concern remaining from the use of antiretrovirals to prevent MTCT is whether the reduction in HIV transmission will be sustained in breastfeeding populations. Nearly all the women in the study were breastfeeding their babies. The consequences for HIV transmission over the longer term are unknown. Sustained administration of antiretrovirals or early weaning may be needed may be needed to avoid a recrudescence in HIV transmission during infancy. A study in west Africa showed that the efficacy of short-course ZDV treatment in preventing MTCT among breastfed babies was sustained only in children of women not suffering from advanced HIV (CD4 cell counts > 500/ml).[69]

Public health policy regarding breastfeeding in areas of high HIV prevalence is a difficult and controversial arena. Breastfeeding in most developing country settings is very important to sustaining child health. It is superior as a nutrient to commercial formula or other alternatives, confers immunization against infections through the transmission of maternal antibodies, prevents infection from contaminated food and water under conditions of exclusive breastfeeding, and supports birth spacing through its anovulatory effect. In general, children who are breastfed, particularly if the mother practices exclusive breastfeeding during the first four to six months of life, have a much lower rate of mortality and serious morbidity than children who are partially or fully weaned in the first months of life. Psychological benefits and cultural significance are also attached to breastfeeding. Hence, medical and public health authorities have acted vigorously to encourage exclusive breastfeeding during the first months of life and partial breastfeeding up to the second birthday.

The protective effect of breastfeeding is, however, being undermined by HIV transmission through breast milk.[70] Among women who are HIV positive during pregnancy, breastfeeding increases the likelihood of maternal to child transmission by 15 to 20 percentage points above that occurring during pregnancy and labor. It appears that transmission is most likely during the days and weeks following birth, perhaps because colostrum tends to hold an especially high level of the virus relative to breast milk. However, transmission can take place at any time, though the probability diminishes as the duration of breastfeeding increases. The risk of transmission through breast milk is highest among women who become infected after delivery but while breastfeeding because of the high viral load typical of new infections. The probability of transmission through breast milk among children of women infected after delivery is estimated at 29 percent.

In most settings, women will not know their HIV status. As a consequence, decisions must be made on an epidemiological rather than individual basis. Where HIV prevalence among pregnant women is relatively low, the risks to child health of discouraging breastfeeding clearly outweigh the gains from reduced maternal to child transmission. As HIV prevalence rises, the relative benefit to reducing the rate of child mortality declines. Nonetheless, the preponderance of evidence still argues for encouraging widespread breastfeeding, except where the mother is known to be HIV positive and safe feeding alternatives are available. Most pregnant women are uninfected and care must be taken not to dissuade breastfeeding in this group. In addition, the majority of children born to HIV positive women will not become infected. Discouraging breastfeeding among HIV positive women in the absence of a safe alternative puts their HIV negative children at risk of malnutrition and other infectious diseases. Breastfeeding promotion therefore remains part of public health policy in developing countries, though the consequences will be tragic for some children.

More individualized decisions will be possible when women have access to testing, counseling and safe alternatives for feeding their children. Pregnant and breastfeeding women who know they are HIV positive can and should be provided with accurate information and child feeding options that are realistic in the local context. Pasteurizing breast milk and use of infant formula are two options, if they are feasible for the family. Even among the children of women known to be HIV positive, the impact of switching to an alternative to breastfeeding is unclear. A randomized clinical trial in Kenya compared two groups of children born to 425 HIV positive women[71]. One group was breastfed and the other received free powdered infant formula, along with instruction in its proper use. The infant formula group had a significantly lower level of HIV infection (44 percent reduction) over the first two years of life, but there was no difference in the over-all rate of child mortality (20–24 percent). It appears that the negative effects of formula feeding simply washed out the gains due to reduced maternal-to-child transmission of HIV.

Syphilis

Syphilis infection among pregnant women is high in some parts of the world, especially in sub-Saharan Africa. The median prevalence of syphilis reported from surveys of pregnant women in sub-Saharan Africa was six percent, with levels in excess of ten percent reported in Kenya, Cameroon, Tanzania, Gabon and Malawi.[72] Approximately 1/3 of children born to women with syphilis will acquire the disease.

The effects of syphilis during pregnancy include fetal demise, intrauterine growth retardation, preterm birth and stillbirth. Syphilis can have a wide range of serious impacts on the child that include damage to the skin, liver, spleen, skeleton, blood, kidneys, central nervous system, eyes, hearing and teeth. Significant excess mortality is associated with congenital syphilis.

Antenatal screening of women for syphilis is the key to preventing maternal to child transmission of syphilis. The RPR test provides a quick, inexpensive, feasible means of making a presumptive diagnosis in the absence of symptoms.

Treatment of pregnant women who have syphilis will prevent congenital syphilis and can alleviate the fetal impacts of the disease[73]. Both acquired and congenital syphilis can be treated with penicillin. One recommended regimen consists of benzanthine benzylpenicillin (a single dose of 2.4 MU by intramuscular injection) or aqueous procaine procaine benzylpenicillin (1.2 MU daily by intramuscular injection for ten days). Eryhtromycin, 500 mg. orally, four times daily for fifteen days can be used in case of penicillin allergy. Congenital syphilis can be treated with a dose of 50,000 U procaine penincillin intramuscularly per kilogram of body weight daily for ten days.

Gonorrhea

Gonorrhea is common among pregnant women in some areas of the developing world. Prevalence rates among women attending prenatal clinics in African range from 1 percent to 15 percent.[74] Gonorrhea has been linked to preterm birth, premature rupture of membranes, chorioamnionitis and postpartum maternal infection. The most common manifestation of gonorrheal infection in children is infection of the eyes (gonococcal opthalmia neonatorum), which can lead to blindness if untreated. Children can also suffer disseminated gonococcal infection, leading to sepsis.

Pregnant women can be treated for gonorrhea using ceftriaxone (250 mg. IM as a single dose) or cefixime (400 mg. as a single oral dose) or spectinomycin (2 g IM as a single dose).[75] All infants should receive ocular prophylaxis at birth.[76] Alternative regimens for ocular prophylaxis are single applications of 1 percent silver nitrate eye drops, 1 percent tetracycline eye ointment or 0.5 percent erythromycin eye ointment.[77] Prophylaxis should be administered within one hour of birth directly into the conjunctival sac, as delays in administration of as little as 4–5 hours significantly delay efficacy. Care must be taken to store silver nitrate in closed, dark bottles to prevent evaporation and potentially excessive concentrations of silver nitrate that can harm the eyes.

Children born to infected, untreated women are at high risk for infection and should therefore receive prophylactic treatment of ceftriaxone 25–50 mg/kg IV or IM, not to exceed 125 mg in a single dose.[78] Children manifesting gonococcal opthalmia neonatorum (reddish, swollen eyelids with purulent discharge) should receive the same regimen.[79] Kanamycin 25 mg/kg IM as a single dose or spectinomycin 25 mg/kg IM as a single dose are alternative treatments.[80] As will be discussed below, purulent conjunctivitis in neonates can also be due to chlamydia, so children should be monitored to ensure that the gonorrhea treatment is having the desired effect. The untreated mother of an infected child, as well as her partner(s) should also be given the normal adult regimen.

Chlamydia

Chlamydia can cause blindness and pneumonia in infants.[81] Pregnant women with chlamydia can be treated with erythromycin base 500 mg orally four times a day for 7 days or amoxicillin 500 mg orally three times a day for 7 days.[82]

Neonatal conjunctivitis that does not respond to treatment for gonorrhea should be assumed to be due to chlamydia. The recommended regimen is erythromycin 50 mg/kg/day orally divided into four doses daily for 10–14 days.[83] Topical antibiotic treatment will not help and is not needed if systemic antibiotic treatment is used. Infant pneumonia due to chlamydia will respond to erythromycin base 50 mg/kg/day orally divided into four doses daily for 10–14 days.[84]

BLOOD SCREENING FOR HIV[85]

About ten percent of all HIV infections to date are due to HIV contaminated blood and blood products.[86] HIV infected blood and blood products continue to account for five to ten percent of new infections.[87] WHO estimates that 80,000–160,000 new HIV infections from contaminated blood occur every year.[88] Children constitute a disproportionate share of those infected through transfusion. The probability of seroconversion after transfusion with infected blood exceeds 90 percent and is usually estimated in the 95 to 100 percent range.[89]

There are major obstacles to preventing HIV infection through blood transfusion in developing countries. Many facilities that accept and use donated blood lack the equipment and supplies to test blood for HIV. The ELISA (enzyme linked immunosorbent assay) test is used to screen blood supply in developed countries and in some developing countries settings, especially major hospitals in large cities. However, developing country health facilities often lack the staff, money, materiel and equipment to carry out the ELISA test. Even where the test is used, staff are often poorly trained and supervised and quality control of screening is weak.

The sources of blood also exacerbate the problem of HIV transmission. Donors who sell blood as a principal source of income are often important sources of blood supply; these individuals are much more likely to engage in risky behavior, such as injecting drug use and multiple sexual partners. One study in Bangladesh of a sample of blood donors found that 61 percent abused drugs, 30 percent suffered from penile ulcers or purulent urethral discharge and the mean number of lifetime sexual partners was 35[90]. Relatively few institutions use behavioral screens to try to reduce donations from individuals practicing risky behaviors, whether the blood is donated or sold. Poorly regulated and monitored commercial blood banks are common in some countries, especially in Asia. The regulatory structure for blood supply is generally poorly developed and enforcement of existing regulations is difficult.

All tests are subject to the window period between infection and seropositivity; i.e., a period of 6 to 18 weeks ensues between infection and the development of antibodies that register on the screening tests. This may yield a significant number of contaminated transfusions in countries where HIV prevalence is high in the general population or in the sub-population of blood donors, especially if behavioral screens are not used.

There are a number of strategies that can be used to reduce the risk of transmission via transfusion of blood or blood products:

1. Reduce the use of transfusion to the minimum needed to protect life and health. Studies in Tanzania and Cote d'Ivoire have shown that many transfusions are not medically necessary, thereby unnecessarily placing patients at risk[91,92,93]. Children receive a disproportionate share of medically unnecessary and risky transfusions. In addition, inadequate use is made of

alternatives to whole blood transfusion, such as plasma substitutes, that could avoid the risk of infection.
2. Behavioral screens to blood supply should be applied. Patients can donate their own blood ahead of time (autologous blood supply) when the need can be predicted; e.g. for surgery that is elective or not carried out on an emergency basis. Use of paid blood donors should be discouraged, though these individuals currently constitute a large proportion of donors in many developing countries. Unpaid volunteers drawn from lower risk groups are generally a safer source than paid donors. The widespread use of simple interview protocols to screen for risky behaviors that increase the likelihood of HIV infection should be encouraged.
3. Much more widespread use should be made of rapid HIV tests that do not require technical sophistication and yield results within a few minutes. These rapid tests use blood, serum, saliva or urine to detect HIV antibodies. The usual procedure is to test the bodily fluid against a strip that has been impregnated with antigens. The HIV antibodies react to the antigen, leaving a visible coding on the strip. The strip remains unaffected if the sample is free of HIV antibodies. The WHO has identified at least 37 rapid tests, most of which have a sensitivity of at least 99 percent and a specificity of at least 95 percent.[94] Most of the tests take less than ten minutes to produce results and few require more than 30 minutes. Widespread application of relatively inexpensive, non-invasive rapid tests could play a major role in screening out HIV positive blood donors.
4. Training and supervision of health staff in blood transfusion and screening methods is essential. Staff are often unaware of simple, practical steps they can take to prevent infection of patients and supervisory systems do not reward or encourage such preventive measures. Moving beyond the issue of blood screening, staff should also be encouraged to apply universal precautions in carrying out medical procedures that carry the risk of transmission via blood.

HPV AND CERVICAL CANCER

Cervical cancer is a sexually transmitted disease attributable to specific strains of the human papillomavirus (HPV), a group of viruses that also cause genital warts. Strains HPV 16, HPV 18, HPV 33, HPV 35 and HPV 45 have been linked to the development of cervical cancer.[95] The progression from infection with a high risk HPV strain, which is quite common, to cancer appears to be triggered by other risk factors that include early onset of sexual intercourse, multiple sexual partners, poor nutrition, smoking and HIV infection. As is the case for the herpes simplex virus, condoms do not protect against HPV, since skin-to-skin contact outside the area covered by the condom can transmit the virus.

Cervical cancer causes 300,000 deaths per year and 450,000 new cases of cervical cancer are reported each year.[96] This almost certainly under-estimates the true incidence, which is estimated at approximately 900,000 new cases per year. Cervical cancer is the leading cause of cancer mortality among women in the developing world. Cervical cancer deaths are highly concentrated in the developing world and among the poor since it is an eminently treatable disease if caught early. Cervical cancer is uncommon among women under the age of 35.

The American Cancer Society "gold standard" for preventing and managing cervical cancer consists of two major elements: (1) reducing exposure to HPV by limiting the number of sexual partners and risk factors that induce the transition to invasive disease; and, (2) preventing the progression from cervical dysplasia (pre-cancerous cells) to invasive disease through universal screening of adult women.

TABLE 8-7. Stages of Cervical Cancer and their Consequence

Stage	Degree of invasion	Treatment	5 year survival rate
0	Lining of cervix	Cryosurgery, laser surgery or electrosurgical excision	Completely curable
IA1	< 3mm deep and < 7mm wide	Simple or radical hysterectomy	95%
IA2	3–5 mm deep and < 7mm wide		
IB	> 5mm deep and .7mm wide	Radical hysterectomy with pelvic lymph node dissection or high dose radiation therapy	85–90%
IB1	< 4 cm in size		
IB2	> 4cm in size		
IIA	Cancer has spread into the upper part of the vagina	Radical hysterectomy with pelvic lymph node dissection or high dose radiation therapy	75–80%
IIB	Cancer has spread to the tissue next to the cervix		
IIIA	Cancer has spread to lower third of vagina	Combined internal and external radiation therapy	65%
IIIB	Cancer extends to the pelvic wall		
IVA	Cancer has spread to bladder or rectum	Combined internal and external radiation therapy	< 20%
IVB	Cancer has spread to organs beyond the pelvic area		Not curable

The Papanicolaou (Pap) test has been the key in developed countries to preventing the progression from pre-cancerous to cancerous cells. The Pap test is a screening test, not a diagnostic tool; it detects abnormalities in the cervical cells, known as squamous intraepithelial lesions (SIL). If the Pap test detects SIL a biopsy is performed to determine whether precancerous or cancerous cells are present. Only about ten percent of cervical dysplasias eventually lead to cancer. However, it is impossible at this time to predict which are true precursors to cancer. Hence, the norm is to treat all positive findings to prevent any possible progression to cancer. In developed countries, screening has radically reduced the incidence of invasive carcinoma.

The importance of early detection and treatment can be seen in Table 8-7.[97] Cancers are staged in accordance with the degree of metastasis. The type of treatment needed and the associated survival rate varies according to the stage of the cancer. Treatment in the early stages is also technically simpler than that needed for later stages.

Table 8-7 shows the importance of early detection and treatment. Radiation therapy will be difficult to access in many resource poor settings, which exacerbates the need to detect potential cancers at an early stage.

The American Cancer Society recommends a Pap test every year for all women beginning at age 18, though the frequency of the test may be reduced to every three years if findings are negative for three years in a row.

Developing countries are clearly at a major disadvantage in trying to apply the strategy that has yielded a major decline in cervical cancer mortality in developed countries. Pap screening reaches only a tiny fraction of the population and the quality is often very poor. There is no realistic prospect of extending Pap screening and subsequent diagnostic testing to a large percentage of the population on a continuing basis. By way of example, a twelve-fold increase in the number of Indian cytologists would still leave 75 percent of the country uncovered.[98] The capacity to carry out biopsies is even more limited than the ability to conduct Pap tests. Even if a proper diagnosis is provided, therapeutic capability and access to advanced therapies is usually quite low.

There are alternative approaches to reducing the incidence of invasive disease that may be better adapted to the realities of the developing world. These include:

- *Behavior change to reduce risk factors*: Increasing knowledge of cervical cancer, delaying initiation of first intercourse and reducing the number of sex partners can all reduce the risk of cervical cancer. The use of condoms, while not protective against HPV, can reduce the spread of HIV, which contributes to the incidence of cervical cancer.
- *Once in a lifetime screening*: Annual screening for a significant percentage of women is not feasible for most developing countries for the foreseeable future. An alternative is to rely on screening all women at a specific age known to capture the highest proportion of precancerous and early stage disease. Data from an Indian study are instructive.[99] Cervical cancer in women under 35 is uncommon and women over 65 typically constitute a very small fraction of the population. Age-specific cervical cancer rates typically peak among women in their early to mid-fifties. The greatest protective effect of screening occurs in the five years after a negative smear is recorded. This suggests screening women once in their mid to late forties would have the greatest impact on the over-all incidence of cervical cancer. The Indian study found that screening all women at age 50 would have the greatest effect on the cumulative incidence of cervical cancer, while screening at age 45 would yield the highest number of years of life saved. The specific age for once-in-a-lifetime screening will be context specific, but it does suggest a strategy for targeting very limited resources so as to optimize the public health impact.
- *Alternative screening procedures*: Pap screening requires a trained cytologist with appropriate equipment. Given the technical difficulties in extending Pap test to large numbers of women, various alternative approaches to screening have been tried. Programs in Thailand[100] and South Africa[101] have experimented with self-collection of swabs by women, which are then brought to clinics for evaluation. This eliminates the need for one contact with a provider and also overcomes the barrier that many women feel to allowing this invasive diagnostic procedure. One alternative to the Pap test is visual inspection on speculum exam by trained non-physicians, who then refer suspect cases to a physician. This has been found to be sensitive but not specific for Stage 0-IIA cancers. A second alternative is visual inspection after painting the cervix with an acetic acid solution. This has been very useful in capturing pre-malignant lesions; e.g., 60 percent of high-grade pre-cancerous lesions were detected in one trial.[102] A third alternative is to equip health providers with a camera that is used to photograph the cervix; a gynecologist then examines the photo for abnormalities.[103]
- *One session case management*: Even when screening is available, many women are lost to follow-up. The South Africa study cited above assessed immediate treatment in a mobile clinic upon positive screening by a trained nurse. The clinicians used loop electrosurgical excision procedure or laser surgery to remove suspected pre-cancerous lesions or Stage 0 carcinoma, though a biopsy was not performed. The advantage of this process was to minimize the risk that women needing treatment would be lost to follow-up. Conversely, this approach risks treating many women needlessly given the low rate of progression from lesions to invasive disease.

Over the long term, the most hopeful strategy for reducing cervical cancer mortality is the development of an HPV vaccine. However, the development of a safe, effective HPV vaccine that will meet the needs of developing countries faces substantial challenges.[104] It must protect against the multiple strains of HPV that cause cervical cancer, provide long lasting protection without booster shots, and be suitable for the limited infrastructure of developing nations; e.g., be able to withstand high temperature and have long shelf life. An HPV vaccine would also have to be administered to children or young adolescents before they became sexually active if it is to be effective, which poses additional social constraints. Hence, it is likely that many years will elapse before an HPV vaccine becomes a useful approach to reducing cervical cancer.

9

Policy and Politics

With this chapter, we complete our examination of the multiple dimensions of reproductive security. The reader will recall that reproductive security depends upon five elements: healthy behaviors, community empowerment, institutional capacity to deliver high-quality, accessible reproductive health services, the use of appropriate health technologies, and supportive public policy. This chapter begins with a brief discussion of why public policy is critical to achieving reproductive health outcomes. Unfortunately, reproductive health is a highly contentious policy arena. Different political actors hold widely varying, and often opposing, views of both the nature of the reproductive health problem and, therefore, the appropriate solution. The chapter explores some of these alternative perspectives on how and why human reproduction creates a social problem worthy of public attention and investment. As we will see, better health is only one lens through which to view reproduction. The chapter concludes with some suggestions about how the reproductive health manager can be a more effective policy advocate.

WHY POLICY MATTERS

Public policy has a very important impact on reproductive health. Public policy sets the agenda, circumscribes the legitimate and illegitimate, and directs resources. The words and actions of decision-makers can affect reproductive security in the following ways:

- *Legitimizing public dialogue and action*: Both the government bureaucracy and the society at large may be unwilling to act on social problems unless the political leadership has sent a clear signal legitimizing intervention. This is all the more true in the controversial arena of reproductive health. Family planning, HIV/AIDS and sexual and gender based violence are all highly charged issues that lower level officials are often unwilling to address without overt indications of support from their political superiors. In authoritarian societies, open discussion, the flow of technical information and programmatic action on reproductive health issues may be severely constrained without the approval of government leaders. Conversely, respected leaders can help encourage more vigorous action by openly and consistently expressing support

for policies, programs and behaviors that support reproductive health. Political leaders can help place and keep an issue on the national agenda.
- *Consciousness raising*: Public awareness of a particular reproductive health problem and/or its causes may be very limited. Government can and does play a critical role in public education about health issues. In fact, the government is usually the only entity that is in a position to do so on a large scale, as there is little incentive for the private, for-profit sector to do so.
- *Legal framework*: Laws and regulations governing access to care, provider behavior, service delivery strategies, contraception, taxation, prices, dissemination of information, sex work and a host of other issues may help or hinder reproductive health programs. In addition, there is often confusion at the service delivery level as to what the law actually requires. A supportive and properly understood legal framework is usually needed for effective programming.
- *Resource allocation:* Reproductive health programs cannot succeed without adequate and properly directed allocation of human, financial and physical resources. Public policy sets the level of government resource allocation, influences the flow of donor funds and creates incentives for the allocation of private sector money.
- *Implementation strategy*: Public policy typically governs both *what* programs will be implemented and *how* they will be implemented. Policy implementation issues in reproductive health typically include the relative priority of different reproductive health issues, the service delivery strategy, the locus of control over programs, the system for quality assurance, the range of permissible technical interventions, the choice of drugs and contraceptives, and the role played by each class of service provider.
- *Holding the bureaucracy accountable*: Simply issuing a decree, mandate or law is not enough to ensure implementation, even if the requisite resources have been allocated and the legal framework is supportive. Political leaders must act firmly to hold the bureaucracy accountable for performance and to change personnel, structure and processes as needed. The incentives and disincentives political leaders create for effective implementation are a vital component of public policy and of ensuring people get access to reproductive health services.

All of these dimensions—legitimizing action, consciousness-raising, setting the legal framework for action, resource allocation, the implementation strategy and accountability—implicitly or explicitly constitute a statement of causality. That is, they together frame the nature of the reproductive health problem, the intervention(s) that are intended to "solve" the problem, and the allocation of authority and resources that will be used to enforce the solution. Public policy can therefore both support and constrain health managers and providers as they try to address the needs of clients.

THE MANY FACES OF THE REPRODUCTIVE "PROBLEM"

This book has argued that the proper unit of analysis is the household and that poor reproductive health is one of the basic threats to the well being of impoverished households. The object of public policy, in this view, is *enhancing reproductive security*, which is defined as the ability to identify, prevent and manage risks to reproductive health. Reproductive insecurity, signifying poor reproductive health, has been used to describe an array of unsatisfactory conditions—the unmet need for family planning, maternal mortality and morbidity, HIV and other STDs, cervical cancer and sexual violence. While linked to a broader development context, the focus has been on reproduction as a *health* concern, demanding a public health response. By thinking of reproduction as a health problem, we have necessarily focused on public health solutions and focused largely on public health actors and health behaviors.

This view of reproduction as a health issue affecting household security is only one of many lenses through which the same phenomenon might be viewed. Reproduction and reproductive behavior might also be viewed as having an impact on political power, economic development, human rights, gender equity or the moral standing of a society. A public health professional, a political leader, an economist, a lawyer, a women's rights activist, an ethicist or a religious leader may view the pattern of reproduction in a given society very differently. Any of these may view the extant reproductive behaviors as satisfactory or problematic, but for very different reasons. Different definitions of the societal problem(s) associated with reproduction will likely yield different policy solutions, as well as varying degrees of urgency as to the need for action.

Reproduction as a Problem of National Power

Historically, the leaders of ethnic groups, tribes and nation-states have tended to view political power as, at least in part, a function of population size. Bigger populations meant more soldiers, greater capacity to occupy and control land, a larger labor force and larger internal markets (not to mention the ego satisfaction of ruling over a larger rather than smaller group). Political scientists have conventionally included population size as a national asset in determining the power of a nation-state.[1] Governments and leaders have therefore encouraged high birth rates and, selectively, immigration, while discouraging emigration. Some governments, such as that of France, offered awards and financial payments as an inducement for women to bear additional children.

The age structure of the population, which derives from the birth rate, is also a factor in military and national power. Countries with a high proportion of young men (and, more recently, young women), hold a double-edged sword. The relatively large youth cohort increases the pool of potential soldiers. Conversely, high percentages of young adults in poor countries are badly educated, even illiterate. This makes for a poor quality soldier unable to handle much in the way of technologically sophisticated weaponry. The military thus often serves primarily as a *de facto* source of public employment for otherwise out of work youth, with little real belief by leaders that this group constitutes an effective fighting force.

Changes in age structure as fertility declines will change the composition of the military and the role of technology. Countries which experience a relative decline in the proportion of young people will have an incentive to provide each soldier with more sophisticated, capital intensive equipment, trading off the quantity of soldiers for a more effective, better equipped warrior.

Rural to urban migration, which is partially driven by the over-all fertility rate, also plays a role in the military calculus. Urbanization increases the likelihood that the locus of combat will move to the cities, which will pose both political and military challenges for leaders.

In short, the politico-military lens on reproduction has tended to focus on population size and structure as a variable in national or ethnic group power. Consequently, the policy prescription has been to encourage high fertility and reduce net losses from migration, especially among those of military age. This view of "population as power", while still held in many quarters, has been largely undermined by the role of technology and economics in national power. Smaller, wealthier, more technologically sophisticated societies are usually at a comparative advantage relative to larger societies hobbled by low per capita incomes and low levels of technological sophistication. Hence, it has become less obvious that increasing population size is the right policy prescription, as opposed to attaining a smaller, but better educated and equipped youth cohort.

Demographic variables are also a significant underlying factor in internal civil conflicts. Ethnic and religious groups have encouraged high birth rates and discouraged losses from migration as a way of maintaining or increasing political power relative to other groups. Ethnic and religious leaders are often acutely conscious of the size of their group relative to rivals and offer powerful sanctions (positive and negative) to sustain fertility.

Population growth is particularly important as an underlying factor in civil conflict when linked to environmental scarcity (e.g., land and water resources).[2] Decreases in critical renewable resources, inequitable access to available resources, and population growth can combine to stimulate violent confrontation, especially when societies lack effective mechanisms for adapting to scarcity. This dynamic appears to be at work in countries as diverse as Haiti, South Africa, Mexico, and the Philippines. The degree to which population growth feeds violent civil conflict is, of course, contextual and depends on the ability and willingness of leaders to cope with environmental scarcity. Unfortunately, population growth also creates a breeding ground for violence when leaders lack these skills or deliberately choose to manipulate and provoke conflict as a political strategy.

For the purposes of this book, the most important inference to draw is that health concerns are essentially irrelevant or marginal to policy makers when reproduction is viewed primarily as a variable in political or military power. A different understanding of the reproductive "problem" yields very different policy preoccupations and prescriptions.

Reproduction as an Economic Problem

For most of human history, population grew at a slow rate. This is because the death rate was typically only slightly below the birth rate. The crude birth rate is the number of birth per thousand per year in a population; the crude death rate is the number of deaths per thousand per year in a population. The rate of natural increase is the difference between the crude birth rate and the crude death rate and gives the population growth rate, exclusive of migration. Thus, a society with a crude birth rate of 40 per thousand and a crude death rate of 30 per thousand, would have a rate of natural increase of 10 per thousand or one percent per year. Rates of natural increase of less than one percent per year were typical of all societies prior to World War II. In today's developed countries, birth and death rates declined slowly and largely in tandem. A rate of natural increase of one percent implies that, exclusive of the effect of migration, the population will double in size about every 70 years.

The post-World War II period saw a phenomenon unique in human history. Developing countries began to experience rapid declines in crude death rates, while the crude birth rate remained largely unaffected. The declines in the death rate were largely attributable to reductions in infant and child mortality, though these levels remained high by the standards of more developed nations. The rate of natural increase rose correspondingly. Rates of natural increase of two percent to four percent became commonplace. A four percent rate of increase, such as that experienced by Kenya or Rwanda, implies a population doubling time of just sixteen years.

Beginning in the 1950s, some economists and national leaders began to view rapid population growth as an important impediment to development.[3] Rapid population growth meant that economies and the social infrastructure—schools, teachers, hospitals, health providers, housing, and access to clean water—must grow even more rapidly to achieve per capita gains in the standard of living. Moreover, since demographic growth is relentless—occurring year after year—and takes many years to slow, economic growth must be equally consistent. Downturns in the business cycle or economic crises automatically create sudden declines in per capita income (and the availability of core social services) as the economy fails to keep pace with population growth. Even more "catch-up" is needed to improve the standard of living. Concerns over the environmental impact of population growth also began to mount in the 1960s, notably with regard to the impact on forests, desertification, water resources, and human encroachment on the land of endangered species. Book such as *The Population Bomb*[4] warned of dire consequences in the face of continued population growth.

More sober economic analyses pointed to a basic structural problem associated with rapid population growth.[5] A situation of high fertility and declining child mortality necessarily leads to a population that has a high proportion of children. Forty to fifty percent of the population of a developing country experiencing this phenomenon will consist of children under the age of fifteen. Though child labor is common, the economic productivity of children tends to be very low. A high proportion of household and national income must be used to meet the basic consumption needs of children (food, medical care, housing), leaving very little for savings and investment, whether in capital goods (plant and equipment for production) or human capital (such as education). As a consequence, economic growth is inherently restrained in poor, high fertility societies that do not have easy access to additional sources of investment capital. There is simply too little capital available to spur economic growth.

It is important to recognize that Western, especially U.S., economists were largely responsible for developing the intellectual underpinnings for this perspective. The constellation of actors supporting expanded family planning services began with a handful of developing nations in Asia and Latin America, U.S. foundations and private organizations, a few European and international entities, such as the International Planned Parenthood Federation, and the U.S. Government.

This analysis of the economic impact of population growth has been challenged from both the right and the left. Many developing nations charged that the emphasis on population growth was essentially a distraction from an inequitable global economic system. They reminded the advocates of fertility reduction that many developing nations were recovering from an oppressive period of colonialism. They argued that the Western nations and a small, dependent elite in the developing world, were profiteering from a system in which the poor nations sold primary products (crops, minerals) at low prices to developed nations, while being forced to purchase high value manufactured goods and technologies from the West. Simultaneously, the developed nations plucked the most valuable intellectual resources of the developing world through the "brain drain". Undue emphasis on fertility as a key economic variable drew attention away from more fundamental issues of global equity. There was understandable resentment at the notion that the West, especially the U.S., should blame poverty on the poor for having too many children. Moreover, it was pointed out that no Western nation had used a deliberate policy of fertility reduction as a means of spurring development. Fertility reduction occurred as a natural consequence of the development process, which entailed lower child mortality, more education for women and greater urbanization. Development, the argument went, is the best contraceptive.

The critics from developing nations were quickly joined by the former Soviet Union and its allies. Population became an ideological wedge issue, through which the Soviets felt they could score points against the U.S. and the Europeans. Because of its opposition to artificial contraception, the Catholic Church also became an outspoken opponent of government and donor sponsorship of family planning programs. By the mid-1970s, there were clear ideological blocs vying for dominance on the population issue. The U.S, a few European countries and a small but growing coterie of developing nations pursued a fertility reduction strategy, against the opposition of much of the Non-Aligned Movement and the Soviet Bloc.

A conservative critique of the economic case for fertility reduction emerged during the 1980s[6]. In essence, this critique argued that the view of rapid population growth failed to take into account the powerful corrective forces of the marketplace. For example, the presumed negative impact of rapid population growth on natural resources was really an instance of failure to properly use market forces. If forests, for example, are privately owned, then declining wood supplies will perforce drive up the price of fuel wood. Rising prices will yield decreased demand, more efficient use of wood through the use of better technologies and switching to alternative fuel sources. The same virtuous circle can, it was argued, be found in every domain; e.g., rising demand for food induces the use of more productive agricultural technologies. More people mean more labor, which generates higher over-all production. Pressure on resources and scarcity are an inducement to the adoption of more productive technologies. The negative consequences purportedly associated with rapid population growth actually reflect government interference in the marketplace that distorts the prices for goods and labor or which otherwise channel resources away from where they can be used most efficiently. Population growth is either neutral or beneficial in its effect once one allows for the corrective effect of market forces. In short, the conservative economists have argued, markets are the best contraceptive.

The conservative economic critique, coupled with religious opposition, helped galvanize new opposition to family planning programs. At the 1984 International Conference on Population, the U.S. delegation, under orders from the Reagan Administration, repudiated the notion that rapid population growth is a barrier to development. In a reversal from previous years, conservatives in the United States became less sympathetic or hostile to supporting family planning programs.

On balance, the economic research indicates that rapid population growth does have negative consequences.[7,8] The degree of impact is contextual, reflecting the resource base, government policy and household adjustments to population pressures. High dependency ratios do tend to depress savings. Reducing fertility does create a "demographic bonus" that permits greater per child investment in education. Slower population growth tends to reduce pressure on land and water resources. High fertility negatively affects both maternal and child health, which has economic repercussions. Family planning programs are a powerful tool for reducing fertility, though fertility is affected by other variables, many of which are less immediately amenable to government intervention.

The treatment of reproduction as an economic variable generates a very particular definition of the problem and the policy solution. If one defines rapid population growth as an important drag on economic growth, then high fertility is the essential problem, with fertility reduction as the preferred policy response. As a practical matter, "fertility reduction" translated into support for family planning programs as the principal means for slowing population growth. The "left wing" economists argued that reproduction is simply not a very important economic variable or that, if population growth is a problem, development is the best contraceptive. Conservative economists claimed that population growth is beneficial or neutral, prescribing free markets as the best policy.

Reproduction as a Health Problem

The health problems associated with reproduction have been detailed at length earlier in this book. These include maternal mortality and morbidity, child mortality, HIV/AIDS and other sexually transmitted diseases, sexual violence and so forth.

The health perspective fundamentally re-frames the same basic phenomenon—reproduction—into an issue of health policy, rather than an economic or politico-military problem. Redefining reproduction as a health problem has the following implications:

- The policy and programmatic solutions tend to be drawn from the domains of public health and medicine. Yet, the roots of many reproductive health problems are to be found in broader issues of poverty, social injustice and gender inequity. Public health interventions are an important but not sufficient means of addressing reproductive insecurity. The focus on reproduction as a health problem may obscure the broader social sources and consequences of reproductive insecurity, leading to only partially effective policy remedies.
- The priority accorded the reproduction "problem" may change, positively or negatively. Political leaders may be more willing to address a health problem, rather than tackle a potentially controversial issue in the name of long run economic benefits. Conversely, reproductive health may be seen as only one of many health concerns and not as an issue of critical importance to national development.
- There are new or different normative implications of policy change. Promoting good health is usually perceived as an unalloyed good. Political leaders may feel more personally comfortable arguing for policies that change sexual behavior or reproductive outcomes for health reasons. They may also find it easier to make the case for improved health to constituents, rather than arguing that fewer (or more) children are needed "for the good of the nation". However, a health perspective does not necessarily imply a respect for human rights. In practice, it may mean that health providers withhold information, constrain options or coerce choice by health providers who "know what is best" for the client. That is why organizations such as the International Planned Parenthood Federation have taken the step of issuing statements of client rights.
- Reproduction as a health problem brings into play a whole new set of constituents and actors, largely drawn from the medical and public health communities. The support of these actors becomes essential for public policy to proceed; protracted consciousness-raising among the health and medical staff has often been a precursor to policy change. Conversely, the support of medial and health professionals can provide the necessary political "cover" for leaders to promote new policies influencing reproduction and sexual behavior.
- Reproductive health must compete with other health problems for resources, without the added impetus of economic or politico-military benefits. Since reproductive health problems disproportionately affect poor, marginalized and rural women, they are less likely to attract the political support needed for significant sustained investment or appropriate targeting of resources.

In sum, framing reproduction as a health problem can work to increase or diminish its political palatability to decision-makers. Reproductive health programs may be viewed as easy to espouse because of their health benefits; conversely, they may simply be seen as one more claimant on an over-stretched health budget.

Reproduction as a Human Rights Problem

All of the foregoing definitions of the reproduction problem—political, economic, and health—tend to treat people, especially women, as *objects* of public policy. That is, some external "expert" or political authority has determined that the current pattern of reproductive behavior is unsatisfactory and needs to be changed. The resources of the states are then brought to bear to induce new behaviors. Alternatively, the government authorities may determine that the current behaviors are desirable and use the powers of government to maintain the status quo.

The treatment of reproduction as an object of public policy can lead to the abuse or ignoring of human rights. This violation of human rights can occur either by denying access to services and information needed for the purpose of constraining choice or by coercing a specific "choice" by individuals or groups. The right of individuals and couples to make free and informed choices about reproduction and health care may be vitiated in the name of some higher good, such as political power, religion or economic growth. People (especially women) have been denied access to reproductive health services and information, such as family planning, because political leaders want to maintain current fertility, control women's sexuality or simply retain the current balance of power between men and women. Conversely, the government may want to precipitate new behaviors and use coercive or abusive means to induce the acceptance of contraception, conformity to norms of sexual conduct or other reproductive behaviors. Family planning programs in China and India have clearly engaged in abuses in the name of reducing fertility and the rate of population growth.[9,10] Many more governments have denied women access to essential reproductive health services.

Hence, an alternative definition of the reproduction problem is the failure to respect or promote human rights in matters of reproduction by dictating or constraining choice and access to information and services.[11] Formal definitions of reproductive rights are grounded in or explicitly articulated in an array of treaties and international accords, including the Universal Declaration of Human Rights, the International Bill of Rights, the World Population Programme of Action, the Convention on the Elimination of All Forms of Discrimination Against Women, and the reports of the International Conferences on Women. The report of the 1994 International Conference on Population and Development (ICPD) includes the following definition of reproductive rights[12]:

> ...reproductive rights embrace certain human rights that are already recognized in national laws, international human rights documents and other consensus documents. These rights rest on the recognition of the basic right of all couples and individuals to decide freely and responsibly the number, spacing and timing of their children and to have the information and means to do so, and the right to attain the highest standard of sexual and reproductive health. It also includes their right to make decisions concerning reproduction free of discrimination, coercion and violence, as expressed in human rights documents. In the exercise of this right, they should take into account the needs of their living and future children and their responsibilities towards the community. The promotion of the responsible exercise of these rights for all people should be the fundamental basis for government- and community-supported policies and programmes in the area of reproductive health, including family planning. As part of their commitment, full attention should be given to

> the promotion of mutually respectful and equitable gender relations and particularly to meeting the educational and service needs of adolescents to enable them to deal in a positive and responsible way with their sexuality.

The reproductive rights perspective provides a fresh look at the reproduction "problem", expressing the need to treat reproduction as one aspect of a broader effort to promote human dignity. Protection and promotion of reproductive rights, in this view, becomes the centerpiece of policy. There may be additional economic or social benefits, but these are the happy by-product and not the purpose of respecting reproductive rights, which are an intrinsic good. Promotion of reproductive rights leads to a fairly broad policy and programmatic prescription, including making available an array of reproductive health services, reducing gender inequity, and addressing the sexual and reproductive health needs of people throughout the life cycle.

Non-governmental organizations, women's groups and feminists have been among the most effective and vocal proponents of the reproductive rights perspective. Their advocacy helped shape the outcome of the 1994 ICPD. By the mid-1990s there was a network of reproductive rights activists spread across many countries.

Reproduction as a Religious or Moral Problem

Reproduction is not a "technical" problem, whose meaning is adequately captured by a set of health, demographic, political or economic variables. Reproduction is inextricably interwoven with our thoughts, feelings and beliefs about sexuality. Our conceptualization of reproduction cannot be divorced from our thinking about sexuality. Sexuality and reproduction are fundamental expressions of who we are as people, the standard of behavior to which we aspire and the type of relationships, family and/or household we are trying to create. As much as any aspect of the human condition, sexuality is inherently a highly charged and complex issue. One need hardly belabor the immense role of sexuality and reproduction in family dynamics, social relations, culture, psychology, the arts and many other aspects of human life.

Every society has evolved a complex set of rules governing reproduction and sexuality. Some of these rules are embodied in laws that can be enforced through the powers of the state, while many others are social conventions that are widely understood or respected. Secular and/or religious moral codes will typically encompass such issues as:

- The moral purposes and boundaries of sexuality
- The relationship between men and women
- Sexual practices and partners
- Childbearing
- Health and health behaviors
- Contraception
- Abortion
- Circumcision
- Sexual violence

Actual behavior may vary from the governing code. However, this does not vitiate the fact that people properly view sexuality and reproduction as *moral* issues. It is therefore not surprising that reproductive politics tend to be highly contentious, since they reflect fundamental debates about deeply held social rules and roles.

From the perspective of virtually every major religion, sexuality is inextricably linked to the experience of the sacred. Religious laws governing reproduction and sexual conduct are usually rooted in a much broader theology.[13] Religious precepts about the nature of God (or gods), the relationship between the deity and humans, the beginning of life, the soul, marital relations and myriad other issues are typically the premises on which the code governing reproduction and sexuality are derived. Challenges to religious laws on reproduction are therefore challenges to basic tenets of belief. For people of faith, religious precepts necessarily take precedence over other concerns, such as the economic, political or even health benefits of new reproductive behaviors. At minimum, people of faith will insist that moral considerations weigh equally in decisions about behavior, programs and policy and that discussions proceeding from an essentially technocratic premise lacking a moral center will inevitably have pernicious social consequences.

In sum, reproduction may be viewed as a moral or religious "problem". That is, the central concern is ensuring or encouraging adherence to a set of beliefs or a code of conduct. Adherence to these norms is an inherent and extremely precious good, as well as serving to produce happier, better people and societies. Religious and secular codes need not conflict with other considerations (such as health or economy), but they must at least be taken into account seriously and explicitly and must be given priority when conflicts arise. Proponents of religious and moral codes will therefore act to support public policies that further their beliefs, while opposing policies that they believe induce immoral or unethical conduct.

Summing Up: Different Definitions, Different Prescriptions

As we have seen, reproduction may be perceived as:

- A source of political and military power;
- A variable having a negative, positive or neutral influence on economic and social development;
- A key determinant of the health status of women and children;
- Ensconced in a set of human rights that must be protected;
- An expression of a code of moral and/or religious conduct.

Each of these perspectives has fervent adherents. The varying definitions of the reproduction "problem" tend to yield quite different policy prescriptions. Those who perceive reproduction primarily as a health issue will focus on medical and public health solutions. Rights advocates will focus on building legal and political protections, as well as the political power of women. Those whose perspective is primarily framed by economics will be more likely to suggest policies and programs that optimize the allocation of scarce resources. Religious adherents will argue for giving primacy to more ethical behavior over other, more technocratic solutions.

The same specific objective conditions—unintended pregnancy or HIV/AIDS—may therefore yield wholly different definitions and solutions, with attendant conflict among the varying proponents. This is not always the case; e.g., the health and human rights perspectives may (but do not necessarily) yield very similar policy outcomes. As will be discussed below, advancing policy change often means putting together a coalition of people and groups who see their diverse interests as overlapping in a particular policy proposal. It is often possible, through negotiation and compromise, to find common ground around a policy proposal.

But the perspectives differ often enough and radically enough to consistently generate bitter clashes over the policies a government should adopt. An advocate of policies to reduce the rate of population growth may clash with a human rights advocate over the limits of government intervention in reproductive choice. An advocate for a specific religious perspective may oppose the policies supported by someone primarily concerned with advancing public health outcomes. Some political actors may reject the notion that reproduction is properly the province of any public policy intervention.

These debates are often highly emotional and contentious. The advocates are usually talking past each other, as they are departing from very different premises about the nature of the "problem".

Public policy derives from the conflict, compromise and consensus among the advocates of these diverse perspectives. Each seeks to assemble a winning coalition that can influence the decision-makers. We now turn our attention to the process by which the reproductive health advocate can seek to influence policy.

THE MANAGER AS POLICY ADVOCATE[14]

The potential array of unsatisfactory conditions facing policy makers is infinite—societies are never, *in toto*, adequately healthy, wealthy or wise. This reality is exacerbated in developing nations; the poorer the country, the more daunting and demanding the set of unsatisfactory conditions. National leaders are constantly struggling with every imaginable issue: political crisis, conflicts, low incomes, bad schools, environmental degradation, water and land shortages, poor health, and so forth. Even within the more restricted arena of health, reproductive insecurity is only one of many conditions, competing for attention with high child mortality, epidemics of infectious disease, environmental health, chronic diseases and other concerns. The agenda of any policy maker is necessarily constrained—only a few items can receive his or her attention. Hence, the effective reproductive health program manager must also understand how and why her concerns might rise onto the agenda of political leaders.

Even if an issue draws the attention of the relevant policy makers, they have limited political and financial capital to spend. Policy proposals must meet a set of tests—technical, financial, political and practical—if they are to merit the expenditure of a politician's scarce resources. The ability to mobilize intellectual, political and financial resources is the key to successful advocacy and largely determines the shape of public policy.

The effectiveness of a reproductive health program manager is often determined by her ability to serve as an effective policy advocate. Building legitimacy, raising awareness, positioning the program to attract key constituencies, securing resources, and achieving favorable conditions for implementation are often an important part of the manager's job. It is therefore useful to have a framework for formulating an advocacy strategy. Policy advocacy usually consists of knowing *what* policy change is needed, *who* has the power to make the decision, *identifying those who can influence the decision-makers* and *tailoring arguments* to the information needs of the concerned audiences.

Clarifying Policy Objectives

The first step in effective policy advocacy is being clear about the advocacy objective. Managers must determine if there is a significant *policy* barrier to effective programming. It is therefore often helpful for managers to make a list of possible causes of the problem they are trying to solve to determine the specific policy issue. What is the specific policy change needed to advance reproductive health? Is it consciousness-raising by government leaders? Legitimization of the program by important public figures? Changes in laws or regulations? Increased allocation of resources? Changes in implementation standards?

To be an effective advocate, a manager must be reasonably certain that the proposed policy change will actually benefit the program. The manager should have an empirically-based, logical reason for believing that a specific policy change will meaningfully contribute to program success.

Moreover, managers are often confronted with multiple policy concerns that are inhibiting program progress. Only rarely can a wide array of policy issues be addressed simultaneously. The manager must make a reasonable judgment about the most important policy change(s) needed at any point in time, as well as the feasibility of achieving change in a given period. Knowing what to ask for is part of the challenge of effective advocacy.

For example, the early stages of program development usually require emphasis on consciousness raising and legitimization, while more mature programs must focus on resource allocation and implementation strategies. The HIV/AIDS pandemic is a good example. Most national governments reacted quite late in acknowledging the magnitude of the problem. Effective policy advocacy would have focused on getting government leaders to acknowledge and champion public action in response to the mounting epidemic. In countries where public awareness is much more widespread, greater emphasis may be needed on getting governments to allocate adequate resources and hold the public bureaucracy accountable for achieving results.

Identifying the Relevant Decision-makers and Political Actors

Once the manager has determined *what* to ask for, she must also determine *whom* to ask. The decision-maker whose support is needed will likely change in light of the specific policy problem needing resolution. Solving a policy problem will often involve multiple decision-makers, including legislators, health officials, budget officers, local government leaders and national figures. Moreover, decision-makers are typically sensitive to the reactions of both allies and adversaries to policy change. Effective advocacy requires systematically identifying the array of actors who will be attempt or could influence a specific policy decision.

The earlier discussion of the multiple definitions of the reproductive health "problem" implicitly pointed to the following political actors:

- Political leaders in the executive office (presidency, prime minister) and in the concerned ministries (health, finance, plan and/or justice)
- Legislators, particularly those who hold leadership positions or relevant committee assignments
- Political party members, leaders and supporters
- Government technocrats
- Issue advocates who maintain an organization devoted to a specific policy domain
- University faculty and other analysts who argue the technical validity of proposed policies and programs
- The medical and public health community
- Women's rights and women's health advocates
- Religious leaders and communities
- Traditional and community leaders
- Journalists, editors, publishers and other important media figures
- Donors and other sources of financial support for programs

In practice, conflict and compromise among concerned actors largely determine public policy. The success of an advocacy effort depends on building a winning coalition. Managers will usually develop an acute sense of the relevant decision-makers in their environment, as well as those who influence decision-makers. A very useful exercise can be explicitly identifying the decision-makers, potential advocates for the manager's position, and those who may wish to oppose the manager's proposal. A judgment can then be made about the relative ability of each constituency to influence the outcome of the political process. Who matters? Who is perceived as really influential by the key decision-makers? The manager is then better positioned to build relations with decision-makers, solicit the support of potential allies and either neutralize the arguments of opponents or negotiate a compromise position.

Different Audiences, Different Arguments

A policy proposal may need the support of key legislators, senior ministerial officials, technocrats, prominent medical leaders, religious leaders and journalists or some other combination of political actors. Each actor is likely to approach the policy issue from a different perspective. The case for the manager's policy proposal must be tailored to meet diverse information needs. There is no point making an economic argument to an actor who is primarily concerned with health or religious issues. Different actors are likely to judge a policy proposal using very different criteria.

Criteria that may be applied by different actors include:

- *The likelihood that the policy will achieve the support or draw the ire of constituencies important to the decision-makers*: The perception by decision-makers of political support from stakeholders and the neutralizing of opponents is usually critical to securing change. They must be reassured that policy change will draw or retain adherents, while alienating few constituencies (and even possibly damaging political enemies). Getting key representatives of the relevant constituencies to speak to political leaders is part of the advocacy process.
- *Evidence of the magnitude of the problem*: The bigger the problem, the more likely it is to move onto the agenda of decision-makers, particularly if feasible solutions are proposed. Demonstrable

trends that the problem is growing worse (such as the HIV/AIDS pandemic) and/or that interventions can change the trend line can also be persuasive. Unfortunately, this line of argument often tends to work against solutions that would prevent major problems from emerging. Policies that aim at early intervention are often at a disadvantage because they are unable to generate a sense of crisis that can capture the decision-makers attention and force the issue onto the political agenda.

- *The perceived link between the policy proposal and catalytic events*: Policy proposals can sometimes be directly linked to a highly publicized or personally meaningful event. The public admission of a well-respected person that he or she has HIV or the death of a prominent figure from AIDS is an example of an event that can help push a policy agenda. A dramatic story in the media can sometimes be used to capture public attention and spur action by political leaders. Policy proposals are sometimes attached to other issues; e.g., reproductive rights proposals can be attached to broader efforts at judicial or constitutional reform.
- *Evidence of demand for services*: Political leaders may be more likely to support reproductive health services if they receive scientific or convincing anecdotal information that there in an unsatisfied, expressed demand by the population. Surveys and visits to the field by decision-makers are often helpful in establishing the demand for services.
- *The technical feasibility of the proposed policy*: i.e., the perceived likelihood that the proposed policy, if implemented, will actually achieve the purported benefits. Pilot projects, evaluations and examples from other, similar locations are often useful in showing technical feasibility.
- *The administrative feasibility of the proposed policy*: Many developing country governments have very weak bureaucracies and decision-makers may be skeptical of the ability of the government to successfully implement the proposed policy. Like technical feasibility, evidence of the capacity to implement will help build support.
- *The cost of the proposed policy*: Budget constraints almost always play a role in policy choice. Estimating the costs, showing how the policy will be paid for and assessing cost-effectiveness will be particularly important in securing the support of some key political actors. In developing countries, donors often help promote policy change by defraying the cost.
- *The language used in presenting the policy proposal*: A policy proposal to advance family planning that is couched in the language of "population control" may be less acceptable than one couched in terms of health benefits. Hence, adjusting the language of discourse may be a necessary part of effective advocacy.
- *The congruence of decision-maker values and norms with the policy proposal*: Policy proposals are more likely to receive support when they can be shown to be consistent with the values of the decision-maker and his or her key constituencies. Dialogue with religious leaders, elders and other respected figures in the community can often serve this purpose.

The style of advocacy that will be most effective can also vary widely. There is a continuum from low-profile, low-key persuasion of key figures to high-profile, highly confrontational approaches. Even allies around a particular issue may choose to use different advocacy strategies. It is clear, for example, that confrontational tactics have helped draw attention and resources to HIV/AIDS programs. However, more subdued, analytic approaches may be better suited to optimal allocation of resources within HIV/AIDS programs.

Both the content and style of advocacy should also be conditioned by a calculation of how decision-makers, allies and opponents will react. Quiet, low profile tactics may suffice, or they may be simply seen as evidence of weakness by political leaders and opponents. Confrontational tactics may push issues onto the public and political agenda, but may also serve to alienate potential supporters. A mixed strategy may signal a willingness to arrive at compromise, while demonstrating the ability to mobilize political support. Choosing a strategy depends on the nature of the issue, and the resources both advocates and opponents can bring to bear.

The reproductive health manager is almost invariably thrust into the role of being a political actor and policy advocate. By having a clear framework and strategy for advocacy, the manager can be more effective in creating a supportive environment for her program. Hence, the manager must consider the objective of advocacy, the identity of the key decision-makers, the constituencies that will influence the decision-makers, the criteria that will be applied by different political actors in judging policy proposals and the style of advocacy that will most effectively advance the desired policy.

Notes

NOTES FOR CHAPTER 1

[1] United Nations *World Population Programme of Action*, New York, United Nations, 1994.
[2] Tannahill, Reay *Sex in History*, Scarborough House, 1992.
[3] Morice, P., P. Josset and J.C. Colau "La Gynecologie et l'Obstetrique en Egypte Antique" *J. Gynecol. Obstet. Biol. Reprod.*, 1994, 23, pp. 131–136.
[4] Sullivan, Richard "Divine and Rational: The Reproductive Health of Women in Ancient Egypt" *Obstetrical and Gynecological Survey*, Volume 52, No. 10, pp. 635–642.
[5] Trueba, Guadelupe "Birth in Pre-Hispanic Mexico" *International Midwife*, Winter 1997, pp. 45–47.
[6] Thompson, Sandra "Obstetrics During the Early Roman Empire" *Midwives Chronicle and Nursing Notes* June, 1987.
[7] Sources for the history of contraception are: Asbell, Bernard *The Pill* New York: Random House, 1995; Djerassi, Carl *The Politics of Contraception* San Francisco: W.H. Freeman, 1981; Himes, Norman *Medical History of Contraception* New York: Gamut Press, 1963; Riddle, John M. *Contraception and Abortion from the Ancient World to the Renaissance* Cambridge: Harvard University Press, 1992; Tannahill, Reay *Sex in History*, Scarborough House, 1992.
[8] Sparling, Frederick P. "Biology of *neissareia gonocrrhae*" in *Sexually Transmitted Diseases, Third Edition*, Holmes, King K., et. al. editors, New York, McGraw Hill, 1999 p. 433.
[9] Kloos Helmut and Zein, Ahmed Zein "AIDS and other STDs in Ethiopia: Historical, social and epidemiological aspects" *Africa Urban Quarterly* Vol. 6, Nos 1 and 2, Feb. and May 1991.
[10] Billstein, Stephen A. "Pubic lice" in *Sexually Transmitted Diseases, Third Edition*, Holmes, King K., et. al. editors, op. cit., p. 641.
[11] Schacter, Julius "Biology of *chlamydia trachomatis*", ibid, p. 391.
[12] Koutsky, Laura A. and Kiviat, Nancy B. "Genital human papillomavirus", ibid., p. 347.
[13] Crosby, Alfred W. "The early history of syphilis: A reappraisal" *American Anthropologist*, 71 (1969) pp. 218–227.
[14] Lyons, Martinez "Sexually transmitted diseases in the history of Uganda" *Genitourinary Medicine*, 70 (1994) pp. 138–145.
[15] Kloos and Zein, op. cit.
[16] Corey, Lawrence and Wald, Anna "Genital herpes" in *Sexually Transmitted Diseases, Third Edition*, Holmes, King K., et. al. editors, p. 285.
[17] Ronald, Allan R. and Albritton, William "Chancroid and *haemophilus ducreyi*" in *Sexually Transmitted Diseases, Third Edition*, Holmes, King K., et. al. editors, p. 515.
[18] Krieger, John M. and Alderete, John F. "*Trichomonas vaginalis* and Trichomoniasis" in *Sexually Transmitted Diseases, Third Edition*, Holmes, King K., et. al. editors, p. 587.
[19] Potts, Malcom and Short, Roger *Ever since Adam and Eve: The evolution of human sexuality* Cambridge: Cambridge University Press, 1999, p. 244.
[20] Riddle, John M. *Contraception and Abortion from the Ancient World to the Renaissance* Cambridge: Harvard University Press, 1992; Riddle, John M. *Eve's Herbs: A History of Contraception and Abortion in the West* Cambridge: Harvard University Press, 1997.

[21] Brandt, Allan "Sexually transmitted diseases" in: *Companion Encyclopedia of the History of Medicine*; W. F. Bynum and Roy Porter (eds.) London ; New York: Routledge, 1993, pp. 578–579.

[22] Rosenfield, A. and Maine, D. "Maternal mortality—neglected tragedy: Where is the M in MCH?" *Lancet*, 2:83–85, 1985.

[23] Paxman, John M., Rizzo, Alberto, Brown, Laura, Benson, Jamie " The clandestine epidemic: The practice of unsafe abortion in Latin America" *Studies in Family Planning*, Vol. 24, No. 4. (Jul.–Aug., 1993), pp. 205–226.

[24] De Browere, Vincent, Rene Tonglet and Wim Van Leberghe "Strategies for Reducing Maternal Mortality in Developing Countries: What Can We Learn from the History of the Industrialized West" *Tropical Medicine and International Health*, Volume 3, No. 10, pp. 771–782 (October, 1998).

[25] Sources for the history of obstetric care are: Barlow, Yvonne "Childbirth: Management of Labour Through the Ages" *Nursing Times*, August 31, 1994, Volume 90, No. 35, pp. 41–43; Cianfrani, Theodore *A Short History of Obstetrics and Gynecology* Springfield: Charles C. Thomas, 1960; O'Dowd, Michael J. and Elliot E. Philipp *The History of Gynaecology and Obstetrics* New York: Parthenon, 1994; Thoms, Herbert *Our Obstetric Heritage: The Story of Safe Childbirth* Hamden, CT: Shoe String Press, 1960.

[26] Parisot, Jeannette *Johnny Come Lately: A short history of the condom* London: Journeyman Press, 1987.

[27] De Brouwere, et. al., op. cit.

[28] Adapted from Chambers, Robert *Rural Development: Putting the Last First* London: Longman, 1983, pp. 111–113.

[29] I am indebted to Dr. Timothy Frankenberger of CARE for his patient and repeated explanations of the livelihood security concept.

[30] See Middleberg, Maurice *"Health Security: A framework for health programming"* Atlanta: CARE, 1997 for a discussion of the health security concept.

[31] See Mason, Karen Oppenheim and Taj, Anju Malhotra "Differences between women's and men's reproductive goals in developing countries" *Population and Development Review*, Vol. 13, No. 4 (Dec. 1987), pp. 611–638.

[32] See Netting, Robert McC.; Wilk, Richard, R. and Arnould, Eric J. *Households: Comparative and Historical Studies of the Domestic Group* Berkely: University of California Press, 1984 for a further discussion of the household concept.

NOTES FOR CHAPTER 2

[1] Upadhyay, U.D. and B. Robey "Why Family Planning Matters" *Population Reports* Series J, No. 49, Baltimore: Johns Hopkins University School of Public Health, Population Information Program, July 1999.

[2] Based data from six countries in Latin America, 20 countries in sub-Saharan Africa and Bangladesh, India and Nepal in Asia. All surveys taken during 1990s.

[3] ibid.

[4] U.S. Bureau of the Census, Report WP/98, *World Population Profile: 1998*, U.S. Government Printing Office, Washington, D.C., 1999, page 50.

[5] McDevitt, Thomas, N. with Arjun Adlakha, Timothy Fowler and Vena Harris-Bourne *Trends in Adolescent Fertility and Contraceptive Use in the Developing World* Washington, D.C.: U.S. Bureau of the Census, 1996.

[6] ibid.; National Research Council *Contraception and Reproduction: Health Consequences for Women and Children in the Developing World*, Washington, D.C.: National Academy Press, 1989; Parnell, Allan M. (editor) *Contraceptive Use and Controlled Fertility: Health Issues for Women and Children*, Washington, D.C.: National Academy Press, 1989.

[7] Ross, John A. and Elizabeth Frankenberger *Findings from Two Decades of Family Planning Research* New York; The Population Council, 1993, page 76.

[8] National Research Council, 1989, op. cit.; Shane, Barbara *Family Planning Saves Lives, Third Edition* Washington, D.C.: Population Reference Bureau, 1996: Tsui, Amy O., Judith Wasserheit and Joahn Haaga, editors *Reproductive Health in Developing Countries: Expanding Dimensions, Building Solutions* Washington, D.C.: National Academy Press, 1997; Upadhyay, U.D. and Robey, B. "Why Family Planning Matters" *Population Reports* Series J, No. 49, Baltimore: Johns Hopkins University School of Public Health, Population Information Program, July 1999.

[9] Rutstein, Shea "Effect of Birth Intervals on Mortality and Health: Multivariate Cross-Country Analysis" (presentation at MACRO International Seminar), 1999.

[10] National Research Council, 1989, op. cit.; Parnell, op. cit.

[11] Ibid.

[12] Tsui, et. al., op. cit.; Institute of Medicine *The Best Intentions: Unintended Pregnancy and the Well-Being of Children and Families* Washington, D.C.: National Academy Press, 1995.

[13] Institute of Medicine, 1995, op. cit.; National Research Council, 1989, op. cit.; Parnell, 1989, op. cit.; Tsui, et. al., op. cit; Ross, Susan Rae *Promoting Quality Maternal and Newborn Care: A Reference Manual for Program Managers* Atlanta: CARE, 1999.

[14] Tsui, et. al., op. cit., page 90.

[15] Ross, op. cit.; Tsui, et. al., op. cit.; World Health Organization *Reduction of Maternal Mortality: A Joint WHO/UNFPA/UNICEF/World Bank Statement* Geneva, 1999.

[16] Tsui, et. al., op. cit., page 117.

[17] Tsui, et. al., op. cit., page 116.

[18] Sources: World Health Organization *Reduction of Maternal Mortality*; Maine, Deborah, Victoria Ward and Abdi Tahir El Tahir *Meeting the Community Half Way: Programming Guidelines for the Reduction of Maternal Mortality* New York, Center for Population and Family Health, Columbia University.

[19] Source: Li, X.F., J.A. Fortney, M. Kotelchuk and L.H. Glover "The post-partum period: the key to maternal mortality: *International Journal of Gynecology and Obstetrics* 54 (1996) 1–10, 1993.

[20] Ross, op. cit., page 11.

[21] Ross, op. cit, page 1.8.

[22] Source: Stewart, M Kathryn, Cynthia K. Stanton, and Omar Ahmed 1997 *Maternal Health Care*, DHS Comparative Studies No. 25, Calverton, MD: Macro International, Inc., p. 5.

[23] ibid, page 3.7.

[24] Source: World Bank *World Development Indicators 1999*.

[25] Source: International Federation of Gynecology and Obstetrics Committee on the Ethical Aspects of Human Reproduction and Women's Health.

[26] Source: Salter, C., Johnson, H.B. and Hengen, N. "Care for Post-abortion Complications: Saving Women's Lives" *Population Reports*, Series L, No. 10. Baltimore: Johns Hopkins School of Public Health, Population Information Program, June 1993.

[27] *World Population Profile*, op. cit., p. A-11.

[28] Source: Henshaw, Stanley K. "Unintended Pregnancy and Abortion: A Public Health Perspective" in Paul, Maureen, et. al. (eds.) *A Clinician's Guide to Medical and Surgical Abortion* New York: Churchill Livingstone, 1999, pp. 13.

[29] Tsui, et. al., op. cit., page 96.

[30] Source: Salter, C., Johnson, H.B. and Hengen, N. "Care for Post-abortion Complications: Saving Women's Lives" *Population Reports*, Series L, No. 10. Baltimore: Johns Hopkins School of Public Health, Population Information Program, June 1993.

[31] ibid.

[32] Benson, Janie, Lori Ann Nicholson, Lynne Gaffikin and Stephen N. Kinoti "Complications of Unsafe Abortion in sub-Saharan Africa: A Review" *Health Policy and Planning*, Volume 11, No. 2, pp. 117–131.

[33] See Mundigo, Axel I and Cynthia Indriso (eds.) *Abortion in the Developing World*, New Yor: Zed Books, 1999, especially Section III for a discussion of quality of care issues.

[34] See Singh, K. and S.S. Ratnam "The Influence of Abortion Legislation on Maternal Mortality" *International Journal of Gynecology and Obstetrics*, 63 Suppl. 1(1998) S123–S129.

[35] See Faundes, A. and E. Hardy "Illegal Abortion: Consequences for Women's Health and the Health Care System" *International Journal of Gynecology and Obstetrics*, 58 (1997) pp. 77–83.

[36] Bankole, Akinrinola, Susheela Singh and Taylor Haas "Reasons Why Women Have Abortions: Evidence from 27 Countries" *International Family Planning Perspectives*, Volume 24, Issue 3 (Sep., 1998) pp. 117–127.

[37] See Mundigo and Indriso, *Abortion in the Developing World*, op. cit, Section I for studies of the relationship between abortion and contraception in seven developing countries.

[38] Source: UNAIDS *AIDS Epidemic Update: December, 2001*.

[39] Source: UNAIDS *AIDS Epidemic Update: December, 2001*.

[40] Sources: Mann, Jonathan and Daniel J. Tarantola *AIDS in the World II: Global Dimensions, Social Roots and Responses*, New York: Oxford University Press, 1996; Chapter 1 in Gibney, Laura, DiClemente, Ralph and Sten H. Vermund *Preventing HIV in Developing Countries*, New York: Kluwer, 1999, Chapter 1.

[41] Source: UNAIDS Epidemiological Fact Sheets: 2000 Update.

[42] Source: U.S. Bureau of the Census *World Population Profile 1998*, U.S. Government Printing Office, Washington, D.C., 1999, pp. 56–57.

[43] UNAIDS *Technical Update: Mother-to-child transmission of HIV*, September 2000.

[44] Source: UNAIDS.

[45] Source: World Health Organization *WHO Initiative on HIV/AIDS and Sexually Transmitted Infections: An Overview of Selected Curable Sexually Transmitted Diseases*, n.d. (online document).

[46] Source: *Demographic and Health Surveys*.

[47] Upadhyay, U.D. and B. Robey, op. cit.

[48] Adapted from Lapham, Robert. J. and George B.Simmons "Overview and Framework" in Lapham, Robert. J. and George B.Simmons, eds., *Organizing for Effective Family Planning Programs*, Washington, D.C., : National Academy Press, 1989, p. 6.

[49] *World Population Profile, 1998*, op. cit.

[50] Bongaarts, John "A simple method for estimating the contraceptive prevalence required to achieve a fertility target" *Studies in Family Planning*, 1984 Jul–Aug; 15(4):184–190.

[51] For a skeptic's perspective see Pritchett, Lant "Desired Fertility and the Impact of Population Policies" *Population and Development Review*, Vol. 20, No. 3, 1994, pp 1–55.

[52] Bulatao, Rodolfo A. *The Value of Family Planning Programs in Developing Countries* Santa Monica, RAND, 1998, p. 31.

[53] Source: U.S. Bureau of the Census, International Data Base.

[54] Maine, D., et. al. "Prevention of Maternal Deaths in Developing Countries: Program Options and Practical Considerations" Paper presented at the International Safe Motherhood Conference, Nairobi, Feb. 10–13, 1987.

[55] Source: ibid.

[56] ibid.

[57] Adapted from Ross, op. cit., p. 1.16.

[58] Source: Anderson, Roy M. "Transmission Dynamic of Sexually Transmitted Infections" in *Sexually Transmitted Diseases, Third Edition*, Holmes, King K., et. al. editors, New York: McGraw-Hill, 1999.

[59] Estimates of transmission probability are from Anderson, op. cit., p. 27.

[60] Adapted from World Bank *Confronting AIDS: Public Priorities in a Global Epidemic*, New York: Oxford University Press, 1998.

[61] Carael, Michel "Sexual Behavior" in *Sexual Behavior and AIDS in the Developing World*, John Cleland and Benoit Ferry, editors, London: Taylor and Francis, 1995, p. 115. U.S. data are from Michael, Robert T, et. al. *Sex in America: A Definitive Survey* Boston: Little, Brown & Company, 1994.

[62] In some sites, the population covered was ages 15–59.

[63] Cleland, John, with Benoit Ferry and Michel Carael "Summary and Conclusions in *Sexual Behavior and AIDS in the Developing World*, p. 111.

[64] Carael, op. cit., p. 116.

NOTES FOR CHAPTER 3

[1] Taken from Prochaska, J. O., Colleen A. Redding and Kerry E. Evers "The Transtheoretical Model and Stages of Change" in *Health Behavior and Health Education* Karen Glanz, et. al. editors, San Francisco: Jossey-Bass, 1997.

[2] I am grateful to Ralph DiClemente for this insight.

[3] See *Health Behavior and Health Education* Karen Glanz, et. al. editors, San Francisco: Jossey-Bass, 1997 for a good overview of approaches to health behavior modification.

[4] Adapted from Miller, William R. and Stephen Rollnick *Motivational Interviewing* New York, Guilford Press, 1991.

[5] Bandura, A. *Social Learning Theory* Englewood Cliffs, NJ: Prentice Hall, 1977.

[6] Hosken, Fran P. *The Hosken Report: Genital and Sexual Mutilation of Females*, Fourth Revised Edition, Women's International Network News, 1993, p. 189.

[7] This section draws from Piotrow Phyllis Tilson, D. Lawrence Kincaid, Jose G. Rimon II and Ward Rinehart *Health Communications: Lessons from Family Planning and Reproductive Health* Westport, CT: Praeger, 1997, especially pages 89–108.

[8] Source: Central Statistical Organization (CSO) and Macro International (MI). 1998. *Yemen Demographic and Health Survey 1997*. Calverton, Maryland: CSO and MI, pp. 163–162.

[9] Piotrow, et. al., op. cit, pp. 101–102.

[10] Taken from Bertrand, Jane, Robert J. Magnani and James C. Knowles *Handbook of Indicators for Family Planning Program Evaluation*, n.d., p. 5.

[11] Fertility indicators are adapted from Bertrand, et. al., op. cit., Chapters 8 and 9. Maternal health indicators are adapted from Koblinsky, Marge, Katie McLaurin, Pauline Russell-Brown and Pamina Gorbach in *Indicators for Reproductive Health Program Evaluation*, Jane Bertrand and Amy Tsui, eds., Carolina Population Center, University of North Carolina, December, 1995. SID/HIV indicators are adapted from Dallabetta, Gina and Susan Hassig "Final Report of the Subcommittee on STD/HIV" in *Indicators for Reproductive Health Program Evaluation*.

NOTES FOR CHAPTER 4

[1] Jewkes, Rachel and Murcott, Anne "Community representatives: Representing the 'community'?" *Social Science and Medicine* Vol. 46, No. 7, pp. 843–858, 1998.

[2] Helfenbein, Saul and Sayeed, Abu "Increasing Community Participation" *Family Planning Manager*, Management Sciences for Health web site (www.msh.org/chs/tools).

[3] Maine, Deborah "Lessons for program design from the Preventing Maternal Mortality projects" *International Journal of Gynecology and Obstetrics* 59 Suppl. 2 (1997) S259–S265, p. S262.

[4] Beeker, Carolyn, Guenther-Grey, Carolyn and Raj, Anita "Community empowerment, paradigm drift and the primary prevention of HIV/AIDS" *Social Science and Medicine*, Vol. 46, No. 7 (1 Apr 1998), pp. 831–842.

[5] Hillery, George A. "Definitions of community: areas of agreement" *Rural Sociology*, Vol. 20, No.11, 1955.

[6] Jewkes, Rachel and Murcott, Anne "Meanings of community" *Social Science and Medicine*, Vol. 43, No. 4, pp. 555–563.

[7] ibid, p. 558.

[8] Aluwalia, Indu and Thomas Schmid *Community Involvement and Community Empowerment: Training of Trainers Manual*, National Center for Chronic Disease Prevention and Health Promotion, Centers for Disease Control and Prevention, Atlanta, n.d.

[9] Asthana, Sheena and Oostvogels, Robert "Community participation in HIV prevention: Problems and prospects for community-based strategies among female sex workers in Madras" *Social Science and Medicine*, Vol. 43, No. 2, pp. 133–147, 1996.

[10] Jewkes, Rachel and Murcott, Anne "Meanings of community", op. cit., p. 557.

[11] Piotrow Phyllis Tilson, D. Lawrence Kincaid, Jose G. Rimon II and Ward Rinehart *Health Communications: Lessons from Family Planning and Reproductive Health*, Wesport, CT: Praeger, 1997, pp. 34–35.

[12] Rifkin, S.B. *Health Planning and Community Participation* London: Croom-Helm, 1985.

[13] Source: Kambou, Sarah Degnan in *Embracing Participation in Development: Wisdom from the Field* Meera Kaul Shah, Sarah Degnan Kambou and Barbara Monahan (eds.), Atlanta:CARE, 1999.

[14] Choguill, Marisa B. Guaraldo "A ladder of community participation for underdeveloped countries" *Habitat International*, Vol. 20, No. 3, pp. 431–444, 1996.

[15] Beeker, Carolyn, Guenther-Grey, Carolyn and Raj, Anita "Community empowerment, paradigm drift and the primary prevention of HIV/AIDS" *Social Science and Medicine*, Vol. 46, No. 7 (1 Apr 1998), pp. 831–842.

[16] Minkler, Meredith and Wallerstein, Nina "Improving Health Through Community organization and Community Building" in *Health Behavior and Health Education: Theory, Research and Practice* Second Edition, Glanz, Karen et. al., eds, op. cit. p. 251.

[17] Ahuwalia and Schmid, op. cit., p. 24.

[18] Askew, Ian "Organizing community participation in family planning projects in South Asia" *Studies in Family Planning*, Vol. 20, No. 4 (Jul.–Aug., 1989) pp. 185–202.

[19] Cleland, John "Community participation in family planning" in *Family Planning, Health and Family Well-Being: Proceedings of the United Nations Expert Group Meeting on Family Planning, Health and Family Well-Being* Banagalore, India 26–30 October 1992. United Nations Population Division, 1996, pp. 245–255 (ST/ESA/SER.R/131).

[20] Askew, Ian and Khan, A.R. "Community participation and national family planning programs: Some organizational issues" *Studies in Family Planning*, Vol. 21, No. 3, (May–June, 1990), pp. 127–142.

[21] Tatar, Mehtap "Community participation in health care: The Turkish case" *Social Science and Medicine*, Vol. 42, No. 11, (1996) pp. 1493–1500.

[22] Purdey, Alice F.; Adhikari, Gyan Bahadur; Robinson, Sheila and Cox, Philip W. "Participatory health development in rural Nepal: Clarifying the process of community empowerment" *Health Education Quarterly* Vol. 21, No. 3 (Fall, 1994) pp. 329–343.

[23] The participatory techniques used in defining community and assessing need are drawn from Shah, Meera Kaul "A step-by-step guide to popular PLA tools and techniques" in *Embracing Participation in Development: Wisdom from the Field* Meera Kaul Shah, Sarah Degnan Kambou and Barbara Monahan (eds.), op. cit. The stories of CARE projects in Zambia are also drawn from this source.

[24] McAllister, Lynn and Fischer, Claude "A procedure for surveying personal networks" *Sociological Methods and Research* Vol. 7, No. 2, No. 1978.

[25] Ferligoj, A. and Hlebec, V. "Evaluation of social network measurement instruments" *Social Networks* Vol. 21 (2) 1999 pp. 111–130.

[26] Bond, Katherine C., Valente, Thomas A. and Kendall, Carl "Social network influences on reproductive behaviors in northern Thailand" *Social Science and Medicine* 49 (1999) pp. 1599–1614.

[27] See Dever, G.E.Alan, *Community Health Analysis*, Gaithersburg, MD: Aspen, 1991 for a discussion of these methods and indicators.

[28] Kanani, Shubhada J. "Application of rapid assessment procedures in the context of women's morbidity" in *Rapid Assessment Procedures: Qualitative Methodologies for Planning and Evaluation of Health Related Programmes* Scrimshaw, Nevin S. and Gleason, Gary r. (eds) Boston: International Nutrition Foundation for Developing Countries, 1992.

[29] Shah, Meera Kaul, op. cit.

[30] Shah, Meera kaul and Nkhama, Gladys "Listening to young voices: Participatory appraisal on adolescent health sexual and reproductive health in peri-urban Lusaka", CARE, 1996.

[31] This process is an adaptation and application of that developed in Kretzmann, John P. and McKnight, John L. *Building Communities from the Inside Out: A Path Toward Finding and Mobilizing a Community's Assets*, Chicago: ACTA Publications, 1993.

[32] Chiwuzie, J., Okojie, O., Okolocho, C, Omorogbe, S., Oronsaye, A., Akpala, W., Ande, B., Onoguwe, B., Oikeh, E. "Emergency loan funds to improve access to obstetric care in Ekpoma, Nigeria" *International Journal of Gynecology and Obstetrics* 59 Suppl. 2 (1997) S259–S265, p. S231–S236.

[33] Essien, E., Ifenne, D., Sabitu, K., Musa, A., Alti-Mu'azu, M., Adidu, V., Golji., N., Muladdus, M. "Community loan funds and transport services for obstetric emergencies in northern Nigeria" *International Journal of Gynecology and Obstetrics* 59 Suppl. 2 (1997) S259–S265, pp. S237–S234.

[34] Source: World Health Organization *World Health Report 2000*, Geneva, 2000, Annex Table 8.

[35] Adapted from Stinson, Wayne *Community Financing of Primary Health Care* Washington, D.C.: American Public Health Association, 1982.

[36] Adapted from Wolff, James A., Suttenfield, Linda J. and Binzen, Susanna, C. (editors) *The Family Planing Manager's Handbook* West Hartford, CT., Kumarian Press, 1991.

[37] See Middleberg, Maurice I. *Assessing Management Capacity Among Non-Governmental Organizations*, CARE, July 1993; Fisher, Andrew, et. al. *Guidelines and Instruments for a Family Planning Situation Analysis* New York: Population Council, 1992; Paul, Samuel *Institutional Development in World Bank Projects: A Cross-Sectoral Review*, World Bank, April 1990 (WPS392).

NOTES FOR CHAPTER 5

[1] World Bank *The Minimum Package of Health Services* (World Bank web site, February 10, 2000).

[2] Heise, L., Ellsberg, M. and Gottemoeller, M. "Ending Violence Against Women" *Population Reports*, Series L, No. 11. Baltimore, Johns Hopkins University School of Public Health, Population Information Program, December 1999.

[1] Mensch, Barbara; Fisher, Andrew; Askew, Ian and Ayorinde Ajayi "Using situation analysis data to assess the functioning of family planning clinics in Nigeria, Tanzania and Zmbabwe" *Studies in Family Planning* Vol. 25, #1 (Jan.–Feb., 199), pp. 18–31.

[2] Lynam, Pamela; Rabinovitz,, Lleslie McNeil and Shobowale, Mofoluka "Using self-assessment to improve the quality of family planning services" *Studies in Family Planning* Vol. 24, #4 (Jul.–Aug., 1993), pp. 252–260.

3. Ayuku, D.; Bentley, M.; Egessa, O.; Maman, S.; Sweat, M.; Moss, W.; Nyarang'o, P.; Chemati, A.; and Halsey, N. "Factors that facilitate and impede STD control in Western Kenya" paper presented at 1996 International Conference on AIDS.
4. U.S. Agency for International Development, Office of Population *PROFIT Project Compendium*, Washington, D.C., n.d.
5. Sheon, Amy, Schellstede, William and Derr, Bonnie "Contraceptive social marketing" in *Organizing for Effective Family Planning Programs*, Robert J. Lapham and George Simmons, eds., Washington, D.C.: National Academy Press, 1987.
6. See Bruce, Judith "Fundamental elements of the quality of care: A simple framework", *Studies in Family Planning* 21(2): 61–91. Mar./Apr. 1990.
7. World Health Organization *Mother-Baby Package*, Geneva: 1998, p. 66.
8. Dallabetta, Gina and Hassig, Susan *Indicators for Reproductive Health Program Evaluation: Final Report of the Subcommittee on STD/HIV* Chapel Hill, NC: Carolina Population Center, 1995, pp. 70–72.
9. The discussion of technical competence draws on Huezo, C.M. and Diaz, S. "Quality of care in family planning: Clients' right and provider needs" in Senanyake P. and Kleinman, R.L. *The Proceedings of the IPPF Family Planning Congress, New Delhi, October 1992*, Pearl River, New York; Parthenon Publishing Group, 1993, pp. 235–244.
10. See Kols, Adrienne J. and Sherman, Jill E. "Family planning programs: Improving quality" *Population Reports* Series J, No. 47, Baltimore, Johns Jopins University School of Public Health, Population Information Program, November 1998 for a summary of research on client expectations.
11. Source: CARE-Bangladesh *Building Capacity of NGOS for Family Planning Activity*, Dhaka: CARE-Bangladesh, May 1999.
12. Couple–year of protection is a measure of the magnitude of contraceptive commodities and services provided; e.g., the distribution of 15 cycles of oral contraceptives is recorded as one couple-year of protection. A conversion factor exists for every contraceptive method.

NOTES FOR CHAPTER 6

1. Key references used for the section on contraceptive technology are: Hatcher, Robert A., James Trussell, Felicia Stewart, Willard Cates, Jr., Gary K. Stewart, Felicia Guest and Deborah Kowal *Contraceptive Technology* New York: Ardent Media, 1998; Centers for Disease Control and Prevention *Family Planning Methods and Practice: Africa* 2nd edition, Atlanta: Centers for Disease Control and Prevention, National Center for Chronic Disease Prevention, Division of Reproductive Health, 1999; Hatcher, Robert A, Ward Rinehart, Richard Blackburn, Judith S. Geller and James D. Shelton *The Essentials of Contraceptive Technology* Baltimore: Johns Hopkins University, School of Public Health, Population Information Program, 1997; JHPIEGO *Pocket-Guide for Family Planning Service Providers. 1996–1998, Second Edition* March, 2000 (web site: www.reproline.jhu.edu/english/6read/6multi/pg/index.htm#Preface); JHPIEGO *Service Delivery Guidelines* March, 2000 (web site: www.reproline.jhu.edu/english/6read/6multi/sdg/index.htm).
2. Source: Trussell, James and Kowal, Deborah "The Essentials of Contraception: Efficacy, Safety and Personal Considerations" in Hatcher, Robert A, et. al. *Contraceptive Technology*, op. cit., p. 230.
3. Kowal, Deborah "Abstinence and the Range of Sexual Expression" in Hatcher, Robert A, et. al. *Contraceptive Technology*, op. cit., pp. 297–301.
4. Centers for Disease Control and Prevention *Family Planning Methods and Practice: Africa*, op. cit., pp. 499–505.
5. Hatcher, Robert A, Ward Rinehart, Richard Blackburn, Judith S. Geller and James D. Shelton *The Essentials of Contraceptive Technology* op. cit., pp. 14-1–14-18.
6. Adapted from Kowal, Deborah "Abstinence and the Range of Sexual Expression" in Hatcher, Robert A, et. al. *Contraceptive Technology*, op. cit., p. 301.
7. Kowal, Deborah "Coitus Interruptus (Withdrawal)" in Hatcher, Robert A, et. al. *Contraceptive Technology*, op. cit. pp. 303–307.
8. Centers for Disease Control and Prevention *Family Planning Methods and Practice: Africa*, op. cit., pp. 491–497.
9. Hatcher, Robert A, Ward Rinehart, Richard Blackburn, Judith S. Geller and James D. Shelton *The Essentials of Contraceptive Technology* op. cit., pp. 14-1–14-18.
10. Jennings, Victoria H., Lamprecht, Virginia M., and Kowal, Deborah "Fertility Awareness Methods" in Hatcher, Robert A, et. al. *Contraceptive Technology*, op. cit., pp. 297–302.

[11] Centers for Disease Control and Prevention *Family Planning Methods and Practice: Africa*, op. cit., pp. 471–490.
[12] Hatcher, Robert A, Ward Rinehart, Richard Blackburn, Judith S. Geller and James D. Shelton *The Essentials of Contraceptive Technology* op. cit., pp. 14-1–14-18.
[13] Warner, D. Lee and Hatcher, Robert A. "Male Condoms" in Hatcher, Robert A, et. al. *Contraceptive Technology*, op. cit., pp. 325–355.
[14] Centers for Disease Control and Prevention *Family Planning Methods and Practice: Africa*, op. cit., pp. 429–442.
[15] Hatcher, Robert A, Ward Rinehart, Richard Blackburn, Judith S. Geller and James D. Shelton *The Essentials of Contraceptive Technology* op. cit., pp. 11-1–11-18.
[16] Cates, Jr., Willard and Raymond, Elizabeth G. "Vaginal Spermicides" in Hatcher, Robert A, et. al. *Contraceptive Technology*, op. cit., pp. 357–369.
[17] Stewart, Felicia "Vaginal Barriers" in Hatcher, Robert A, et. al. *Contraceptive Technology*, op. cit., pp. 371–404.
[18] Hatcher, Robert A, Ward Rinehart, Richard Blackburn, Judith S. Geller and James D. Shelton *The Essentials of Contraceptive Technology* op. cit., pp. 13-1–13-19.
[19] Source: Stewart, Felicia "Vaginal Barriers" in Hatcher, Robert A, et. al. *Contraceptive Technology*, op. cit., p. 377.
[20] Hatcher, Robert A. and John Guillebaud "The Pill: Combined Oral Contraceptives" in Hatcher, Robert A, et. al. *Contraceptive Technology*, op. cit., pp. 405–466.
[21] Centers for Disease Control and Prevention *Family Planning Methods and Practice: Africa*, op. cit., pp. 295–339.
[22] Hatcher, Robert A, Ward Rinehart, Richard Blackburn, Judith S. Geller and James D. Shelton *The Essentials of Contraceptive Technology* op. cit., pp. 5-1–5-28.
[23] Van Look, Paul F.A. and Stewart, Felicia "Emergency Contraception" in Hatcher, Robert A, et. al. *Contraceptive Technology*, op. cit., pp. 277–295.
[24] Taken from Hatcher, Robert A. and John Guillebaud "The Pill: Combined Oral Contraceptives" in Hatcher, Robert A, et. al. *Contraceptive Technology*, op. cit., p. 457.
[25] Hatcher, Robert A. "Depo-Provera, Norplant and Progestin-Only Pills (Minipills)" in in Hatcher, Robert A, et. al. *Contraceptive Technology*, op. cit., pp. 467–509.
[26] Centers for Disease Control and Prevention *Family Planning Methods and Practice: Africa*, op. cit., pp. 341–386.
[27] Hatcher, Robert A, Ward Rinehart, Richard Blackburn, Judith S. Geller and James D. Shelton *The Essentials of Contraceptive Technology* op. cit., pp. 6-1–6-18.
[28] Hatcher, Robert A. "Depo-Provera, Norplant and Progestin-Only Pills (Minipills)" in Hatcher, Robert A, et. al. *Contraceptive Technology*, op. cit., pp. 467–509.
[29] Centers for Disease Control and Prevention *Family Planning Methods and Practice: Africa*, op. cit., pp. 341–386.
[30] Hatcher, Robert A, Ward Rinehart, Richard Blackburn, Judith S. Geller and James D. Shelton *The Essentials of Contraceptive Technology* op. cit., pp. 7-1–7-21.
[31] Sivin, Irving, Nash, Harold and Waldman, Sandra *Jadelle® Levonorgestrel Rod Implants: A Summary of Scientific Data and Lessons Learned from Programmatic Experience* New York: Population Council, 2002.
[32] Hatcher, Robert A. "Depo-Provera, Norplant and Progestin-Only Pills (Minipills)" in Hatcher, Robert A, et. al. *Contraceptive Technology*, op. cit., pp. 467–509.
[33] Centers for Disease Control and Prevention *Family Planning Methods and Practice: Africa*, op. cit., pp. 341–386.
[34] Hatcher, Robert A, Ward Rinehart, Richard Blackburn, Judith S. Geller and James D. Shelton *The Essentials of Contraceptive Technology* op. cit., pp. 8-1–8-24.
[35] Stewart, Gary K. "Intrauterine Devices (IUD)" in Hatcher, Robert A, et. al. *Contraceptive Technology*, op. cit., pp. 511–543.
[36] Centers for Disease Control and Prevention *Family Planning Methods and Practice: Africa*, op. cit., pp. 387–428.
[37] Hatcher, Robert A, Ward Rinehart, Richard Blackburn, Judith S. Geller and James D. Shelton *The Essentials of Contraceptive Technology* op. cit., pp. 12-1–12-28.
[38] Stewart, Gary K. and Carignan, Charles S. "Female and Male Sterilization" in Hatcher, Robert A, et. al. *Contraceptive Technology*, op. cit., pp. 545–588.
[39] Centers for Disease Control and Prevention *Family Planning Methods and Practice: Africa*, op. cit., pp. 507–546.
[40] Hatcher, Robert A, Ward Rinehart, Richard Blackburn, Judith S. Geller and James D. Shelton *The Essentials of Contraceptive Technology* op. cit., pp. 9-1–9-23.
[41] Peterson H.B.; Xia Z.; Hughes J.M.; Wilcox L.S.; Tylor L.R.; Trussell J.; Grimes D.A.; Hammond C.B.; Gibbs R.S.; Rosenfield A.; Soper D.P. "The risk of pregnancy after tubal sterilization: findings from the U.S. collaborative review of sterilization" *American Journal of Obstetrics and Gynecology* Volume 174, Issue 4 1996 p. 1161–1170.
[42] Stewart, Gary K. and Carignan, Charles S. "Female and Male Sterilization" in Hatcher, Robert A, et. al. *Contraceptive Technology*, op. cit., pp. 545–588.

[43] Centers for Disease Control and Prevention *Family Planning Methods and Practice: Africa*, op. cit., pp. 507–546.

[44] Hatcher, Robert A, Ward Rinehart, Richard Blackburn, Judith S. Geller and James D. Shelton *The Essentials of Contraceptive Technology* op. cit., pp. 10-1–10-19.

NOTES TO CHAPTER 7

[1] Source: May, Katharyn A. and Laura R. Mahlmeister *Maternal and Neonatal Nursing: Family Centered Care* 3rd Edition, Philadelphia: J.P. Lippincott, 1994.

[2] ibid.

[3] Yuster, E.A., "Rethinking the role of the risk approach and antenatal care in maternal mortality reduction" *International Journal of Gynecology and Obstetrics* 50 Suppl. 2 (1995) S59–S61.

[4] McDonagh, Marilyn "Is antenatal care effective in reducing maternal mortality?" *Health Policy and Planning* 11 (1): 1–15 (1996).

[5] De Brouwere, Vincent, Tonglet, Rene and Van Leberghe, Win "Strategies for reducing maternal mortality in developing countries: what can we learn from the history of the industrialized West?" *Tropical Medicine and International Health* Volume 3 No. 10 pp. 771–782, October 1998.

[6] Maine, Deborah, Ward, Victoria and ElTahir, Abdel *Meeting the community half way: Programmatic guidelines for the reduction of maternal mortality* New York, UNICEF, December 1993.

[7] Maine, Deborah, McCarthy, James and Ward, Victoria, M. *Guidelines for monitoring progress in the reduction of maternal mortality* New York, UNICEF, 1992.

[8] Sources: World Health Organization, *Mother-Baby Package: Implementing safe motherhood in developing countries* Geneva, 1998; Ross, Susan Rae *Promoting Quality Maternal and Newborn Care: A Reference Manual for Program Managers* Atlanta: CARE, 1999; Neuberg, Roger *Obstetrics: A Practical Manual* Oxford, Oxford University Press, 1995; May and Mahlmeister, op. cit.

[9] World Health Organization *Antenatal Care: Report of a Technical Working Group* Geneva, 31 October–4 November 1994.

[10] Sources for this section are May and Mahlmeister, op. cit., pp. 341–387; Neuberg, op. cit., pp. 55–114; Ross, op. cit., pp. 5-29–5-52 ; WHO *Mother–Baby Package*, op. cit., pp. 33–50; WHO *Antenatal Care*, op. cit., pp. 19–23.

[11] Estimates of the proportion of pregnancies ending in spontaneous abortion vary widely.

[12] Centers for Disease Control *Global AIDS Program: Strategies* web site http://www.cdc.gov/nchstp/od/gap/strategies/1_overview.htm.

[13] Schultz, Linda J., Steketee, Richard W., Chitsulo, Lester, Macheso, Alan, Kazembe, Peter and Wirima, Jack J. "Evaluation of maternal practices, efficacy and cost-effectiveness of alternative antimalarial regimens for use in pregnancy: chloroquine and sulfadoxine-pyremethamine" Supplement to *The American Journal of Tropical Medicine & Hygiene* Vol. 55, No. 1, pp. 87–94.

[14] Source: Stolzfus, Rebecca J and Michele L. Dreyfuss *Guidelines for the Use of Iron Supplementation to Prevent and Treat Iron Deficiency Anemia* Washington, D.C.: ILSI Press, 1998.

[15] May and Mahlmeister, op. cit., p. 391.

[16] Taken from May and Mahlmestier, op. cit., p. 406.

[17] Ross, op. cit., p. 2.7.

[18] Ross, Susan Rae, op. cit., p. 5.45.

[19] Ramakrishnan, Usha, Renu Majrekar, Juan Rivera, Teresa Gonzales-Gossio and Reynaldo Martorell "Micronutrients and pregnancy outcome: A review of the literature" *Nutrition Research*, Vol. 19, No. 1, pp. 103–159, 1999.

[20] ibid.

[21] May and Mahlmeister, op. cit., p. 392.

[22] Ramakrishnan, Usha, et. al., op. cit.

[23] Koblinsky, M.A. "Beyond maternal mortality – magnitude, interrelationship and consequences of women's health, pregnancy-related complications and nutritional status on pregnancy outcomes *International Journal of Gynecology and Obstetrics* 48 Suppl. (1995) s21–s32.

[24] Stolzfus, Rebecca J and Michele L. Dreyfuss *Guidelines for the Use of Iron Supplementation to Prevent and Treat Iron Deficiency Anemia* Washington, D.C.: ILSI Press, 1998.

[25] West, Keith P. Jr., et. al. "Double blind, cluster randomised trial of low dose supplementation with Vitamin A or beta-carotene on mortality related to pregnancy in Nepal" *British Medical Journal* Volume 318 (7183) 27 February 1999, pp. 570–575.

[26] International Vitamin A Consultative Group *IVACG Statement: Safe Uses of Vitamin A During Pregnancy and Lactation*, 1998.

[27] Maberly, Glenn "Iodine deficiency" *Bulletin of the World Health Organization* 76 Suppl 2:118–120, 1998.

[28] Maberly, Glenn F. "Iodine deficiency disorders: contemporary scientific issues" *Journal of Nutrition* 124 (8 Suppl): 1473S–1478S, 1994 Aug.

[29] Ramakrishnan, Usha, et. al., op. cit.

[30] ibid.

[31] May and Mahlmeister, op. cit., p. 394.

[32] ibid.,

[33] Ramakrishnan, Usha, et. al., op. cit.

[34] ibid.

[35] May and Mahlmeister, op. cit., p. 393.

[36] Ramakrishnan, Usha, et. al., op. cit.

[37] ibid.

[38] Source: National Academy of Sciences *Recommended Dietary Allowances, 10th edition* Washington, 1989.

[39] Sources for this section are May and Mahlmeister, op. cit., pp. 415–597; Marshall, Margaret Ann and Sandra Tebben Buffington *Life Saving Skills Manual for Midwives* Washington, D.C.: American College of Nurse-Midwives, 1991; Neuberg, op. cit., pp. 138–231; Ross, op. cit., pp. 5.52–5.67; World Health Organization *Care in Normal Birth: Report of a Technical Working Group* Geneva, 1999; WHO *Mother-Baby Package*, op. cit.

[40] Some authors refer to a fourth stage of labor, which includes the immediate post-partum period; see, for example, May and Mahlmeister, Chapters 19 and 21, op. cit.

[41] Wold Health Organization *Care in Normal Birth*, op. cit.

[42] May and Mahlmeister, op. cit., pp. 661–725; Marshall, and Buffington, op. cit.; Neuberg, op. cit., pp. 143–149, 186–223; Ross, op. cit., pp. 5.58–5.67; WHO *Mother-Baby Package*, op. cit.

[43] There is an alternative procedure for use in emergencies under conditions where a Cesarean section is impossible. This procedure is known as a symphisiotomy and involves cutting through the symphisis (public bone) in order to allow passage of the fetus.

[44] Sources: May and Mahlmeister, op. cit., pp. 781–875; Neuberg, op. cit., pp. 158–159, 225–231, 250–259; Ross, op. cit., pp. 5.67–5.74.

[45] Ross, op. cit., p. 5.68; American College of Nurse-Midwives *Healthy Mother and Healthy Newborn Care: A Guide for Caregivers* Washington, D.C.: ACNM, 1998.

[46] Ross, Susan Rae, op. cit., p. 5.69.

[47] Sources: May and Mahlmeister, op. cit., pp. 837–875; Marshall, and Buffington, op. cit.; Neuberg, op. cit., pp. 225–231, 250–259; Ross, op. cit., pp. 5.72–5.74.

[48] Ross, op. cit, following WHO, suggests as a criterion "soaking one pad/cloth every hour in the first 8 hours, soaking 1 pad/cloth every 2 hours in the second 8 hours." Burns, et. al., op. cit, suggests "more than two cupfuls" or "enough to soak through 2 thick rags in an hour" immediately after birth or soaking "more than one thick rag an hour after the first day."

[49] Sources: Cates, Willard and Charlotte Ellerston, "Abortion" In Hatcher, et. al., *Contraceptive Technology*, op. citi, pp. 679–700; Winkler, Judith, Paul D. Blumenthal and Forrest C. Greenslade "Early Abortion Services: New Choices for Providers and Women" *Advances in Abortion Care*, Volume 5, No. 2; Ewart, Wendy R. and Beverly Winikoff "Towards Safe and Effective Medical Abortion" *Science* Volume 281 (5376), 24 July 1998, pp. 520–521; Population Council *Medical Methods of Early Abortion in Developing Countries: Consensus Statement*, 1998.

[50] Sources: Cates and Ellertson, op. cit., p. 697; World Health Organization *Post abortion family planning: A practical guide for managers* Geneva: World Health Organization, 1997.

[51] Source: Ross, op. cit., p. 1.11.

[52] ibid.

[53] ibid.

[54] Werner, David *Where There is No Doctor*, Palo Alto, California: Hesperian Foundation, 1992, p. 184.

[55] Centers for Disease Control and Prevention *1998 Guidelines for the Treatment of Sexually Transmitted Diseases* MMWR 1998; 47 (No. RR-1), p. 67.

[56] World Health Organization and UNICEF *Management of Childhood Illnesses*, p. 22.
[57] Ross, op. cit., p. 5.90.
[58] World Health Organization and UNICEF *Management of Childhood Illnesses*, p. 26.
[59] Werner, David *Where There is No Doctor,* Palo Alto, California: Hesperian Foundation, 1992, p. 185.
[60] ibid., p. 275.

NOTES TO CHAPTER 8

[1] Source: Centers for Disease Control and Prevention *1998 Guidelines for the Treatment of Sexually Transmitted Diseases* MMWR 1998; 47 (No. RR-1).
[2] Chart is adapted from Holmes, King K. and Ryan, Caroline, A. "STD Care Management" in *Sexually Transmitted Diseases, Third Edition*, Holmes, King K., et. al. editors, op. cit., p. 658.
[3] For a discussion of STD drugs and their management, see Brasseur, Olivier, Allan Ronald and Peter Piot "STD Drugs" in Dallabetta, Gina, Marie Laga and Peter Humphrey (editors) *Control of Sexually Transmitted Diseases*, Family Health International, n.d.
[4] Centers for Disease Control and Prevention *Global AIDS Program Technical Strategies*.
[5] Oberzaucher, Nicola and Baggaley *HIV Voluntary Counselling and Testing: A gateway to prevention and care* UNAIDS, 2002.
[6] The Voluntary HIV-1 Counseling and Testing Efficacy Study Group "Efficacy of voluntary HIV-1 counselling and testing in individuals and couples in Kenya, Tanzania, and Trinidad: a randomised trial" *Lancet* 356 (9224): 103–112, 8 July 2000.
[7] Michael Sweat, Steven Gregorich, Gloria Sangiwa, Colin Furlonge, Donald Balmer, Claudes Kamenga, Olga Grinstead, Thomas Coates "Cost-effectiveness of voluntary HIV-1 counselling and testing in reducing sexual transmission of HIV-1 in Kenya and Tanzania" *Lancet* 356 (9224): 113–121, 8 July 2000.
[8] Philippe Van de Perre "HIV voluntary counselling and testing in community health services" *Lancet* 356 (9224): 113–121, 8 July 2000.
[9] Wolitski RJ, MacGowan RJ, Higgins DL, Jorgensen CM. "The effects of HIV counseling and testing on risk-related practices and help-seeking behavior" *AIDS Educ Prev* 1997; 9 (suppl): 5267.
[10] Limpakarnjanarat, Khanchit. Mastro, Timothy D. Saisorn, Supachai. Uthaivoravit, Wat. Kaewkungwal, Jaranit. Korattana, Supaporn. Young, Nancy L. Morse, Stephen A. Schmid, D Scott. Weniger, Bruce G. Nieburg, Phillip. "HIV-1 and other sexually transmitted infections in a cohort of female sex workers in Chiang Rai, Thailand." *Sexually Transmitted Infections*. 75(1):30–35, February 1999.
[11] Steen, Richard PA, MPH; Vuylsteke, Bea MD, MSC ; Decoito, Tony MD; Ralepeli, Stori SPN; Fehler, Glenda MSC; Conley, Jacci BA; Bruckers, Liesbeth MSC ; Dallabetta, Gina MD; Ballard, Ron Mibiol, Ph.D. "Evidence of Declining STD Prevalence in a South African Mining Community Following a Core-Group Intervention" *Sexually Transmitted Diseases* 27(1):1–8, January 2000.
[12] CARE-Togo, for example, implemented a program aimed at educating truck and taxi drivers about HIV and STD, as well as promoting condom use.
[13] Mwakagile, D., Mmari, E., Makwaya, C., Mbwana, J., Biberfeld, G., Mhalu, F. Sandstrom, E. "Sexual behaviour among youths at high risk for HIV-1 infection in Dar es Salaam, Tanzania" *Sexually Transmitted Infections* 77(4):255–259, August 2001.
[14] Rekart, M L. "Sex in the city: sexual behaviour, societal change, and STDs in Saigon" *Sexually Transmitted Infections* 78 Supplement 1:i47–i54, April 2002.
[15] Wilson, David. Cawthorne, Paul. "'Face up to the truth': helping gay men in Vietnam protect themselves from AIDS" *International Journal of STD & AIDS* 10(1):63–66, January 1999; CARE-Bolivia also ran a program targeting gay men in Tarija, Bolivia.
[16] Adapted from Curtis, J. Randall and King K. Holmes "Individual-Level Risk Assessment for STD/HIV Infection" in *Sexually Transmitted Diseases, Third Edition*, Holmes, King K., et. al. editors, op. cit., pp. 669–683.
[17] Mayaud, Philippe. Uledi, Elizabeth. Cornelissen, Jan. ka-Gina, Gina. Todd, James. Rwakatare, Medard. West, Beryl. Kopwe, Lilian. Manoko, Domitilia. Grosskurth, Heiner. Hayes, Richard. Mabey, David. "Risk scores to detect cervical infections in urban antenatal clinic attenders in Mwanza, Tanzania" *Sexually Transmitted Infections* 74(1S) Supplement 1:139S–146S, June 1998.

[18] Toomey, Kathleen E., Ahmed S. Latif and Richard C. Steen "Partner Management" in *Control of Sexually Transmitted Diseases*, Dallabetta, Gina et. al., op. cit., 211–224.

[19] Rothenberg, Richard B and John J. Potterat "Partner Notification for Sexually Transmitted Diseases and HIV Infection" in *Sexually Transmitted Diseases, Third Edition*, Holmes, King K., et. al. editors, op. cit., pp. 745–752.

[20] Steen, Richard PA, MPH. and Dallabetta, Gina MD, "The Use of Epidemiologic Mass Treatment and Syndrome Management for Sexually Transmitted Disease Control" *Sexually Transmitted Diseases*. 26(4) Supplement:S12–S20, April 1999.

[21] These criteria are taken from Tam, Milton R. "Laboratory Diagnosis of Sexually Transmitted Diseases in Resource Poor Settings" in *Sexually Transmitted Diseases, Third Edition*, Holmes, King K., et. al. editors, op. cit., p. 1410.

[22] See World Health Organization *Management of Patients with Sexually Transmitted Diseases: Report of a WHO Study Group*, WHO Technical Report Series #810, Geneva, 1991, Annex 1.

[23] ibid., adapted from pages 72–73.

[24] Centers for Disease Control and Prevention *1998 Guidelines for the Treatment of Sexually Transmitted Diseases* MMWR 1998; 47 (No. RR-1).

[25] WHO *Management of Patients with Sexually Transmitted Diseases*, op. cit.

[26] Vuylsteke, Bea and Marie Laga "Approach to Management of STDs in Developing Countries" in *Sexually Transmitted Diseases, Third Edition*, Holmes, King K., et. al. editors, op. cit., pp. 1399–1409.

[27] WHO *Management of Patients with Sexually Transmitted Diseases*, op. cit., p. 14.

[28] Holmes and Ryan, op. cit.

[29] Vuylsteke, Bea and Mehelus, Andre "STD Syndrome Management" in *Control of Sexually Transmitted Diseases*, Dallabetta, Gina et. al., op. cit., p. 157.

[30] *Control of Sexually Transmitted Diseases*, Dallabetta, Gina et. al., op. cit., p. 166.

[31] Steen, Richard PA, MPH. and Dallabetta, Gina MD, "The Use of Epidemiologic Mass Treatment and Syndrome Management for Sexually Transmitted Disease Control" *Sexually Transmitted Diseases*. 26(4) Supplement: S12–S20, April 1999.

[32] Grosskurth H., Gray R., Hayes R., Mabey D., Wawer M. "Control of sexually transmitted diseases for HIV-1 prevention: understanding the implications of the Mwanza and Rakai trials" *Lancet* 355(9219):1981–1987, 2000 Jun 3.

[33] Stamm WE., Handsfield HH., Rompalo AM., Ashley RL., Roberts PL., Corey L. "The association between genital ulcer disease and acquisition of HIV infection in homosexual men" *JAMA*. 260(10):1429–1433, 1988 Sep 9.

[34] Cameron DW., Simonsen JN., D'Costa LJ., Ronald AR., Maitha GM., Gakinya MN., Cheang M. Ndinya-Achola JO., Piot P., Brunham RC. "Female to male transmission of human immunodeficiency virus type 1: risk factors for seroconversion in men" *Lancet*. 2(8660):403–407, 1989 Aug 19.

[35] Plummer FA., Simonsen JN., Cameron DW., Ndinya-Achola JO., Kreiss JK., Gakinya MN., Waiyaki P., Cheang M., Piot P., Ronald AR. "Cofactors in male–female sexual transmission of human immunodeficiency virus type 1" *Journal of Infectious Diseases*. 163(2):233–239, 1991 Feb.

[36] Laga M., Manoka A., Kivuvu M., Malele B., Tuliza M., Nzila N., Goeman J., Behets F., Batter V., Alary M. "Non-ulcerative sexually transmitted diseases as risk factors for HIV-1 transmission in women: results from a cohort study" *AIDS*. 7(1):95–102, 1993 Jan.

[37] Cohen MS., Hoffman IF., Royce RA., Kazembe P., Dyer JR., Daly CC., Zimba D., Vernazza PL., Maida M., Fiscus SA., Eron JJ Jr. "Reduction of concentration of HIV-1 in semen after treatment of urethritis: implications for prevention of sexual transmission of HIV-1" AIDSCAP Malawi Research Group. *Lancet* 349(9069):1868–1873, 1997 Jun 28.

[38] Ghys PD., Fransen K., Diallo MO., Ettiegne-Traore V., Coulibaly IM., Yeboue KM., Kalish ML., Maurice C., Whitaker JP., Greenberg AE., Laga M. "The associations between cervicovaginal HIV shedding, sexually transmitted diseases and immunosuppression in female sex workers in Abidjan, Cote d'Ivoire" *AIDS* 11(12): F85–93, 1997 Oct.

[39] Grosskurth H., Mosha F., Todd J., Mwijarubi E., Klokke A., Senkoro K., Mayaud P., Changalucha J., Nicoll A., ka-Gina G. "Impact of improved treatment of sexually transmitted diseases on HIV infection in rural Tanzania: randomised controlled trial" *Lancet* 346(8974):530–536, 1995 Aug 26.

[40] Wawer MJ. Sewankambo NK., Serwadda D., Quinn TC., Paxton LA., Kiwanuka N., Wabwire-Mangen F., Li C., Lutalo T., Nalugoda F., Gaydos CA., Moulton LH., Meehan MO., Ahmed S., Gray RH. "Control of sexually transmitted diseases for AIDS prevention in Uganda: a randomised community trial" *Lancet* 353(9152): 525–535, 1999 Feb 13.

[41] Grosskurth H., Gray R., Hayes R., Mabey D., Wawer M. "Control of sexually transmitted diseases for HIV-1 prevention: understanding the implications of the Mwanza and Rakai trials" *Lancet* 355(9219):1981–1987, 2000 Jun 3.

[42] Sources for this section include World Bank *Confronting AIDS: Public Priorities in a Global Epidemic* New York: Oxford University Press, 1997 (especially chapter 4) and De Cock, Kevin and Elly T. Katabira "Approach to the management of HIV/AIDS in developing countries" in *Sexually Transmitted Diseases, Third Edition*, Holmes, King K., et. al. editors, op. cit., pp. 1391–1397.

[43] Source: World Bank *World Development Indicators 2000* (web site) Table 2.14.

[44] Adapted from Greenberg Judith and Peggy Clarke "Support groups for people with HIV, HPV and HSV infections" in *Sexually Transmitted Diseases, Third Edition*, Holmes, King K., et. al. editors, op. cit., pp. 753–759.

[45] See O'Malley, Jeffrey, Vinh Kim Nguyen and Sarah Lee "Non-governmental organizations" in Mann and Tarantola, *AIDS in the World II*, op. cit., pp. 341–361 for a good discussion of the role and dynamics of NGOs.

[46] *Confronting AIDS* op. cit., pp. 176–177.

[47] De Cock and Katabira, op. cit., p. 1393.

[48] Adapted from De Cock and Katabira, op. cit., p. 1395.

[49] Karon, John M. PhD; Fleming, Patricia L. PhD; Steketee, Richard W. MD; De Cock, Kevin M. MD "HIV in the United States at the Turn of the Century: An Epidemic in Transition" *American Journal of Public Health* 2001; 91:1060–1068.

[50] Centers for Disease Control and Prevention HIV Mortality: L285 Slide Series (through 2000).

[51] Medecins dans Frontieres *Untangling the Web of Price Reductions: A pricing guide for the purchase of ARVs for developing countries, 2nd edition* Geneva: June 2002.

[52] ibid.

[53] McGreevy William, Berozzi, Stefano and Izazola, Jose-Antonio "Current and Future Resources for HIV/AIDS" in *State of the Art: AIDS and Economics* Washington: The Futures Group, 2002.

[54] Sources for this section are Ward, Darrell E. *The AmFAR AIDS Handbook* London: W.W. Norton and Co., 1999; Eron, Joseph J and Hirsch, Martin "Antiviral Therapy of Human Immunodeficiency Virus Infection" in *Sexually Transmitted Diseases, Third Edition*, Holmes, King K., et. al. editors, op. cit., pp. 1009–1030; Panel on Clinical Practices for Treatment of HIV Infection *Guidelines for the Use of Antiretroviral Agents in HIV-Infected Adults and Adolescents* February 4, 2002 (Updated recommendations available at www.hivatis.org).

[55] Panel on Clinical Practices for Treatment of HIV Infection *Guidelines for the Use of Antiretroviral Agents in HIV-Infected Adults and Adolescents* February 4, 2002, p. 8.

[56] Paul Farmer, Fernet Léandre, Joia Mukherjee, Rajesh Gupta, Laura Tarter, & Jim Yong Kim "Community-based treatment of advanced HIV disease: introducing DOT-HAART (directly observed therapy with highly active antiretroviral therapy)" *Bulletin of the World Health Organization*, 2001, 79 (12) pp. 1145–1151.

[57] Watts, Heather D. and Robert C. Brunham "Sexually Transmitted Diseases, Including HIV Infection in Pregnancy" in *Sexually Transmitted Diseases, Third Edition*, Holmes, King K., et. al. editors, op. cit., pp. 1117–1118.

[58] Andiman, Warren A. MD. "Transmission of HIV-1 from mother to infant" *Current Opinion in Pediatrics* 14(1): 78–85, February 2002.

[59] Connor, Edward, M., Sperling RS. Gelber R. Kiselev P. Scott G. O'Sullivan MJ. VanDyke R. Bey M. Shearer W. Jacobson RL "Reduction Of Maternal-Infant Transmission Of Human Immunodeficiency Virus Type 1 With Zidovudine Treatment" *New England Journal of Medicine* 331:1173–1180, 1994.

[60] "Administration of Zidovudine During Late Pregnancy and Delivery to Prevent Perinatal Transmission—Thailand, 1996–1998, *Morbidity and Mortality Weekly Report* 1998; 47:151–154.

[61] Dabis, Francois, Msellati P. Meda N. Welffens-Ekra C. You B. Manigart O. Leroy V. Simonon A. Cartoux M. Combe P. Ouangre A. Ramon R. Ky-Zerbo O. Montcho C. Salamon R. Rouzioux C. Van de Perre P. Mandelbrot L. "6-month efficacy tolerance and acceptability of a short regimen of zidovudine to reduce verical transmission of HIV in breastfed children in Cote d'Ivoire and Burkina Faso: a double-blind placebo-controlled multicentre trial" *The Lancet* 353 (9155) pp. 786–792, 6 March 1999.

[62] Wiktor, Stefan, Ekpini E. Karon JM. Nkengasong J. Maurice C. Severin ST. Roels TH. Kouassi MK. Lackritz EM. Coulibaly IM. Greenberg AE. "Short course oral zidovudine for prevention of mother-to-child transmission of HIV-1 in Abidjan, Cote d'Ivoire: a randomised trial" *The Lancet* 353 (9155) pp. 781–785, 6 March 1999.

[63] Shaffer, Nathan; Chuachoowong, Rutt; Mock, Philip A; Bhadrakom, Chaiporn; Siriwasin, Wimol; Young, Nancy L; Chotpitayasunondh, Tawee; Chearskul, Sanay; Roongpisuthipong, Anuvat; Chinayon, Pratharn; Karon, John;

Mastro, Timothy D; Simonds, R J. "Short-course zidovudine for perinatal HIV-1 transmission in Bangkok, Thailand: a randomised controlled trial" *The Lancet* 353 (9155) pp. 773–780, 6 March 1999.

[64] Panel on Clinical Practices for Treatment of HIV Infection *Guidelines for the Use of Antiretroviral Agents in HIV-Infected Adults and Adolescents* February 4, 2002 (convened by the U.S. Department of Health and Human Services and the Henry J. Kaiser Family Foundation).

[65] Andiman, Warren A. MD. "Transmission of HIV-1 from mother to infant" *Current Opinion in Pediatrics* 14(1): 78–85, February 2002.

[66] Shaffer, Nathan; Chuachoowong, Rutt; Mock, Philip A; Bhadrakom, Chaiporn; Siriwasin, Wimol; Young, Nancy L; Chotpitayasunondh, Tawee; Chearskul, Sanay; Roongpisuthipong, Anuvat; Chinayon, Pratharn; Karon, John; Mastro, Timothy D; Simonds, R J. "Short-course zidovudine for perinatal HIV-1 transmission in Bangkok, Thailand: a randomised controlled trial" *The Lancet* 353 (9155) pp. 773–780, 6 March 1999.

[67] Guay, Laura A., Musoke, Philippa. Fleming, Thomas. Bagenda, Danstan. Allen, Melissa. Nakabiito, Clemensia. Sherman, Joseph. Bakaki, Paul. Ducar, Constance. Deseyve, Martina. Emel, Lynda. Mirochnick, Mark. Fowler, Mary Glenn. Mofenson, Lynne. Miotti, Paolo. Dransfield, Kevin. Bray, Dorothy. Mmiro, Francis. Jackson, J Brooks "Intrapartum and neonatal single-dose nevirapine compared with zidovudine for prevention of mother-to-child transmission of HIV-1 in Kampala, Uganda: HIVNET 012 randomised trial" *The Lancet* 354: pp. 795–802, 4 September 1999.

[68] Marseille, Elliot :Cost-effectiveness of single-dose nevirapine regimen for mothers and babies to decrease vertical HIV-1 transmission in sub-Saharan Africa" *The Lancet* 354: pp. 803–809, 4 September 1999.

[69] Leroy V. Karon JM. Alioum A. Ekpini ER. Meda N. Greenberg AE. Msellati P. Hudgens M. Dabis F. Wiktor SZ. West Africa PMTCT Study Group. "Twenty-four month efficacy of a maternal short-course zidovudine regimen to prevent mother-to-child transmission of HIV-1 in West Africa. [Clinical Trial. Journal Article. Randomized Controlled Trial" *AIDS*. 16(4):631–641, 2002 Mar 8.

[70] Le Coeur Sophie and Marc Lallemant "Breast-feeding and HIV/AIDS" in Mann & Tarantola *AIDS in the World II*, op. cit., p. 274.

[71] Nduati, Ruth, John G. Mbori-Ngacha D. Richardson B. Overbaugh J. Mwatha A. Ndinya-Achola J. Bwayo J. Onyango FE. Hughes J. Kreiss J "Effect of breastfeeding and formula feeding on transmission of HIV-1: A randomized clinical trial" *Journal of the American Medical Association* Vol. 238 (9), 1 March 2000, pp. 1167–1174.

[72] Radolf, Jusitn D., Pablo J. Sanchez, Kenneth F. Schulz and F. Kevin Murphy "Congenital Syphilis" in *Sexually Transmitted Diseases, Third Edition*, Holmes, King K., et. al. editors, op. cit., p. 1168.

[73] Recommended treatment regimens are taken from Temmerman, Marleen, Subash Hira and Marie Laga "STDs and Pregnancy" in *Control of Sexually Transmitted Diseases*, Dallabetta, Gina et. al., op. cit., pp. 174–175.

[74] *ibid* p. 178.

[75] Recommended treatment regimens are taken from Vuylsteke, Bea and Meheus, Andre "STD Syndrome Management" in *Control of Sexually Transmitted Diseases*, Dallabetta, Gina et. al., op. cit., p. 166.

[76] Temmerman, Marleen, Subash Hira and Marie Laga "STDs and Pregnancy" in *Control of Sexually Transmitted Diseases*, Dallabetta, Gina et. al., op. cit., p. 184.

[77] *ibid.*, p. 180.

[78] Centers for Disease Control and Prevention *1998 Guidelines for the Treatment of Sexually Transmitted Diseases*, op. cit., p. 67.

[79] ibid., p. 66.

[80] Temmerman, Marleen, Subash Hira and Marie Laga "STDs and Pregnancy" in *Control of Sexually Transmitted Diseases*, Dallabetta, Gina et. al., op. cit., p. 181.

[81] Centers for Disease Control and Prevention *1998 Guidelines for the Treatment of Sexually Transmitted Diseases*, op. cit., p. 57.

[82] *ibid.*, p. 56.

[83] *ibid.*, p. 57.

[84] *ibid.*, p. 58.

[85] Other sexually transmissible diseases, such as syphilis and hepatitis can also be transmitted via blood transfusion. This section focuses on HIV because of its unique gravity.

[86] Gibney, Laura, Choudhury P. Khawaja Z. Sarker M. Islam N. Vermund SH "HIV/AIDS in Bangladesh: An Assessment of Biomedical Risk Factors for Transmission" *International Journal of STD and AIDS* Vol 10 (5) May 1999, pp. 338–346.

[87] Foster, Susan "Benefits of HIV Screening of Blood Transfusions in Zambia" *The Lancet* Volume 346 (8969) 22 July 1995 pp. 225–227.

[88] Larkin, Marilynn "WHO's Blood-Safety Initiative: A Vain Effort?" *The Lancet* Volume 355 (9211) 8 April 2000 p. 1245.

[89] Foster, S., op. cit.

[90] Gibney, L., et. al., op. cit.

[91] Vos J., Gumodoka B. Ng'weshemi JZ. Kigadye FC. Dolmans WM. Borgdorff MW "Are some blood transfusions avoidable? A hospital record analysis in Mwanza Region Tanzania" *Tropical and Geographic Medicine* 45 (6): 301–303, 1993.

[92] Gumodoka B., Ng'weshemi JZ. Kigadye FC. Dolmans WM. Borgdorff MW "Blood transfusion practices in Mwanza Region, Tanzania" *AIDS* 7(3):387–392, March, 1993.

[93] Lackritz, E.M., Djommand G., Vetter KM, Zadi, F., Diaby L., DeCock KM "Beyond blood screening: reducing unnecessary transfusions and improving laboratory services in Cote d'Ivoire" *International Conference on AIDS* 9(1): 92 (abstract no. WS-C11-2), June 6–11, 1993.

[94] Source: WHO Programme on Blood Safety web site: www.who.int/pht/blood_safety/hivkits.html.

[95] Source: American Cancer Society Cervical Cancer Resource Center web site: *http://www.cancer.org/eprise/main/docroot/CRI/content/CRI242X* What are the risk factors for cervical cancer?

[96] Nazeer, S. "Cervical cancer control in developing countries: Memorandum from a WHO meeting" *Bulletin of the World Health Organization* 74 (4): 345–351.

[97] Source: American Cancer Society web site, 10/12/99.

[98] Murthy NS. Agarwal SS. Prabhakar AK. Sharma S. Das DK. "Estimation of reduction of life-time risk of cervical cancer through one life-time screening" *Neoplasma.* 40(4):255–258, 1993.

[99] ibid.

[100] Pengsaa P. Vatanasapt V. Sriamporn S. Sanchaisuriya P. Schelp FP. Noda S. Kato S. Kongdee W. Kanchanawirojkul N. Aranyasen O. "A self-administered device for cervical cancer screening in northeast Thailand" *Acta Cytologica*. 41(3):749–754, 1997 May–Jun.

[101] Thomas C. Wright, Jr, MD; Lynette Denny, MMED, FCOG; Louise Kuhn, PhD; Amy Pollack, MD; Attila Lorincz, PhD "HPV DNA Testing of Self-collected Vaginal Samples Compared With Cytologic Screening to Detect Cervical Cancer" *JAMA* 283 (1) January 5, 2000, p. 81.

[102] Megevand E. Denny L. Dehaeck K. Soeters R. Bloch B. "Acetic acid visualization of the cervix: an alternative to cytologic screening" *Obstetrics & Gynecology* 88(3):383–386, 1996 Sep.

[103] Richart, E.M. "Screening: the next century" *Cancer* 76 (10) Suppl. Pp. 1919–1927.

[104] Kols, Adrienne and Sherris, Jacqueline *HPV Vaccines: Promise and Challenges* Seattle: PATH, July 2000.

NOTES TO CHAPTER 9

[1] See Nichiporuk, Brian *The Security Dynamics of Demographic Factors*, Rand Corporation, MR-1088-WFHF/RF/DLPF/A, 2000 for a discussion of political power, security issues and population.

[2] Homer-Dixon, Thomas. "Environmental Scarcities and Violent Conflict: Evidence from Cases." *International Security*, vol. 19, no. 1 (Summer 1994) pp. 5–40.

[3] Coale, Ansley and Hoover, Edgar *Population Growth and Economic Development in Low Income Countries* Princeton, N.J.: Princeton University Press, 1958.

[4] Erlich, Paul R *The Population Bomb* Buccaneer Books, 1971.

[5] National Academy of Sciences *Rapid Population Growth: Consequences and Policy Implications* Baltimore: Johns Hopkins University Press, 1971.

[6] See Simon, Julian L. *Theory of Population and Economic Growth* Blackwell Publishers, 1986.

[7] Bulatao, Rodolfo A. *The Value of Family Planning Programs in Developing Countries* Santa Monica, RAND, 1998, pp. 9–20.

[8] World Bank *Population and Development: Implications for the World Bank* Washington: World Bank, 1994.

[9] Hesketh, T. and Zhu, WX "The one child family policy: the good, the bad, and the ugly" *British Medical Journal* 314 (7095): 1685–1687, 1997 June 7.

[10] Landman LC. "Birth control in India: the carrot and the rod?" *Family Planning Perspectives*, 9(3):101–110, 1977 May–Jun.

[11] See Sen, Gita; Germaine, Adrienne; and Lincoln C. Chen (eds.) Population *Policies Reconsidered: Health, Empowerment and Rights*, Cambridge: Harvard University Press, 1994 for a discussion of this perspective.

[12] UNFPA *Report of the International Conference on Population and Development* (Cairo 5–13 September 1994), section 7.3.

[13] See, for example, Musallam, Basim F. *Sex and Society in Islam : Birth control before the nineteenth century* Cambridge: Cambridge University Press, 1983; Feldman, David M. *Birth Control in Jewish Law* Northvale, New Jersey: Jason Aronson Inc., 1998; Sacred Congregation for the Doctrine of the Faith *Persona Humana: Declaration on Certain Questions Concerning Sexual Ethics* December 29, 1975.

[14] Sources for this section are Lindenberg, Marc and Crosby, Benjamin *Managing Development: The Political Dimension* Hartford, Connecticut: Kumarian Press, 1981 and Kingdon, John W. *Agendas, Alternatives and Public Policies* Boston: Little, Brown and Co., 1984.

References

BOOKS AND MONOGRAPHS

Aluwalia, Indu and Thomas Schmid *Community Involvement and Community Empowerment: Training of Trainers Manual*, National Center for Chronic Disease Prevention and Health Promotion, Centers for Disease Control and Prevention, Atlanta, n.d.

American College of Nurse-Midwives *Healthy Mother and Healthy Newborn Care: A Guide for Caregivers* Washington, D.C.: ACNM, 1998.

Asbell, Bernard *The Pill* New York: Random House, 1995.

Bandura, A. *Social Learning Theory* Englewood Cliffs, NJ: Prentice Hall, 1977.

Bertrand, Jane and Tsui, Amy (editors) *Indicators for Reproductive Health Program Evaluation*, Carolina Population Center, University of North Carolina, December, 1995.

Bertrand, Jane, Robert J. Magnani and James C. Knowles *Handbook of Indicators for Family Planning Program Evaluation* Carolina Population Center, University of North Carolina, n.d.

Bulatao, Rodolfo A. *The Value of Family Planning Programs in Developing Countries* Santa Monica, RAND, 1998.

Burns, August A.; Lovitch, R.; Maxwell, J.; and Shapiro, K. *Where Women Have No Doctor* Berkeley, CA: The Hesperian Foundation, 1997.

CARE-Bangladesh *Building Capacity of NGOS for Family Planning Activity*, Dhaka: CARE-Bangladesh, May 1999.

Centers for Disease Control and Prevention *1998 Guidelines for the Treatment of Sexually Transmitted Diseases* MMWR 1998; 47 (No. RR-1).

Centers for Disease Control and Prevention *Family Planning Methods and Practice: Africa 2nd edition*, Atlanta: Centers for Disease Control and Prevention, National Center for Chronic Disease Prevention, Division of Reproductive Health, 1999.

Centers for Disease Control and Prevention *HIV Mortality: L285 Slide Series (through 2000)*.

Centers for Disease Control and Prevention *Global AIDS Program: Strategies* web site http://www.cdc.gov/nchstp/od/gap/strategies/1_overview.htm

Central Statistical Organization (CSO) and Macro International (MI). *Yemen Demographic and Health Survey 1997*. Calverton, Maryland: CSO and MI, 1998.

Chambers, Robert *Rural Development: Putting the Last First* London: Longman, 1983.

Cianfrani, Theodore *A Short History of Obstetrics and Gynecology* Springfield: Charles C. Thomas, 1960.

Cleland, John and Ferry, Benoit (editors) *Sexual Behavior and AIDS in the Developing World*, London: Taylor and Francis, 1995.

Coale, Ansley and Hoover, Edgar *Population Growth and Economic Development in Low Income Countries* Princeton, N.J.: Princeton University Press, 1958.

Dallabetta, Gina and Hassig, Susan *Indicators for Reproductive Health Program Evaluation: Final Report of the Subcommittee on STD/HIV* Chapel Hill, NC: Carolina Population Center, 1995.

Dallabetta, Gina, Marie Laga and Peter Humphrey (editors) *Control of Sexually Transmitted Diseases*, Family Health International, n.d.

Dever, G.E. Alan, *Community Health Analysis*, Gaithersburg, MD: Aspen, 1991.

Djerassi, Carl *The Politics of Contraception* San Francisco: W.H. Freeman, 1981.

Erlich, Paul R *The Population Bomb* Buccaneer Books, 1971.

Feldman, David M. *Birth Control in Jewish Law* Northvale, New Jersey: Jason Aronson Inc., 1998.
Fisher, Andrew, et. al. *Guidelines and Instruments for a Family Planning Situation Analysis* New York: Population Council, 1992.
Forsythe, Steven (editor) *State of the Art: AIDS and Economics* Washington: The Futures Group, 2002.
Gibney, Laura, DiClemente, Ralph and Sten H. Vermund *Preventing HIV in Developing Countries*, New York: Kluwer, 1999.
Glanz, Karen; Lewis, Frances M.; and Rimer, Barbara K. (editors) *Health Behavior and Health Education* San Francisco: Jossey-Bass, 1997.
Hatcher, RA; Pluhar, E.; Zieman, M.; et. al. *A Personal Guide to Managing Contraception for Men and Women* Decatur, GA., Bridging the Gap Communications, Inc., 2000.
Hatcher, RA; Trussell, J.; Stewart, F.; Howells, S.; Russell, C.; Kowal, D. *Emergency Contraception: The Nation's Best Kep Secret* Atlanta: Bridging the Gap Communications, Inc., 1995.
Hatcher, Robert A, Ward Rinehart, Richard Blackburn, Judith S. Geller and James D. Shelton *The Essentials of Contraceptive Technology* Baltimore: Johns Hopkins University, School of Public Health, Population Information Program, 1997.
Hatcher, Robert A., James Trussell, Felicia Stewart, Willard Cates, Jr., Gary K. Stewart, Felicia Guest and Deborah Kowal *Contraceptive Technology* New York: Ardent Media, 1998.
Himes, Norman *Medical History of Contraception* New York: Gamut Press, 1963.
Holmes, King K.; Sparling, Frederick P.; Mardh, Per-Anders; Lemon, Stanley M.; Stamm, Walter E.; Piot, Peter; Wasserheit, Judith M. *Sexually Transmitted Diseases, Third Edition* New York: McGraw-Hill, 1999.
Hosken, Fran P. *The Hosken Report: Genital and Sexual Mutilation of Females*, Fourth Revised Edition, Women's International Network News, 1993.
Institute of Medicine *The Best Intentions: Unintended Pregnancy and the Well-Being of Children and Families* Washington, D.C.: National Academy Press, 1995.
International Vitamin A Consultative Group *IVACG Statement: Safe Uses of Vitamin A During Pregnancy and Lactation*, 1998.
JHPIEGO *PocketGuide for Family Planning Service Providers 1996 • 1998, Second Edition* March, 2000 (web site: www.reproline.jhu.edu/english/6read/6multi/pg/index.htm#Preface).
JHPIEGO *Service Delivery Guidelines* March, 2000 (web site: www.reproline.jhu.edu/english/6read/6multi/sdg/index.htm).
Kingdon, John W. *Agendas, Alternatives and Public Policies* Boston: Little, Brown and Co., 1984.
Kols, Adrienne and Sherris, Jacqueline *HPV Vaccines: Promise and Challenges* Seattle: PATH, July 2000.
Kretzmann, John P. and McKnight, John L. *Building Communities from the Inside Out: A Path Toward Finding and Mobilizing a Community's Assets*, Chicago: ACTA Publications, 1993.
Lapham, Robert. J. and George B.Simmons, (editors)., *Organizing for Effective Family Planning Programs*, Washington, D.C., : National Academy Press, 1989.
Lindenberg, Marc and Crosby, Benjamin *Managing Development: The Political Dimension* Hartford, Connecticut: Kumarian Press, 1981.
Maine, Deborah, McCarthy, James and Ward, Victoria, M. *Guidelines for monitoring progress in the reduction of maternal mortality* New York, UNICEF, 1992.
Maine, Deborah, Victoria Ward and Abdi Tahir El Tahir *Meeting the Community Half Way: Programming Guidelines for the Reduction of Maternal Mortality* New York, Center for Population and Family Health, Columbia University.
Mann, Jonathan and Daniel J. Tarantola *AIDS in the World II: Global Dimensions, Social Roots and Responses*, New York: Oxford University Press, 1996.
Marshall, Margaret Ann and Sandra Tebben Buffington *Life Saving Skills Manual for Midwives* Washington, D.C.: American College of Nurse-Midwives, 1991.
May, Katharyn A. and Laura R. Mahlmeister *Maternal and Neonatal Nursing: Family Centered Care* 3rd Edition, Philadelphia: J.P. Lippincott, 1994.
McDevitt, Thomas, N. with Arjun Adlakha, Timothy Fowler and Vena Harris-Bourne *Trends in Adolescent Fertility and Contraceptive Use in the Developing World* Washington, D.C.: U.S. Bureau of the Census, 1996.
Medecins dans Frontieres *Untangling the Web of Price Reductions: A pricing guide for the purchase of ARVs for developing countries, 2nd edition* Geneva: June 2002.
Michael, Robert T; Gagnon, John H.; Laumann, Edward O.; and Kolata, Gina *Sex in America: A Definitive Survey* Boston: Little, Brown & Company, 1994.
Middleberg, Maurice I. *Assessing Management Capacity Among Non-Governmental Organizations*, Atlanta: CARE, July 1993.

REFERENCES

Miller, William R. and Stephen Rollnick *Motivational Interviewing* New York, Guilford Press, 1991.

Mundigo, Axel I and Cynthia Indriso (eds.) *Abortion in the Developing World*, New Yor: Zed Books, 1999.

Musallam, Basim F. *Sex and Society in Islam : Birth control before the nineteenth century* Cambridge: Cambridge University Press, 1983.

National Academy of Sciences *Rapid Population Growth: Consequences and Policy Implications* Baltimore: Johns Hopkins University Press, 1971.

National Academy of Sciences *Recommended Dietary Allowances, 10th edition* Washington, 1989.

National Research Council *Contraception and Reproduction: Health Consequences for Women and Children in the Developing World*, Washington, D.C.: National Academy Press, 1989.

Netting, Robert McC.; Wilk, Richard, R. and Arnould, Eric J. *Households: Comparative and Historical Studies of the Domestic Group* Berkely: University of California Press, 1984.

Neuberg, Roger *Obstetrics: A Practical Manual* Oxford, Oxford University Press, 1995.

Nichiporuk, Brian *The Security Dynamics of Demographic Factors*, Rand Corporation, MR-1088-WFHF/RF/DLPF/A, 2000 for a discussion of political power, security issues and population.

O'Dowd, Michael J. and Elliot E. Philipp *The History of Gynaecology and Obstetrics* New York: Parthenon, 1994.

Oberzaucher, Nicola and Baggaley *HIV Voluntary Counselling and Testing: A gateway to prevention and care* UNAIDS, 2002.

Panel on Clinical Practices for Treatment of HIV Infection *Guidelines for the Use of Antiretroviral Agents in HIV-Infected Adults and Adolescents* February 4, 2002.

Parisot, Jeannette *Johnny Come Lately: A short history of the condom* London: Journeyman Press, 1987.

Parnell, Allan M. (editor) *Contraceptive Use and Controlled Fertility: Health Issues for Women and Children*, Washington, D.C.: National Academy Press, 1989.

Paul, Maureen, et. al. (editors.) *A Clinician's Guide to Medical and Surgical Abortion* New York: Churchill Livingstone, 1999.

Paul, Samuel *Institutional Development in World Bank Projects: A Cross-Sectoral Review*, World Bank, April 1990 (WPS392).

Piotrow Phyllis Tilson, D. Lawrence Kincaid, Jose G. Rimon II and Ward Rinehart *Health Communications: Lessons from Family Planning and Reproductive Health* Westport, CT: Praeger, 1997.

Potts, Malcom and Short, Roger *Ever Since Adam and Eve: The evolution of human sexuality* Cambridge: Cambridge University Press, 1999.

Riddle, John M. *Contraception and Abortion from the Ancient World to the Renaissance* Cambridge: Harvard University Press, 1992.

Riddle, John M. *Eve's Herbs: A History of Contraception and Abortion in the West* Cambridge: Harvard University Press, 1997.

Rifkin, S.B. *Health Planning and Community Participation* London: Croom-Helm, 1985.

Ross, John A. and Elizabeth Frankenberger *Findings from Two Decades of Family Planning Research* New York; The Population Council, 1993.

Ross, Susan Rae *Promoting Quality Maternal and Newborn Care: A Reference Manual for Program Managers* Atlanta: CARE, 1999.

Sacred Congregation for the Doctrine of the Faith *Persona Humana:Declaration on Certain Questions Concerning Sexual Ethics* December 29, 1975.

Sen, Gita; Germaine, Adrienne; and Lincoln C. Chen (editors.) *Population Policies Reconsidered: Health, Empowerment and Rights*, Cambridge: Harvard University Press, 1994 for a discussion of this perspective.

Shah, Meera Kaul; Kambou, Sarah Degnan; and Monahan, Barbara (editors.) in *Embracing Participation in Development: Wisdom from the Field*, Atlanta: CARE, 1999.

Shane, Barbara *Family Planning Saves Lives, Third Edition* Washington, D.C.: Population Reference Bureau, 1996.

Simon, Julian L. *Theory of Population and Economic Growth* Blackwell Publishers, 1986.

Sivin, Irving, Nash, Harold and Waldman, Sandra *Jadelle® Levonorgestrel Rod Implants: A Summary of Scientific Data and Lessons Learned from Programmatic Experience* New York: Population Council, 2002.

Stewart, M Kathryn, Cynthia K. Stanton, and Omar Ahmed 1997 *Maternal Health Care*, DHS Comparative Studies No. 25, Calverton, MD: Macro International, Inc.

Stinson, Wayne *Community Financing of Primary Health Care* Washington, D.C.: American Public Health Association, 1982.

Tannahill, Reay *Sex in History*, Scarborough House, 1992.

Thoms, Herbert *Our Obstetric Heritage: The Story of Safe Childbirth* Hamden, CT: Shoe String Press, 1960.

Tsui, Amy O., Judith Wasserheit and Joahn Haaga, editors *Reproductive Health in Developing Countries: Expanding Dimensions, Building Solutions* Washington, D.C.: National Academy Press, 1997.

U.S. Agency for International Development, Office of Population *PROFIT Project Compendium*, Washington, D.C., n.d.

U.S. Bureau of the Census, Report WP/98, *World Population Profile: 1998*, U.S. Government Printing Office, Washington, D.C., 1999, page 50.

UNAIDS *AIDS Epidemic Update: December, 1999*.

UNAIDS *Epidemiological Fact Sheets: 2000 Update*.

UNAIDS *Technical Update: Mother-to-child transmission of HIV*, September 2000.

UNFPA *Report of the International Conference on Population and Development* (Cairo 5–13 September 1994).

Ward, Darrell E. *The AmFAR AIDS Handbook* London: W.W. Norton and Co., 1999.

Werner, David *Where There is No Doctor*, Palo Alto, California: Hesperian Foundation, 1992.

Wolff, James A., Suttenfield, Linda J. and Binzen, Susanna, C. (editors) *The Family Planing Manager's Handbook* West Hartford, CT., Kumarian Press, 1991.

World Bank *Confronting AIDS: Public Priorities in a Global Epidemic*, New York: Oxford University Press, 1998.

World Bank *Population and Development: Implications for the World Bank* Washington: World Bank, 1994.

World Bank *The Minimum Package of Health Services* (World Bank web site, February 10, 2000).

World Bank *World Development Indicators 1999*.

World Bank *World Development Indicators 2000* (web site).

World Health Organization *Care in Normal Birth: Report of a Technical Working Group* Geneva, 1999.

World Health Organization and UNICEF *Management of Childhood Illnesses*.

World Health Organization *Antenatal Care: Report of a Technical Working Group* Geneva, 31 October–4 November 1994.

World Health Organization *Management of Patients with Sexually Transmitted Diseases: Report of a WHO Study Group*, WHO Technical Report Series #810, Geneva, 1991.

World Health Organization *Mother-Baby Package: Implementing safe motherhood in developing countries* Geneva, 1998.

World Healvth Organization *Post abortion family planning: A practical guide for managers* Geneva: World Health Organization, 1997.

World Health Organization *Reduction of Maternal Mortality: A Joint WHO/UNFPA/UNICEF/World Bank Statement* Geneva, 1999.

World Health Organization *WHO Initiative on HIV/AIDS and Sexually Transmitted Infections: An Overview of Selected Curable Sexually Transmitted Diseases*, n.d. (online document).

World Health Organization *World Health Report 2000*, Geneva, WHO, 2000.

ARTICLES AND BOOK CHAPTERS

"Administration of Zidovudine During Late Pregnancy and Delivery to Prevent Perinatal Transmission—Thailand, 1996–1998, *Morbidity and Mortality Weekly Report* 1998; 47:151–154.

Andiman, Warren A. MD. "Transmission of HIV-1 from mother to infant" *Current Opinion in Pediatrics* 14(1):78–85, February 2002.

Andiman, Warren A. MD. "Transmission of HIV-1 from mother to infant" *Current Opinion in Pediatrics* 14(1):78–85, February 2002.

Askew, Ian "Organizing community participation in family planning projects in South Asia" *Studies in Family Planning*, Vol. 20, No. 4 (Jul.–Aug., 1989) pp. 185–202.

Askew, Ian and Khan, A.R. "Community participation and national family planning programs: Some organizational issues" *Studies in Family Planning*, Vol. 21, No. 3, (May–June, 1990), pp. 127–142.

Asthana, Sheena and Oostvogels, Robert "Community participation in HIV prevention: Problems and prospects for community-based strategies among female sex workers in Madras" *Social Science and Medicine*, Vol. 43, No. 2, pp. 133–147, 1996.

Ayuku, D.; Bentley, M.; Egessa, O.; Maman, S.; Sweat, M.; Moss, W.; Nyarang'o, P.; Chemati, A.; and Halsey, N. "Factors that facilitate and impede STD control in Western Kenya" paper presented at 1996 International Conference on AIDS.

REFERENCES

Bankole, Akinrinola, Susheela Singh and Taylor Haas "Reasons Why Women Have Abortions: Evidence from 27 Countries" *International Family Planning Perspectives*, Volume 24, Issue 3 (Sep., 1998) pp. 117–127.

Barlow, Yvonne "Childbirth: Management of Labour Through the Ages" *Nursing Times*, August 31, 1994, Volume 90, No. 35, pp. 41–43.

Beeker, Carolyn, Guenther-Grey, Carolyn and Raj, Anita "Community empowerment, paradigm drift and the primary prevention of HIV/AIDS" *Social Science and Medicine*, Vol. 46, No. 7 (1 Apr 1998), pp. 831–842.

Beeker, Carolyn, Guenther-Grey, Carolyn and Raj, Anita "Community empowerment, paradigm drift and the primary prevention of HIV/AIDS" *Social Science and Medicine*, Vol. 46, No. 7 (1 Apr 1998), pp. 831–842.

Benson, Janie, Lori Ann Nicholson, Lynne Gaffikin and Stephen N. Kinoti "Complications of Unsafe Abortion in sub-Saharan Africa: A Review" *Health Policy and Planning*, Volume 11, No. 2, pp. 117–131.

Blackburn, R.D., Cunkelman, J.A., and Zlidar, V.M. "Oral Contraceptives—An Update" *Population Reports*, Series A, No. 9. Baltimore, Johns Hopkins University School of Public Health, Population Information Program, Spring 2000.

Bond, Katherine C., Valente, Thomas A. and Kendall, Carl "Social network influences on reproductive behaviors in northern Thailand" *Social Science and Medicine* 49 (1999) pp. 1599–1614.

Bongaarts, John "A simple method for estimating the contraceptive prevalence required to achieve a fertility target" *Studies in Family Planning*, 1984 Jul–Aug; 15(4):184–190.

Brandt, Allan "Sexually transmitted diseases" in: *Companion Encyclopedia of the History of Medicine*; W. F. Bynum and Roy Porter (eds.) London ; New York: Routledge, 1993.

Bruce, Judith "Fundamental elements of the quality of care: A simple framework", *Studies in Family Planning* 21(2): 61–91. Mar./Apr. 1990.

Cameron DW., Simonsen JN., D'Costa LJ., Ronald AR., Maitha GM., Gakinya MN., Cheang M. Ndinya-Achola JO., Piot P., Brunham RC. "Female to male transmission of human immunodeficiency virus type 1: risk factors for seroconversion in men" *Lancet*. 2(8660):403–407, 1989 Aug 19.

Chiwuzie, J., Okojie, O., Okolocho, C, Omorogbe, S., Oronsaye, A., Akpala, W., Ande, B., Onoguwe, B., Oikeh, E. "Emergency loan funds to improve access to obstetric care in Ekpoma, Nigeria" *International Journal of Gynecology and Obstetrics* 59 Suppl. 2 (1997) S259–S265, p. S231–S236.

Choguill, Marisa B. Guaraldo "A ladder of community participation for underdeveloped countries" *Habitat International*, Vol. 20, No. 3, pp. 431–444, 1996.

Cleland, John "Community participation in family planning" in *Family Planning, Health and Family Well-Being: Proceedings of the United Nations Expert Group Meeting on Family Planning, Health and Family Well-Being* Banagalore, India 26–30 October 1992. United Nations Population Division, 1996, pp. 245–255 (ST/ESA/SER.R/131).

Cohen MS., Hoffman IF., Royce RA., Kazembe P., Dyer JR., Daly CC., Zimba D., Vernazza PL., Maida M., Fiscus SA., Eron JJ Jr. "Reduction of concentration of HIV-1 in semen after treatment of urethritis: implications for prevention of sexual transmission of HIV-1" AIDSCAP Malawi Research Group. *Lancet* 349(9069):1868–1873, 1997 Jun 28.

Connor, Edward, M., Sperling RS. Gelber R. Kiselev P. Scott G. O'Sullivan MJ. VanDyke R. Bey M. Shearer W. Jacobson RL "Reduction Of Maternal-Infant Transmission Of Human Immunodeficiency Virus Type 1 With Zidovudine Treatment" *New England Journal of Medicine* 331:1173–1180, 1994.

Crosby, Alfred W. "The early history of syphilis: A reappraisal" *American Anthropologist*, 71 (1969) pp. 218–227.

Dabis, Francois, Msellati P. Meda N. Welffens-Ekra C. You B. Manigart O. Leroy V. Simonon A. Cartoux M. Combe P. Ouangre A. Ramon R. Ky-Zerbo O. Montcho C. Salamon R. Rouzioux C. Van de Perre P. Mandelbrot L. "6-month efficacy tolerance and acceptability of a short regimen of zidovudine to reduce verical transmission of HIV in breastfed children in Cote d'Ivoire and Burkina Faso: a double-blind placebo-controlled multicentre trial" *The Lancet* 353 (9155) pp. 786–792, 6 March 1999.

De Browere, Vincent, Rene Tonglet and Wim Van Leberghe "Strategies for Reducing Maternal Mortality in Developing Countries: What Can We Learn from the History of the Industrialized West" *Tropical Medicine and International Health*, Volume 3, No. 10, pp. 771–782 (October, 1998).

Essien, E., Ifenne, D., Sabitu, K., Musa, A., Alti-Mu'azu, M., Adidu, V., Golji, N., Muladdus, M. "Community loan funds and transport services for obstetric emergencies in northern Nigeria" *International Journal of Gynecology and Obstetrics* 59 Suppl. 2 (1997) S259–S265, pp. S237–S234.

Ewart, Wendy R. and Beverly Winikoff "Towards Safe and Effective Medical Abortion" *Science* Volume 281 (5376), 24 July 1998, pp. 520–521.

Faundes, A. and E. Hardy "Illegal Abortion: Consequences for Women's Health and the Health Care System" *International Journal of Gynecology and Obstetrics*, 58 (1997) pp. 77–83.

Ferligoj, A. and Hlebec, V. "Evaluation of social network measurement instruments" *Social Networks* Vol. 21(2) 1999 pp. 111–130.

Foster, Susan "Benefits of HIV Screening of Blood Transfusions in Zambia" *The Lancet* Volume 346 (8969) 22 July 1995 pp. 225–227.

Ghys PD., Fransen K., Diallo MO., Ettiegne-Traore V., Coulibaly IM., Yeboue KM., Kalish ML., Maurice C., Whitaker JP., Greenberg AE., Laga M. "The associations between cervicovaginal HIV shedding, sexually transmitted diseases and immunosuppression in female sex workers in Abidjan, Cote d'Ivoire" *AIDS* 11(12):F85–93, 1997 Oct.

Gibney, Laura, Choudhury P. Khawaja Z. Sarker M. Islam N. Vermund SH "HIV/AIDS in Bangladesh: An Assessment of Biomedical Risk Factors for Transmission" *International Journal of STD and AIDS* Vol 10(5) May 1999, pp. 338–346.

Grosskurth H., Gray R., Hayes R., Mabey D., Wawer M. "Control of sexually transmitted diseases for HIV-1 prevention: understanding the implications of the Mwanza and Rakai trials" *Lancet* 355(9219):1981–1987, 2000 Jun 3.

Grosskurth H., Gray R., Hayes R., Mabey D., Wawer M. "Control of sexually transmitted diseases for HIV-1 prevention: understanding the implications of the Mwanza and Rakai trials" *Lancet* 355(9219):1981–1987, 2000 Jun 3.

Grosskurth H., Mosha F., Todd J., Mwijarubi E., Klokke A., Senkoro K., Mayaud P., Changalucha J., Nicoll A., ka-Gina G. "Impact of improved treatment of sexually transmitted diseases on HIV infection in rural Tanzania: randomised controlled trial" *Lancet* 346(8974):530–536, 1995 Aug 26.

Guay, Laura A., Musoke, Philippa. Fleming, Thomas. Bagenda, Danstan. Allen, Melissa. Nakabiito, Clemensia. Sherman, Joseph. Bakaki, Paul. Ducar, Constance. Deseyve, Martina. Emel, Lynda. Mirochnick, Mark. Fowler, Mary Glenn. Mofenson, Lynne. Miotti, Paolo. Dransfield, Kevin. Bray, Dorothy. Mmiro, Francis. Jackson, J Brooks "Intrapartum and neonatal single-dose nevirapine compared with zidovudine for prevention of mother-to-child transmission of HIV-1 in Kampala, Uganda: HIVNET 012 randomised trial" *The Lancet* 354: pp. 795–802, 4 September 1999.

Gumodoka B., Ng'weshemi JZ. Kigadye FC. Dolmans WM. Borgdorff MW "Blood transfusion practices in Mwanza Region, Tanzania" *AIDS* 7(3):387–392, March, 1993.

Heise, L., Ellsberg, M. and Gottemoeller, M. "Ending Violence Against Women" *Population Reports*, Series L, No. 11. Baltimore, Johns Hopkins University School of Public Health, Population Information Program, December 1999.

Helfenbein, Saul and Sayeed, Abu "Increasing Community Participation" *Family Planning Manager*, Management Sciences for Health web site (www.msh.org/chs/tools).

Henshaw, Stanley K. "Unintended Pregnancy and Abortion: A Public Health Perspective" in Paul, Maureen, et. al. (eds.) *A Clinician's Guide to Medical and Surgical Abortion* New York: Churchill Livingstone, 1999.

Hesketh, T. and Zhu, WX "The one child family policy: the good, the bad, and the ugly" *British Medical Journal* 314 (7095): 1685–1687, 1997 June 7.

Hillery, George A. "Definitions of community: areas of agreement" *Rural Sociology*, Vol. 20, No. 11, 1955.

Homer-Dixon, Thomas "Environmental scarcities and violent conflict: Evidence from cases" *International Security* Vol. 19, no. 1 (Summer 1994), pp. 5–40.

Huezo, C.M. and Diaz, S. "Quality of care in family planning: Clients' right and provider needs" in Senanyake P. and Kleinman, R.L. *The Proceedings of the IPPF Family Planning Congress, New Delhi, October 1992*, Pearl River, New York; Parthenon Publishing Group, 1993, pp. 235–244.

Jewkes, Rachel and Murcott, Anne "Community representatives: Representing the 'community'?" *Social Science and Medicine* Vol. 46, No. 7, pp. 843–858, 1998.

Jewkes, Rachel and Murcott, Anne "Meanings of community" *Social Science and Medicine*, Vol. 43, No. 4, pp. 555–563.

Kanani, Shubhada J. "Application of rapid assessment procedures in the context of women's morbidity" in *Rapid Assessment Procedures: Qualitative Methodologies for Planning and Evaluation of Health Related Programmes* Scrimshaw, Nevin S. and Gleason, Gary r. (eds) Boston: International Nutrition Foundation for Developing Countries, 1992.

Karon, John M. PhD; Fleming, Patricia L. PhD; Steketee, Richard W. MD; De Cock, Kevin M. MD "HIV in the United States at the Turn of the Century: An Epidemic in Transition" *American Journal of Public Health* 2001; 91:1060–1068.

Kloos Helmut and Zein, Ahmed Zein "AIDS and other STDs in Ethiopia: Historical, social and epidemiological aspects" *Africa Urban Quarterly* Vol. 6, Nos 1 and 2, Feb. and May 1991.

Koblinsky, M.A. "Beyond maternal mortality—magnitude, interrelationship and consequences of women's health, pregnancy-related complications and nutritional status on pregnancy outcomes *International Journal of Gynecology and Obstetrics* 48 Suppl. (1995) s21–s32.

Kols, Adrienne J. and Sherman, Jill E. "Family planning programs: Improving quality" *Population Reports* Series J, No. 47, Baltimore, Johns Jopins University School of Public Health, Population Information Program, November 1998.

Lackritz, E.M., Djommand G., Vetter KM, Zadi, F., Diaby L., DeCock KM "Beyond blood screening: reducing unnecessary transfusions and improving laboratory services in Cote d'Ivoire" *International Conference on AIDS* 9(1): 92 (abstract no. WS-C11-2), June 6–11, 1993.

Laga M., Manoka A., Kivuvu M., Malele B., Tuliza M., Nzila N., Goeman J., Behets F., Batter V., Alary M. "Non-ulcerative sexually transmitted diseases as risk factors for HIV-1 transmission in women: results from a cohort study"*AIDS*. 7(1):95–102, 1993 Jan.

Lande, R. E. "New era for injectables" *Population Reports*, Series K, No. 5. Baltimore, Johns Hopkins School of Public Health, Population Information Program, August 1995.

Landman LC. "Birth control in India: the carrot and the rod?" *Family Planning Perspectives*, 9(3):101–110, 1977 May–Jun.

Larkin, Marilynn "WHO's Blood-Safety Initiative: A Vain Effort?" *The Lancet* Volume 355 (9211) 8 April 2000 p. 1245.

Leroy V. Karon JM. Alioum A. Ekpini ER. Meda N. Greenberg AE. Msellati P. Hudgens M. Dabis F. Wiktor SZ. West Africa PMTCT Study Group. "Twenty-four month efficacy of a maternal short-course zidovudine regimen to prevent mother-to-child transmission of HIV-1 in West Africa. [Clinical Trial. Journal Article. Randomized Controlled Trial" *AIDS*. 16(4):631–641, 2002 Mar 8.

Li, X.F., J.A. Fortney, M. Kotelchuk and L.H. Glover "The post-partum period: the key to maternal mortality: *International Journal of Gynecology and Obstetrics* 54 (1996) 1–10, 1993.

Limpakarnjanarat, Khanchit. Mastro, Timothy D. Saisorn, Supachai. Uthaivoravit, Wat. Kaewkungwal, Jaranit. Korattana, Supaporn. Young, Nancy L. Morse, Stephen A. Schmid, D Scott. Weniger, Bruce G. Nieburg, Phillip. "HIV-1 and other sexually transmitted infections in a cohort of female sex workers in Chiang Rai, Thailand." *Sexually Transmitted Infections*. 75(1):30–35, February 1999.

Lynam, Pamela; Rabinovitz,, Lleslie McNeil and Shobowale, Mofoluka "Using self-assessment to improve the quality of family planning services" *Studies in Family Planning* Vol. 24, #4 (Jul.–Aug., 1993), pp. 252–260.

Lyons, Martinez "Sexually transmitted diseases in the history of Uganda" *Genitourinary Medicine*, 70 (1994) pp. 138–145.

Maberly, Glenn "Iodine deficiency" *Bulletin of the World Health Organization* 76 Suppl 2:118–20, 1998.

Maberly, Glenn F. "Iodine deficiency disorders: contemporary scientific issues" *Journal of Nutrition* 124 (8 Suppl): 1473S–1478S, 1994 Aug.

Maine, D., et. al. "Prevention of Maternal Deaths in Developing Countries: Program Options and Practical Considerations" Paper presented at the International Safe Motherhood Conference, Nairobi, Feb. 10–13, 1987.

Maine, Deborah "Lessons for program design from the Preventing Maternal Mortality projects" *International Journal of Gynecology and Obstetrics* 59 Suppl. 2 (1997) S259–S265, p. S262.

Marseille, Elliot "Cost-effectiveness of single-dose nevirapine regimen for mothers and babies to decrease vertical HIV-1 transmission in sub-Saharan Africa" *The Lancet* 354: pp. 803–809, 4 September 1999.

Mayaud, Philippe. Uledi, Elizabeth. Cornelissen, Jan. ka-Gina, Gina. Todd, James. Rwakatare, Medard. West, Beryl. Kopwe, Lilian. Manoko, Domitilia. Grosskurth, Heiner. Hayes, Richard. Mabey, David. "Risk scores to detect cervical infections in urban antenatal clinic attenders in Mwanza, Tanzania" *Sexually Transmitted Infections* 74(1S) Supplement 1:139S–146S, June 1998.

McAllister, Lynn and Fischer, Claude "A procedure for surveying personal networks" *Sociological Methods and Research* Vol. 7, No. 2, No. 1978.

McDonagh, Marilyn "Is antenatal care effective in reducing maternal mortality?" *Health Policy and Planning* 11(1): 1–15 (1996).

Megevand E. Denny L. Dehaeck K. Soeters R. Bloch B. "Acetic acid visualization of the cervix: an alternative to cytologic screening" *Obstetrics & Gynecology* 88(3):383–386, 1996 Sep.

Mensch, Barbara; Fisher, Andrew; Askew, Ian and Ayorinde Ajayi "Using situation analysis data to assess the functioning of family planning clinics in Nigeria, Tanzania and Zmbabwe" *Studies in Family Planning* Vol. 25, #1 (Jan.–Feb., 199), pp. 18–31.

Middleberg, Maurice "Health Security: A framework for health programming" paper prepared for the CARE Health and Population Unit, Atlanta: CARE, 1997.

Mishell, Daniel R. "Intrauterine Devices: Mechanisms of Action, Safety and Efficacy" *Contraception* 58 (453–53S), 1998.

Morice, P., P. Josset and J.C. Colau "La Gynecologie et l'Obstetrique en Egypte Antique" *J. Gynecol. Obstet. Biol. Reprod.*, 1994, 23, pp. 131–136.

Murthy NS. Agarwal SS. Prabhakar AK. Sharma S. Das DK. "Estimation of reduction of life-time risk of cervical cancer through one life-time screening" *Neoplasma.* 40(4):255–258, 1993.

Mwakagile, D., Mmari, E., Makwaya, C., Mbwana, J., Biberfeld, G., Mhalu,F. Sandstrom, E. "Sexual behaviour among youths at high risk for HIV-1 infection in Dar es Salaam, Tanzania" *Sexually Transmitted Infections* 77(4):255–259, August 2001.

Nazeer, S. "Cervical cancer control in developing countries: Memorandum from a WHO meeting" *Bulletin of the World Health Organization* 74 (4): 345–351.

Nduati, Ruth, John G. Mbori-Ngacha D. Richardson B. Overbaugh J. Mwatha A. Ndinya-Achola J. Bwayo J. Onyango FE. Hughes J. Kreiss J "Effect of breastfeeding and formula feeding on transmission of HIV-1: A randomized clinical trial" *Journal of the American Medical Association* Vol. 238 (9), 1 March 2000, pp. 1167–1174.

Nelson, Anita "Intrauterine Device Practical Guidelines: Medical Conditions" *Contraception* 58 (59S–63S), 1998.

Paul Farmer, Fernet Léandre, Joia Mukherjee, Rajesh Gupta, Laura Tarter, & Jim Yong Kim "Community-based treatment of advanced HIV disease: introducing DOT-HAART (directly observed therapy with highly active antiretroviral therapy)" *Bulletin of the World Health Organization*, 2001, 79(12) pp. 1145–1151.

Paxman, John M., Rizzo, Alberto, Brown, Laura, Benson, Jamie " The clandestine epidemic: The practice of unsafe abortion in Latin America" *Studies in Family Planning*, Vol. 24, No. 4. (Jul.–Aug., 1993), pp. 205–226.

Pengsaa P. Vatanasapt V. Sriamporn S. Sanchaisuriya P. Schelp FP. Noda S. Kato S. Kongdee W. Kanchanawirojkul N. Aranyasen O. "A self-administered device for cervical cancer screening in northeast Thailand" *Acta Cytologica.* 41(3):749–754, 1997 May–Jun.

Peterson H.B.; Xia Z.; Hughes J.M.; Wilcox L.S.; Tylor L.R.; Trussell J.; Grimes D.A.; Hammond C.B.; Gibbs R.S.; Rosenfield A.; Soper D.P. "The risk of pregnancy after tubal sterilization: findings from the U.S. collaborative review of sterilization" *American Journal of Obstetrics and Gynecology* Volume 174, Issue 4 1996 p. 1161–1170.

Plummer FA., Simonsen JN., Cameron DW., Ndinya-Achola JO., Kreiss JK., Gakinya MN., Waiyaki P., Cheang M., Piot P., Ronald AR. "Cofactors in male-female sexual transmission of human immunodeficiency virus type 1" *Journal of Infectious Diseases.* 163(2):233–239, 1991 Feb.

Population Council *Medical Methods of Early Abortion in Developing Countries: Consensus Statement*, 1998.

Pritchett, Lant "Desired Fertility and the Impact of Population Policies" *Population and Development Review*, Vol. 20, No. 3, 19994, pp 1–55.

Purdey, Alice F.; Adhikari, Gyan Bahadur; Robinson, Sheila and Cox, Philip W. "Participatory health development in rural Nepal: Clarifying the process of community empowerment" *Health Education Quarterly* Vol. 21, No. 3 (Fall, 1994) pp. 329–343.

Ramakrishnan, Usha, Renu Majrekar, Juan Rivera, Teresa Gonzales-Gossio and Reynaldo Martorell "Micronutrients and pregnancy outcome: A review of the literature" *Nutrition Research*, Vol. 19, No. 1, pp. 103–159, 1999.

Rekart, M L. "Sex in the city: sexual behaviour, societal change, and STDs in Saigon" *Sexually Transmitted Infections* 78 Supplement 1:i47–i54, April 2002.

Richart, E.M. "Screening: the next century" *Cancer* 76 (10) Suppl. Pp. 1919–1927.

Rosenfield, A. and Maine, D. "Maternal mortality—neglected tragedy: Where is the M in MCH?" *Lancet*, 2:83–85, 1985.

Rutstein, Shea "Effect of Birth Intervals on Mortality and Health: Multivariate Cross-Country Analysis" (presentation at MACRO International Seminar), 1999.

Salter, C., Johnson, H.B. and Hengen, N. "Care for Post-abortion Complications: Saving Women's Lives" *Population Reports*, Series L, No. 10. Baltimore: Johns Hopkins School of Public Health, Population Information Program, June 1993.

Schultz, Linda J., Steketee, Richard W., Chitsulo, Lester, Macheso, Alan, Kazembe, Peter and Wirima, Jack J. "Evaluation of maternal practices, efficacy and cost-effectiveness of alternative antimalarial regimens for use in pregnancy: chloroquine and sulfadoxine-pyremethamine" Supplement to *The American Journal of Tropical Medicine & Hygiene* Vol. 55, No. 1, pp. 87–94.

See Mason, Karen Oppenheim and Taj, Anju Malhotra "Differences between women's and men's reproductive goals in developing countries" *Population and Development Review*, Vol. 13, No. 4 (Dec. 1987), pp. 611–638.

REFERENCES

Shaffer, Nathan; Chuachoowong, Rutt; Mock, Philip A; Bhadrakom, Chaiporn; Siriwasin, Wimol; Young, Nancy L; Chotpitayasunondh, Tawee; Chearskul, Sanay; Roongpisuthipong, Anuvat; Chinayon, Pratharn; Karon, John; Mastro, Timothy D; Simonds, R J. "Short-course zidovudine for perinatal HIV-1 transmission in Bangkok, Thailand: a randomised controlled trial" *The Lancet* 353 (9155) pp. 773–780, 6 March 1999.

Shaffer, Nathan; Chuachoowong, Rutt; Mock, Philip A; Bhadrakom, Chaiporn; Siriwasin, Wimol; Young, Nancy L; Chotpitayasunondh, Tawee; Chearskul, Sanay; Roongpisuthipong, Anuvat; Chinayon, Pratharn; Karon, John; Mastro, Timothy D; Simonds, R J. "Short-course zidovudine for perinatal HIV-1 transmission in Bangkok, Thailand: a randomised controlled trial" *The Lancet* 353 (9155) pp. 773–780, 6 March 1999.

Singh, K. and S.S. Ratnam "The Influence of Abortion Legislation on Maternal Mortality" *International Journal of Gynecology and Obstetrics*, 63 Suppl. 1(1998) S123–S129.

Sivin, Irving; Osborn V.; Campodonico, I.; Diaz, S.; Pavez, M.; Wan, L.; Koetsawang. S.; Orawan, K.; Anaant, MP.; Holma, P.; Kamal, A.; Stern, J. "Clinical performance of a new two rod levonogorgestrel contraceptive implant: A three-year randomized study with Norplant implants as controls" *Contraception* 55(73–80), 1997.

Stamm W.E., Handsfield HH., Rompalo AM., Ashley RL., Roberts PL., Corey L. "The association between genital ulcer disease and acquisition of HIV infection in homosexual men" *JAMA*. 260(10):1429–1433, 1988 Sep 9.

Steen, Richard PA, MPH. and Dallabetta, Gina MD, "The Use of Epidemiologic Mass Treatment and Syndrome Management for Sexually Transmitted Disease Control" *Sexually Transmitted Diseases*. 26(4) Supplement:S12–S20, April 1999.

Steen, Richard PA, MPH; Vuylsteke, Bea MD, MSC ; Decoito, Tony MD; Ralepeli, Stori SPN; Fehler, Glenda MSC; Conley, Jacci BA; Bruckers, Liesbeth MSC ; Dallabetta, Gina MD; Ballard, Ron Mibiol, Ph.D. "Evidence of Declining STD Prevalence in a South African Mining Community Following a Core-Group Intervention" *Sexually Transmitted Diseases* 27(1):1–8, January 2000.

Stolzfus, Rebecca J and Michele L. Dreyfuss *Guidelines for the Use of Iron Supplementation to Prevent and Treat Iron Deficiency Anemia* Washington, D.C.: ILSI Press, 1998.

Sullivan, Richard "Divine and Rational: The Reproductive Health of Women in Ancient Egypt" *Obstetrical and Gynecological Survey*, Volume 52, No. 10, pp. 635–642.

Sweat, Michael; Steven Gregorich, Gloria Sangiwa, Colin Furlonge, Donald Balmer, Claudes Kamenga, Olga Grinstead, Thomas Coates "Cost-effectiveness of voluntary HIV-1 counselling and testing in reducing sexual transmission of HIV-1 in Kenya and Tanzania" *Lancet* 356 (9224): 113–121, 8 July 2000.

Tatar, Mehtap "Community participation in health care: The Turkish case" *Social Science and Medicine*, Vol. 42, No. 11, (1996) pp. 1493–1500.

Technical Guidance/Competence Working Group and World Health Organization/Family Planning and Population Unit. "Family planning methods: New guidance" *Population Reports*, Series J, No. 44. Baltimore, Johns Hopkins School of Public Health, Population Information Program, October 1996.

The Voluntary HIV-1 Counseling and Testing Efficacy Study Group "Efficacy of voluntary HIV-1 counselling and testing in individuals and couples in Kenya, Tanzania, and Trinidad: a randomised trial" *Lancet* 356 (9224): 103–112, 8 July 2000.

Thomas C. Wright, Jr, MD; Lynette Denny, MMED, FCOG; Louise Kuhn, PhD; Amy Pollack, MD; Attila Lorincz, PhD "HPV DNA Testing of Self-collected Vaginal Samples Compared With Cytologic Screening to Detect Cervical Cancer" *JAMA* 283 (1) January 5, 2000, p. 81.

Thompson, Sandra "Obstetrics During the Early Roman Empire" *Midwives Chronicle and Nursing Notes* June, 1987.

Treiman, K., Liskin, L. Kols, A., and Rinehart, W. "IUDs—An Update" *Population Reports*, Series B, No. 6. Baltimore, Johns Hopkins School of Public Health, Population Information Program, December 1995.

Trueba, Guadalupe "Birth in Pre-Hispanic Mexico" *International Midwife*, Winter 1997, pp. 45–47.

Upadhyay, U.D. and B. Robey "Why Family Planning Matters" *Population Reports* Series J, No. 49, Baltimore: Johns Hopkins University School of Public Health, Population Information Program, July 1999.

Van de Perre, Philippe "HIV voluntary counselling and testing in community health services" *Lancet* 356(9224): 113–121, 8 July 2000.

Vos J., Gumodoka B. Ng'weshemi JZ. Kigadye FC. Dolmans WM. Borgdorff MW "Are some blood transfusions avoidable? A hospital record analysis in Mwanza Region Tanzania" *Tropical and Geographic Medicine* 45(6): 301–303, 1993.

Wawer MJ. Sewankambo NK., Serwadda D., Quinn TC., Paxton LA., Kiwanuka N., Wabwire-Mangen F., Li C., Lutalo T., Nalugoda F., Gaydos CA., Moulton LH., Meehan MO., Ahmed S., Gray RH. "Control of sexually transmitted diseases for AIDS prevention in Uganda: a randomised community trial" *Lancet* 353(9152):525–535, 1999 Feb 13.

West, Keith P. Jr., et. al. "Double blind, cluster randomised trial of low dose supplementation with Vitamin A or beta-carotene on mortality related to pregnancy in Nepal" *British Medical Journal* Volume 318 (7183) 27 February 1999, pp. 570–575.

Wiktor, Stefan, Ekpini E. Karon JM. Nkengasong J. Maurice C. Severin ST. Roels TH. Kouassi MK. Lackritz EM. Coulibaly IM. Greenberg AE. "Short course oral zidovudine for prevention of mother-to-child transmission of HIV-1 in Abidjan, Cote d'Ivoire: a randomised trial" *The Lancet* 353 (9155) pp. 781–785, 6 March 1999.

Wilson, David. Cawthorne, Paul. "'Face up to the truth': helping gay men in Vietnam protect themselves from AIDS" *International Journal of STD & AIDS* 10(1):63–66, January 1999.

Winkler, Judith, Paul D. Blumenthal and Forrest C. Greenslade "Early Abortion Services: New Choices for Providers and Women" *Advances in Abortion Care*, Volume 5, No. 2.

Wolitski RJ, MacGowan RJ, Higgins DL, Jorgensen CM. "The effects of HIV counseling and testing on risk-related practices and help-seeking behavior" *AIDS Educ Prev* 1997; 9 (suppl): 5267.

Yuster, E.A., "Rethinking the role of the risk approach and antenatal care in maternal mortality reduction" *International Journal of Gynecology and Obstetrics* 50 Suppl. 2 (1995) S59–S61.

Zlidar, V.M. "Helping Women Use the Pill" *Population Reports*, Series A, No. 10. Baltimore, Johns Hopkins University School of Public Health, Population Information Program, Summer 2000.

Index

Abortifacient drugs, 186–187
Abortion, 32–36
  complications of, 187–188
  contraception, post-abortion, 188–189
  death caused by, 30–33
  induced abortion, defined, 32
  legal status and rate of, 35
  maternal reasons for, 35–36
  rate by geographic region, 35
  unsafe, complications of, 28, 30, 33–34, 188–189
  unsafe, defined, 32–33, 35
Abortion methods
  abortifacient drugs, 186–187
  dilation and curettage (D&C), 186
  saline abortion, 187
  surgical abortion, 187
  vacuum aspiration, 186
Abstinence, 136–137
  guidelines for clients, 137
  pros/cons of, 137
Access to services, 106–112
  clinical services, 111–112
  community health worker (CHW) contribution to, 115
  mapping locations of providers, 106–107
  provider to service match, 108–111
  and quality assessment, 119
Adolescent pregnancy, and infant mortality, 26–27
Advocacy, of health program manager, 231–235
Africa, HIV/AIDS epidemic, 37, 39
AIDS: *see* HIV/AIDS
Albendazole, 168
Allbutt, Henry A., 9
Alma-Alta Declaration (1978), 75
Anangaranga, 4
Anemia
  causes of, 171
  in pregnancy, 171
  treatment of, 171
Aristotle, on reproductive health, 3–4
Aseptic methods, six cleans, 175
Asia, HIV/AIDS epidemic, 37

Asset accumulation approach, elements of, 13–14
Assets mapping, community assessment, 92–94
Attention-grabbers, communication campaign, 68
Avicenna, 4
Aztecs, pregnancy/childbirth, 3

Bacterial vaginosis
  management of, 195
  signs/symptoms of, 195
Barrier methods: *see* Spermicides and barrier methods
Basal body temperature, 138; *see also* Fertility awareness methods
Behavioral indicators, 72–74
  definitions of, 73–74
  matrix of indicators, 73
Behavior change
  action/maintenance stage, 61–62
  assessment of, 72–74
  audience segmentation, 64
  behavioral indicators of, 72–74
  communication campaign, 65–72
  contemplation stage, 58–60
  data collection/analysis for program, 63
  goals/domains for, 54
  implementation of program, 71–72
  objective setting, 66–67
  population analysis, 62–65
  pre-contemplative stage, 57–58
  preparation/action stage, 60–61
  programs, elements of, 14–15
  and role models, 60
  and self-efficacy, 56, 60
  SMART objective, 66
  sustaining over long-term, 61–62
  theoretical basis for, 55–56
  Transtheoretical Model of, 55–57
Benzalkonium chloride, 141
Berlin Papyrus, 4
Bes, god, 3
Bible, on birth control, 4
Birth intervals, and infant mortality, 27
Blood screening, for HIV/AIDS, 216–217

261

Blood transfusion, and HIV/AIDS prevention, 216–217
Body maps, community assessment, 88
Body Mass Index (BMI), weight gain in pregnancy, 170
Brandt, Allan, 6
Breastfeeding, and maternal-to-child STD transmission management, 213–214
Breech birth, 178
Budgeting/financial management, tasks in, 127

Cesarean delivery
 historical view, 8
 and obstructed/prolonged labor, 178
Calcium
 deficiency, 171
 supplementation, 172
Calendar method, 138; *see also* Fertility awareness methods
Cancer, cervical cancer, 217–220
Canon, The (Avicenna), 4, 5
Capacity building: *see* Institutional capacity building
CARE Management Capacity Assessment Tool, 128
CARE project: *see* Community empowerment
Caribbean, HIV/AIDS epidemic, 38
Cartooning, community assessment, 89
Catholic Church, population policy of, 226
Celebrities, as role models, 60
Census mapping, process of, 85
Cervical cancer
 alternatives to screening, 219
 early detection, importance of, 218
 and human papillomavirus (HPV), 196, 217
 incidence of, 217
 once-in-a-lifetime screening, 219
 one session case management, 219
 Pap screening, 217–219
 stages of, 218
Cervical cap, 142
 historical view, 8–9
Cervical disorders
 cancer: *see* Cervical cancer
 cervical failure, 178–179
 prenatal complications, 165
Cervical mucus method, 138; *see also* Fertility awareness methods
Chancroid
 management of, 193
 signs/symptoms of, 193
Childbirth
 assistance by trained attendant, locations for, 34
 average duration of, 179
 complications of: *see* Childbirth complications; Maternal mortality; Obstetrical emergencies
 essential interventions during, 174–175

Childbirth (*cont.*)
 maternal survival pathway, 46
 normal labor, features of, 173–174
 postpartum period, 181–186
 and psychosocial support, 174
 trained birth attendant, role of, 175–176
Childbirth complications, 176–181
 cervical failure, 178–179
 chorioamnionitis, 177
 constriction rings, 178
 disseminated intravascular coagulation (DIC), 180
 emergencies: *see* Obstetrical emergencies
 from fetal anomalies, 180–181
 fetal dystocia, 177–178
 hypotonic/hypertonic labor, 178
 and multiple gestation, 180
 pelvic dystocia, 178
 post-term gestation, 181
 premature rupture of the membrane, 176–177
 retained/incomplete placenta, 179
 shock, 179–180
 umbilical cord abnormalities, 180–181
 uterine rupture, 180
 uterine structural anomalies, 178
China
 HIV/AIDS epidemic, 37
 reproductive health in history of, 3, 4
Chlamydia
 incidence/prevalence by location, 39
 management of, 194, 216
 maternal-to-child transmission, 167, 215–216
 signs/symptoms of, 194
Chorioamnionitis, 177
Clinical services, assessment of, 111–112
Coitus interruptus: *see* Withdrawal (*coitus interruptus*)
Collective action; *see also* Community empowerment
 impediments to, 83
 reproductive health related, 80–81
Combined oral contraceptives (COCs), 144–147
 efficacy of, 144–145
 guidelines to clients, 146–147
 mechanism of action, 144
 pros/cons of, 145–146
Commercial sector
 contributions to reproductive health services, 116–117
 issues in working with, 116–117
 providers, types of, 116
Commercial sex, and sexually transmitted disease (STD) transmission, 48, 50–51
Commodity management, elements of, 127
Communication campaign
 attention-grabbers, 68
 benefits-costs as topic, 68
 dialogue versus one-way message, 67–68

INDEX

Community campaign (cont.)
  emotional response, evoking, 68–69
  media and methods in, 69–70
  pre-testing message, 70–71
Community, 76–78
  characteristics of, 76
  definition of, 76
  health program roles, 78–79
  ladder of community participation, 79
  participation, terms related to, 78–79
  participation levels, 79
  population groups within, 77
  provider/services matrix, 110
  and reproductive security approach, 21–22, 75–76
  shared characteristics approach to, 77
  as shifting social construct, 77–78
Community assessment
  assets mapping, 92–94
  body maps, 88
  cartooning, 89
  census mapping, 85
  flow diagrams, 87–88
  focus groups, 89–91
  freelisting, 86–87
  participatory sex census, 88–89, 90
  pile sorting, 86–87
  ranking and scoring, 87
  social mapping, 84
  social network analysis, 85–86
  story telling, 89
  transect walk, 85
  wealth and well-being ranking, 85
Community empowerment, 80–102
  actions related to, 15
  agenda for action from, 91
  assessment of, 101–102
  capacity building, 99–100
  cash resources, mobilization, 96–98
  cycle of empowerment, 82
  definition of, 80
  external sources of resources, 98–99
  facilitation team, 84
  impediments to community action, 83
  leadership development, 100
  multiple techniques, rationale for, 83–84
  needs analysis: see Community assessment
  optimal participation, conditions for, 83
  organization/individuals relationship building, 94–96
  outcomes of, 81
  reproductive health, collective actions, 80–81
  resource mobilization, 91–92
  versus specific health outcomes, 81–82
  target community, definition of, 84–86
Community health workers, 113–116

Community health workers (cont.)
  and client access to services, 115
  drugs/commodities distributed by, 114
  record keeping by, 115
  recruitment of, 113
  retention of, 115–116
  service delivery variations, 114–115
  tasks of, 114
  training and supervision of, 113–114
Community liaison, functions of, 125
Condoms
  female condom, 142
  male condom, 140–141
Constriction rings, 178
Contact tracing, STD management, 200
Contraception methods
  abstinence, 136–137
  contraceptive implants, 151–153
  female sterilization, 156–158
  fertility awareness methods, 138–140
  intrauterine devices, 153–156
  male condoms, 140–141
  oral contraceptives, 144–150
  progestin injection contraceptives, 150–151
  spermicides and barrier methods, 141–143
  vasectomy, 159–160
  withdrawal (coitus interruptus), 137–138
Contraceptive implants, 151–153
  guidelines to clients, 153
  mechanism of action, 152
  pros/cons of, 152–153
Contraceptives/birth control, 40–41
  contraception, 188–189
  with family planning program, 43
  historical view, 4–5, 8–9
  method of: see Contraception methods
  mortality risk, 136
  physiological aspects, 133–135
  post-abortion, 188–189
  provider assessment of, 135–136
  use and age, 40
  use by region, 41
Contractions of childbirth, 173–174
Convention on the Elimination on All Forms of Discrimination Against Women, 228
COPE Self-Assessment Procedure, 112
Copper deficiency, 172
Counseling
  in quality program, 119
  STD management, 198–199, 202
Cowper's gland, 135

Decision-making
  client involvement, 119
  management function, 125

Demographic and Health Survey (DHS), 25
Depression, postpartum, 182
Development programming
   asset accumulation approach, 13–14
   elements of, 13–14
Diabetes, during pregnancy, 169
Diaphragm, 142
   historical view, 8–9
Dilapan, 187
Dilation and curettage (D&C) abortion, 186, 188
Discorides, 4–5
Disseminated intravascular coagulation (DIC), 180
Down's syndrome, 28
Dystocia, 177–179
   cervical failure, 178–179
   fetal dystocia, 177–178
   and maternal death, 30
   pelvic dystocia, 178
   uterine dystocia, 178

Ebers papyrus, 3
Eclampsia
   delivery as cure of, 167
   postpartum period, 183
   prenatal period, 166–167
   signs of, 166–167
Economic perspective, of reproduction as problem, 224–227
Ectopic pregnancy, 165
Egypt, ancient
   birth control, 4
   pregnancy/childbirth, 3
Ehrlich, Paul, 9
ELISA, for HIV/AIDS, 216
Epidemiology: *see* Reproductive health epidemiology
Epididymitis
   signs of, 196
   treatment of, 196
Estrogen, 133–134
Evaluation Project, 118
   list of indicators, 72
Extra-marital sex, factors related to, 51

Facilitation team, community empowerment program, 84
Facilities/equipment management, tasks in, 127–128
Family planning, 42–43
   contraception availability, 43
   impact, measurement difficulties, 43
   socioeconomic factors, 43
   stage theory of, 57
Female condoms, 142
Female genital cutting (FGC), communication campaign against, 65–66
Female reproductive system, 133–134

Female sterilization, 156–158
   efficacy of, 157
   guidelines to clients, 158
   laparoscopy, 157
   minilaparotomy, 156–157
   pros/cons of, 157–158
Feminine hygiene products, historical view, 8–9
Fertility awareness methods, 138–140
   efficacy, 139
   guidelines to clients, 139–140
   types of, 138
Fertility control
   contraceptives, 40–41
   demand for, 41
   economic need for, 225–227
   family planning, 42–43
   government programs, 42
   proximate determinates, 40
   reproductive health interventions, 40–43
   and status of women, 42
   and unintended pregnancy, 25–26
Fertility rate, and maternal mortality ratio, 29
Fetal development, phases of, 162
Fetal dystocia, 177–178
Flow diagrams, community assessment, 87–88
Focus groups, community assessment, 89–91
Folic acid
   deficiencies involving, 171
   and neural tube defects, 172
   supplementation of, 171, 172
Follicle stimulating hormone (FSH), 133–135
Follow-up, in quality programs, 120
4 Cs approach, STD management, 203
Freelisting, community assessment, 86–87
Fruits of Philosophy (Knowlton), 8

Gender, effects on reproductive health, 17–18
Gender discrimination, and poor, 17–18
Gender equality, and fertility control, 42
Genital herpes
   management of, 193
   signs/symptoms of, 193
Genital prolapse, and maternal death, 32
Genital warts; *see also* Human papillomavirus (HPV)
   management of, 195
   signs of, 195
Gonadotropin releasing hormone (GnRH), 133, 161
Gonorrhea
   incidence/prevalence by location, 39
   maternal-to-child transmission, 194, 215
   signs/symptoms of, 194
   treatment of, 194, 215
Grafenberg, Ernst, 9
Granuloma inguinale
   management of, 193

INDEX

Granuloma inguinale (*cont.*)
  signs/symptoms of, 193
Greece, ancient
  pregnancy/childbirth, 3–4
  sexually transmitted diseases (STD), 5

Hathor, goddess, 3
Health district, provider/services matrix, 110–111
Health perspective, of reproduction as problem, 227–228
Helminthic infections, during pregnancy, 168
Hematoma, postnatal bleeding, 185
Hemorrhage
  and maternal death, 30, 31
  postpartum, causes of, 184–185
  prenatal, causes of, 165–166
Hepatitis A and B
  signs/symptoms of, 196
  treatment of, 196
Higher order pregnancy
  and infant mortality, 27–28
  and maternal mortality, 28
Highly active antiretroviral treatment (HAART), 209–212
  adherence, importance of, 211
  complications of, 211
  cost issues, 210
  diagnosis/monitoring in, 211
  drugs used, 210
  effectiveness of, 209–210
  lifetime use, 211
High risk pregnancy, 26–28
Hippocrates, on reproductive health, 3–5
HIV/AIDS
  AIDS orphans, 39
  child mortality statistics, 38
  children infected by, 36
  core transmitters, 48
  homophobia as reaction to, 6
  life expectancy statistics, 38
  maternal-to-child transmission, 212–214, 212–216
  in pregnancy, 167–168
  prevalence and other STDs, 206–207
  regional patterns, 36–38
  signs/symptoms of, 192
  transmission methods, 36–38
  worldwide incidence, 36
HIV/AIDS management
  blood screening, 216–217
  and blood transfusion, 216–217
  highly active antiretroviral treatment (HAART), 209–212
  for opportunistic infections, 208–209
  social support, 207–208
  stigma alleviation, 207

Holland, Edward, 8
Hookworms
  during pregnancy, 168
  treatment of, 168
Hormones
  of combined oral contraceptives (COCs), 144
  of female reproductive system, 133–134
  of male reproductive system, 135
  of pregnancy, 161–162
  of progestin injection contraceptives, 150
  of progestin-only oral contraceptives (POP), 147
Hospital, provider/services matrix, 110
Household
  defined, 17
  and reproductive security approach, 20
  and risk management, 16–17
Hsieh Chi, 4
Human papillomavirus (HPV), 217–220
  and cervical cancer, 196, 217
Human reproduction
  female reproductive system, 133–134
  male reproductive system, 134–135
Human resources management, tasks in, 126
Human rights
  treaties/accords related to, 228
  violations and population control, 228–229
Human rights perspective, of reproduction as problem, 228–229
Hydatidiform mole, 164, 165
Hydrocephalus, 178
Hyperemesis gravidarum, 165
Hypertension; *see also* Eclampsia
  calcium and reduction of, 172
  and maternal death, 30
Hypertonic labor, 178
Hypotonic labor, 178

Ibn Abbas al-Majusi, Ali, 4
Ibn Zakariya al Razi, Muhammed, 4
I Ching, 4
Immunization, of newborn, 190
India, ancient
  birth control in, 4
  pregnancy/childbirth in, 3, 4
India, HIV/AIDS epidemic in, 37
Individual, and reproductive security approach, 20
Individualized birth plan, for high-risk pregnancies, 169–170
Induced abortion: *see* Abortion
Infant mortality, 26–28
  and adolescent pregnancy, 26–27
  and fertility regulation, 25–26
  and higher order pregnancy, 27–28
  and older maternal age, 28
  reducing with newborn care, 189–190

Infant mortality (*cont.*)
  and short birth intervals, 27
  and unintended pregnancy, 28
Infections
  intrapartum period, 176–177
  of newborn, 189–190
  postpartum period, 185–186
  prenatal period, 167–168
Information management, tasks in, 127
Injecting drug users (IDU), HIV/AIDS transmission, 37–38
Inquisition, 5
Institution, and reproductive security approach, 22
Institutional capacity building
  access to services, 106–112
  and commercial sector, 116–117
  community empowerment, 99–100
  community health workers, 113–116
  elements of, 15
  management development, 124–131
  quality of care, 118–124
  services mix, 104–106
Inter alia, unsafe abortion, 34
International Bill of Rights, 228
International Conference on Population and Development (ICPD), 2, 228–229
Interpersonal relations, in quality program, 120
Intrauterine device (IUD), 153–156
  efficacy of, 154
  guidelines to clients, 156
  historical view, 9
  mechanism of action, 154
  pros/cons of, 154–156
  types of, 154
Iodine deficiency, 171
Iron deficiency anemia, 171
Iron supplementation, 171
Ishihama, Atsui, 9

Jadelle rods: *see* Contraceptive implants

Kahun papyrus, 3
Kerr, John, 8
Kielland forceps, 8
Knowlton, Charles, 8
Kountche, Seyni, 69

Labor: *see also* Childbirth
  phases of, 173–174
Lamicel, 187
Laparoscopy, 157
  historical view, 9
Latin America, HIV/AIDS epidemic, 37–38
Lavamisole, 168
Leadership development, elements of, 100

Livelihood security, defined, 12
Living with AIDS Project, 208
Lochia, postpartum, 182
Lungren, S.S., 9
Luteinizing hormone (LH), 133–135
Lymphogranuloma venereum
  management of, 193
  signs/symptoms of, 193

Magnesium deficiency, 171
Maine, Deborah, 6
Malaria
  during pregnancy, 168
  treatment of, 168
Male condoms, 140–141
  efficacy of, 140
  guidelines to clients, 141
  pros/cons of, 141
Male reproductive system, 134–135
Malnutrition: *see* Nutritional deficiencies
Management Capacity Assessment Tool, 99–100
Management development, 124–131
  case example, 128–131
  management capacity assessment, 128
  management systems assessment, 129
  management tasks, 125–128
  plan for, 128
Management Sciences for Health, 128
Management tasks
  budgeting and financial management, 127
  commodity management, 127
  community liaison, 125
  facilities/equipment management, 127–128
  human resources management, 126
  information management, 127
  planning, 125–126
Mass treatment approach, for sexually transmitted disease (STD), 200–201, 206–207
Maternal age, and infant mortality, 26–27, 28
Maternal disability, as consequence of pregnancy, 31–32
Maternal health care: *see* Postpartum care; Prenatal care
Maternal mortality, 28–32
  decreased, reproductive health interventions, 43–46
  geographic locations, 29–30
  and higher order pregnancy, 28
  and high fertility, 28
  lifetime risk, 29
  and limited prenatal care, 32
  maternal death, defined, 29
  maternal health conditions as cause, 28, 29–30
  and maternal medical conditions, 28
  and obstetrical emergencies, 29–30, 43–45

INDEX

Maternal mortality (*cont.*)
  postpartum period, 31
  reducing, methods for, 44–46
  and surviving children, 29, 39
  unsafe abortion, 28, 30, 33–34
Maternal mortality ratio, meaning of, 29
Mebendazole, 168
Medical center, provider/services matrix, 110
Meningitis, of newborn, 190
Menstrual cycle, physiological aspects, 133–134
Menstruation, 134
Methotrexate, as abortifacient, 187
Midwifery, historical view, 3–4
Mifepristone, as abortifacient, 186–187
Minilaparotomy, 156–157
Misoprostol, as abortifacient, 186–187, 187
Moir, J. Chassar, 8
Monetary resources, for community empowerment program, 96–98
Moral perspective, of reproduction as problem, 229–230
Morning sickness, 165
Multiple gestation, risks of, 180
Museveni, Yoweri, 69
Muslim writings, on birth control, 4

National power perspective, of reproduction as problem, 223–234
Neural tube defects, and folic acid deficiency, 172
Nevirapine, in maternal-to-child HIV transmission, 212–213
Newborn care, 189–190
  neonatal mortality, role in reduction of, 189–190
Non-Governmental Organization Services Project (NGO-SP), 128–131
Nonoxynol-9, 141
Norplant: *see* Contraceptive implants
Nutritional deficiencies
  calcium deficiency, 171
  copper deficiency, 172
  folic acid deficiency, 171
  iodine deficiency, 171
  iron deficiency anemia, 171
  magnesium deficiency, 171
  selenium deficiency, 172
  Vitamin A deficiency, 171
  Vitamin C deficiency, 172
  Vitamin D deficiency, 171
  zinc deficiency, 171
Nutritional support, prenatal, 170–173

Obstetrical emergencies: *see also* Childbirth complications
  interval of time, 44–45
  and maternal mortality, 29–30, 43–45

Obstetrical emergencies (*cont.*)
  maternal survival pathway, 46
  pre-delivery planning, 169–170
  pre-natal period, high-risk situations, 163–164
  prevention of, 44–46
  types of, 29–30, 43–45
Obstetric fistula, and maternal death, 31–32
Octoxynol, 141
Ocular infection, newborn and STDs, 190, 215–216
Older mothers, and infant mortality, 28
Once-in-a-lifetime screening, cervical cancer, 219
One session case management, cervical cancer, 219
Opportunistic infections, HIV/AIDS, palliative care, 208–209
Oral contraceptives, 144–150
  combined oral contraceptives (COCs), 144–147
  historical view, 9
  progestin-only oral contraceptives (POP), 147–150
Ota, T., 9
Outcomes, of community empowerment, 81
Ovulation, 133–134
Oxytocin, in labor, 175, 177

Pap test, cervical cancer detection, 217–219
Participatory sex census, community assessment, 88–89, 90
Partner notification, STD management, 200
Paxman, John, 7
Pediculosis publis
  signs of, 195
  treatment of, 195
Pelvic dystocia, 178
Pelvic inflammatory disease (PID)
  and intrauterine device (IUD), 155
  signs/symptoms of, 196
  treatment of, 196
Pile sorting, community assessment, 86–87
Placenta
  delivery of, 175
  retained/incomplete placenta, 179
Placenta abruptio, 166
Placenta previa, 166
Planning
  elements of, 125–126
  SWOT Analysis, 125–126
Pneumonia, newborn, 190
Pomeroy, Ralph, 9
Population analysis
  behavior change program, 62–65
  census mapping, 85
  community empowerment program, 84–86
  for dynamics of STD transmission, 48–51
  social mapping, 84
  social network analysis, 85–86
  wealth and well-being ranking, 85

Population growth, as economic problem, 225–226
Porro, Eduardo, 8
Postpartum care, 182–183
  goals of, 182–183
  scope of, 183
Postpartum period, 181–186
  danger signs, 184
  eclampsia during, 183
  hemorrhage during, 184–185
  infections of, 185–186
  maternal mortality, 31, 44
  physiological changes during, 181–182
  stages of, 181
Post-term gestation, risks of, 181
Poverty
  and gender discrimination, 17–18
  and malnutrition, 170–171
  vulnerabilities of poor, 11–12
Pregnancy: *see also* Childbirth; Prenatal care; Prenatal complications
  abortion, 32–36
  danger signs during, 164
  infant mortality, 26–28
  maternal health conditions, 28, 29–30, 163
  maternal mortality, 28–32
  prenatal period, 161–162
  STDs, maternal-to-child transmission, 212–216
  and teens: *see* Adolescent pregnancy
  unintended, causes of, 25–26
  weight gain recommendations, 170
Premature rupture of the membrane (PROM), 176–177
Prenatal care, 162–164
  locations for non/minimum care, 33
  and maternal mortality, 32
  minimum number of visits, 164
  nutritional, 170–173
  objectives of, 162–163
Prenatal complications, 164–172; *see also* Obstetrical emergencies
  cervical disorders, 165
  diabetes, 169
  eclampsia, 166–167
  ectopic pregnancy, 165
  helminthic infections, 168
  hemorrhage, 165–166
  hydatidiform mole, 164, 165
  hyperemesis gravidarum, 165
  individualized birth plan, 169–170
  malaria, 168
  maternal malnutrition, forms of, 171–172
  placenta abruptio, 166
  placenta previa, 166
  sexually transmitted disease (STD), 167–168
  spontaneous abortion, 165

Prenatal complications (*cont.*)
  teratogenic infections, 168
  tetanus, 168
  urinary tract infections, 167
  vasa previa, 166
Prenatal period
  danger signs, 164
  and health risks, 28, 29–30, 163
  normal pregnancy/fetal growth, 161–162
  phases of, 162
Problem-solving, to sustain behavior change, 61
Progestin injection contraceptives, 150–151
  efficacy of, 150
  guidelines to clients, 151
  mechanism of action, 150
  pros/cons of, 150–151
Progestin-only oral contraceptives (POP), 147–150
  guidelines to clients, 149–150
  mechanism of action, 148
  pros/cons of, 148–149
Prostate gland, 135
Provider map, 106–107
Provider to service match, 108–111
Proximate determinates, fertility control, 40
Psychosocial support, during childbirth, 174
Public health, and reproductive health, 10–11
Public policy
  advocacy, effects of, 15
  functions of, 221–222
  health program manager advocacy, 231–235
  and reproductive security approach, 21
Puerperal infection, and maternal death, 30

Quality of care, 118–124
  in context of standards, 121–123
  quality improvement plan, 123–124
  quality of care indicators, 122
  quality processes, 121–124
  quality standards, 118–120
  reproductive health standards, 118
  sustaining over time, 124
Quality of life, and community empowerment, 81

Ranking and scoring, community assessment, 87
Rapid plasma reagin (RPR) test, 167
Ratirahasya, 4
Record keeping, by community health workers, 115
Relationship building, in community empowerment, 94–96
Religious perspective, of reproduction, 229–230
Reproductive health
  asset accumulation approach, 13–14
  development programming, 13–14
  focus of interventions, 16–17
  and gender, 17–18

INDEX

Reproductive health (*cont.*)
  historical view, 3–6
  medical advances, 7–10
  and poverty, 11–12
  and public health, 10–11
  reproductive security approach, 14–15
  risk analysis, 18–23
  risk management, 16–17
  as social phenomenon, 11
  suppression of, 5–7, 16–17
Reproductive health epidemiology
  induced abortion, 32–36
  infant mortality, 26–28
  maternal mortality, 28–32
  sexually transmitted disease (STD), 36–40
  unintended pregnancy, 25–26
Reproductive health interventions
  and decreased fertility, 40–43
  and decreased maternal mortality, 43–46
  sexually transmitted disease (STD) prevention, 46–51
Reproductive health managers, roles/responsibilities, 103–104
Reproductive medical advances, 7–10
Reproductive medicine, historical view, 7–10
Reproductive politics
  economic perspective, 224–225
  health problem perspective, 227–228
  human rights perspective, 228–229
  national power perspective, 223–224
  public policy, importance of, 221–222
  religious/moral perspective, 229–230
Reproductive rights, 228–229
Reproductive risk, message to raise awareness of, 57–58
Reproductive risk analysis, 18–23
  purpose of, 14
  questions related to, 18–19
  steps in, 14
Reproductive security
  essential services for, 104–106
  meaning of, 14
Reproductive security approach, 14–15
  community elements, 21–22
  flowchart of elements, 19
  individual/household elements, 20
  institutional elements, 22
  policy elements, 21
  technology elements, 21
Risk avoidance, to sustain behavior change, 62
Risk management, focus of interventions, 16–17
Role models, as behavior change agent, 60
Rome, ancient
  pregnancy/childbirth, 4
  sexually transmitted diseases (STD), 5

Rosenfield, Allan, 6
Royal Book, 4
Rural dispensary, provider/services matrix, 110

Saline abortion, 187
Salt, iodized, 172
Sanger, Max, 8
Scabies
  symptoms of, 195
  treatment of, 195
Selenium deficiency, 172
Self-efficacy
  and behavior change, 56, 60
  meaning of, 15, 56
Septicemia, of newborn, 190
Service providers, mapping, 106–107
Sexually transmitted disease (STD), 36–40
  bacterial vaginosis, 195
  chancroid, 193
  chlamydia, 194
  and commercial sex, 48, 50–51
  curable, regional distribution, 39–40
  duration of infectious period, 47–48
  epididymitis, 196
  extra-marital sex, factors related to, 51
  genital herpes, 193
  genital warts, 195
  gonorrhea, 194
  granuloma inguinale, 193
  Hepatitis A and B, 196
  historical view, 5, 9–10
  HIV/AIDS, 36–39, 206–214
  human papillomavirus (HPV), 195, 196, 217–220
  lymphogranuloma venereum, 193
  and number of sexual partners, 48, 50
  pediculosis publis, 195
  pelvic inflammatory disease (PID), 196
  during pregnancy, 167–168
  prevalence and HIV/AIDS risk, 206–207
  probability of transmission, factors in, 47
  repression connected with, 6
  scabies, 195
  stigma of, 6
  syndromes/causative agents, 203
  syndromes/treatments, 205
  syphilis, 192
  vulvovaginal candidiasis, 195
Sexually transmitted disease (STD) management, 46–51
  contact tracing, 200
  core transmitters, focus on, 49–50, 199
  detection of disease, 197–201
  dynamics of transmission assessment, 48–51
  flowcharts, use of, 203–204
  4 Cs approach, 203

Sexually transmitted disease (STD) management (*cont.*)
  mass treatment approach, 200–201, 206–207
  patient management, 201–202
  in resource poor settings, 201–202
  risk assessment protocols, 199–200
  syndromic management, 202–205
  treatment-seeking, factors related to, 198–201
  voluntary counseling and testing (VCT), 198–199
Shock
  causes of, 179–180
  during childbirth, 179–180
  signs of, 180
Situation Analysis Methodology, 112
Six cleans, 175
SMART objective, behavior change campaign, 66
Social mapping, process of, 84
Social network analysis, process of, 85–86
Social support, and HIV/AIDS, 207–208
Soranus, on reproductive health, 4
Spermicides and barrier methods, 141–143
  cervical cap, 142
  diaphragm, 142
  efficacy of, 142
  female condom, 142
  guidelines to clients, 143–144
  historical view, 8–9
  pros/cons of, 142–143
  sponge, 142
Sponge, contraceptive, 142
Spontaneous abortion, 165
Sterilization
  female sterilization, 156–158
  historical view, 9
Stigma, and sexually transmitted diseases (STD), 6
Story telling, community assessment, 89
Stroganoff, Vasilii, 7
Sulfadoxine-pyrimethamine (SP), 168
Sun Ssu-mo, 4
Support groups
  HIV/AIDS, 208
  for sustaining behavior change, 61–62
SWOT Analysis, 125–126
Symptothermal method, 138; *see also* Fertility awareness methods
Syndromic management, of STDs, 202–205
Syphilis
  fetal damage from, 214
  historical view, 5–6
  incidence/prevalence by location, 39, 214
  maternal-to-child transmission, 167, 214–215
  signs/symptoms of, 192
  stages of, 192
  treatment of, 192, 215

Talmud, on birth control, 4
Technology, and reproductive security approach, 21
Teratogenic infections
  effects of, 168
  interventions for, 168
Testes, 134
Testosterone, 134
Tetanus
  during pregnancy, 168, 189
  treatment of, 189
Ticitl, 3
Trained birth attendant, role of, 175–176
Transect walk, community assessment, 85
Transtheoretical Model, 55–57; *see also* Behavior change
Trichomoniasis
  incidence/prevalence by location, 39
  management of, 195
  signs/symptoms of, 195
Tung-hsuan, 4

Umbilical cord abnormalities, 180–181
  cord length anomalies, 181
  umbilical cord prolapse, 180–181
Unintended pregnancy, and infant mortality, 28
Universal Declaration of Human Rights, 228
Urinary tract infections, in pregnancy, 167
Uterine atony, 184
Uterine dystocia, forms of, 178
Uterine inversion, postpartum, 185
Uterine involution, 182
Uterine rupture, 180

Vacuum aspiration abortion, 186
Vaginal tears, and childbirth, 184
Vasa previa, 166
Vas deferens, 134–135
Vasectomy, 159–160
  efficacy of, 159
  guidance to clients, 160
  pros/cons of, 159
Venn diagram, asset mapping, 93
Vitamin deficiencies, types in pregnancy, 172
Vitamin supplementation, guidelines in pregnancy, 173
Voluntary counseling and testing (VCT), 198–199
Vomiting, in pregnancy, 165
Vulvovaginal candidiasis
  management of, 195
  signs/symptoms of, 195

Wealth and well-being ranking, population analysis, 85
Wife's Handbook (Allbutt), 9
Wilde, F.A., 8

Witchcraft, and Inquisition, 5
Withdrawal (*coitus interruptus*), 137–138
   efficacy of, 138
   guidelines for clients, 138
   pros/cons of, 138

World Population Programme of Action, 186, 228

Zidovudine (ZDV), in maternal-to-child HIV transmission, 212–213
Zinc deficiency, 171